T0210803

Catastrophic Diseases: Who Decides What?

Catastrophic Diseases: Who Decides What?

*A Psychosocial and Legal Analysis
of the Problems Posed by Hemodialysis
and Organ Transplantation*

Jay Katz and Alexander Morgan Capron

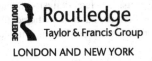
Routledge
Taylor & Francis Group

LONDON AND NEW YORK

First published 1982 by Transaction Publishers

Published 2017 by Routledge
2 Park Square, Milton Park, Abingdon, Oxon OX14 4RN
605 Third Avenue, New York, NY 10017

Routledge is an imprint of the Taylor and Francis Group, an informa business

Copyright © 1975 Russell Sage Foundation, New York

This study was originally supported by Russell Sage Foundation

Library of Congress Catalog Number: 80-21899

Library of Congress Cataloging-in-Publication Data

Katz, Jay, 1922-
    Catastrophic diseases.

    Reprint of the 1975 ed. published by Russell Sage Foundation, New York.
    Bibliography: p.
    Includes index.
    1. Medical innovations—Social aspects. 2. Transplantation of organs, tissues, etc.—Social aspects. 3. Hemodialysis—Social aspects. 4. Medical ethics. 5. Human experimentation in medicine. 6. Medical policy—United States. I. Capron, Alexander Morgan, joint author. II. Title.

RA418.5.M4K37   1982   362.1'9795   80-21899
ISBN 13: 978-0-87855-686-1 (pbk)

Contents

Diseases desperate grown
By desperate appliance are relieved,
Or not at all.

William Shakespeare, *Hamlet*
Act IV, Scene 3

Preface

Some years ago the National Center for Health Services Research and Development asked us to undertake a study of the impact on the immediate participants and on society of novel and expensive research and treatment modalities, such as organ transplantation and hemodialysis. This book is the result of that project.* Through an intense and rewarding collaboration, crisscrossing disciplinary lines, we have gone beyond the scope originally contemplated and have attempted not only to identify the problems raised in the catastrophic diseases process but also to construct a framework for the analysis of these problems. We hope that this model will not only be useful to scholars and decisionmakers in other areas of medical and societal decisionmaking but will also stimulate them to improve on it; for the discussions of the issues posed by modern medicine have suffered from the lack of an analytic framework which permits a confrontation of these problems in a systematic and all-encompassing fashion.

In our work we were immeasurably aided by our consultants from many disciplines—George Baker, Jr. (medicine), Bernard Barber (sociology), Guido Calabresi (law), Carl Fellner (psychiatry), Renée C. Fox (sociology), Dwight E. Harken (surgery), Al Katz (law), Charles E. Lindblom (political science), H. Harrison Sadler (psychiatry), Belding H. Scribner (medicine), Judith P. Swazey (history of science), Paul Terasaki (immunology), and Richard Zeckhauser (economics). Most of these consultants prepared detailed memoranda, commented on drafts of our work, and attended a two-day conference during which the issues examined in this book were scrutinized in great detail. Our debt to our consultants is

---

* The project was performed pursuant to Contract No. HSM 110-69-213 with the Health Services and Mental Health Administration, Department of Health, Education, and Welfare. We also wish to acknowledge the support of the National Science Foundation through a grant (GS38499) made to Jay Katz during the final stages of manuscript revision.

great, though, of course, the responsibility for the final document must rest entirely on our shoulders.

This study was undertaken during a period when the general subject area—the social, ethical, and legal ramifications of medical progress—was receiving a great deal of attention. Some of the scrutiny took the form of scholarly analysis and some was undertaken by persons empowered to promulgate new rules for biomedical research and treatment. Through our work we were able to participate in both parts of this process of scrutiny and reformulation. While immersed in this study we reworked together the final draft of the casebook *Experimentation with Human Beings,* which was funded by Russell Sage Foundation. Both books, though written for different purposes, benefited greatly from one another. Our work on this project is also reflected in the recommendations of the Tuskegee Syphilis Study *Ad Hoc* Advisory Panel on which Jay Katz served and in the advice we gave to the Senate Subcommittee on Health concerning H. R. 7724 in the Ninety-third Congress. That statute, the National Research Act, was subsequently enacted in modified form by Congress, and it provides for the establishment of a national commission, which has recently begun a two-year study of the principles that ought to govern the human experimentation process. Similarly, other aspects of our study are reflected in revised guidelines for experimentation formulated by the National Institutes of Health for which Alexander Capron acted as consultant.

Many of the most significant developments have occurred since our manuscript was submitted to the National Center in the summer of 1973. In preparing the book for publication we have attempted to update the facts presented with the latest data. We have not revised all parts of the book to reflect new thoughts or formulations that we have arrived at since completing the manuscript; that would have been an endless task. Rather, we regard the ideas expressed here as building blocks in the overall process of reexamination of decisionmaking about catastrophic diseases (and biomedical innovation in general). We hope these ideas will stimulate others, as they have us, to further refinements of the concepts and rules in this important area.

We thank our deans, Abraham S. Goldstein and Bernard Wolfman, for providing additional support as well as agreeable academic surroundings in which we could pursue our exploration with minimum distraction. Willys Silvers of the genetics department at the University of Pennsylvania kindly reviewed Chapter Four and provided helpful comments for which we are thankful. We also are grateful to Sam Foley and Eric Frank for assistance in preparing the manuscript for publication and to our secretaries Kathy Lewis, Ruth Pitts, and Carol Yorgey for their expert and cheerful typing of our numerous drafts. We owe a great deal to the assistance of the staff of the Yale Law School Library, particularly Robert E. Brooks, Arthur A. Charpentier, James M. Golden, Isaiah Shein, Solomon C. Smith, and Iris Wildman, as well as to Richard Sloane and Nancy Arnold of the Biddle Law Library at the University of Pennsylvania.

We wish to express our appreciation to the National Center for Health Services Research and Development for funding the project and to its staff, particularly the late Dr. Nathaniel H. Barish and Dr. Laurence R. Tancredi, for their interest in the topic which got the project underway and for their patient assistance which saw it through to completion. We are sad that Dr. Barish who was most eager to have this book published did not live to see it in print. We are grateful to Elisabeth Krabisch for her copyediting and to Jean Yoder and William Bennett of Russell Sage Foundation for the care they gave the book's production. Finally, we thank our families for their loving support and sustenance during the seemingly endless period that this work so deeply absorbed our attention.

J. K. & A. M. C.

New Haven, Connecticut
Philadelphia, Pennsylvania
January 1975

Technical Note

When we submitted our original report on "Social Factors Affecting the Modern Treatment of Catastrophic Diseases" (HSM 110-69-213) to the National Center for Health Services Research we included as appendices the memoranda drafted by our consultants. The appendices were as follows:

A. Guido Calabresi, *Memorandum* (1970)
B. Renée C. Fox, *The Courage to Fail* (1970)
C. C. E. Lindblom, *New Decision-Making Procedures Governing Research on the Treatment of Catastrophic Diseases* (1970)
D. Bernard Barber, *The Structure, Functions and Efficacy of Peer Review Committees in the Experimental and Allocative Phases of Clinical Treatment* (1972)
E. Carl Fellner, *The Genetically Unrelated Living Kidney Donor: Unemployed and Unwanted* (1972)
F. Dwight E. Harken, *Clinical Moratoria Related to Catastrophic Illness* (1972)
G. Al Katz, *Process Design for Selection of Hemodialysis and Organ Transplant Recipients* (1972)
H. H. Harrison Sadler, *Summary Notes on a Clinical Decision-Making Model* (1972)
J. Belding H. Scribner, *The Problem of Patient Selection for Treatment with an Artificial Kidney* (1972)
K. Paul Terasaki, *Organ Transplantation* (1972)
L. Richard Zeckhauser, *Catastrophic Illness* (1972)

In this book references to the consultants' reports are identified according to the foregoing list of appendices. Although they are not included here, all except the one by Fox are on file with the National Center and available (for the cost of duplication). The work by Fox was incorporated into R. C.

Fox & J. Swazey, The Courage To Fail published in 1974 by the University of Chicago Press. In addition, revised versions of the memoranda by Katz and Zeckhauser were published in 22 Buffalo Law Review 373 (1973) and 21 Public Policy 149 (1973), respectively.

The footnotes in this book follow A Uniform System Of Citation used by legal publications. In this system, the volume number for case reports, periodicals and multi-volume books appears *before* the name of the work, which is *followed* by the page cited to and, in parenthesis, the date of publication. In citing articles, only the last name of the author(s) is given, but initials are included in citing books. Footnotes are numbered consecutively within each chapter, and internal references are indicated by *supra* and *infra* citations to other footnotes within the same chapter or, where indicated, to other chapters.

Introduction

People do not choose to suffer from catastrophic diseases, but considerable human choice is involved in the ways in which the participants in the process treat and conduct research on these illnesses. Throughout this report we shall therefore again and again return to one overall question: Who should have the authority to make the decisions which have such far-reaching consequences for those affected by catastrophic diseases and for society as a whole? This question gains urgency as well as importance from the fact that catastrophic disease research and treatment illustrate well a number of more general phenomena. First, decisions about these diseases exemplify the "tragic choices"[1] which face society in many areas of scarcity besides medical care. The tragedy is particularly pronounced because the threat involved is death and the persons competing for the life-saving resources are identifiable individuals, not all of whom will be saved. Second, catastrophic diseases, like lightning, strike rarely but when they do anyone can be their victim. Thus, they concern society not only because of the *known* individual tragedies they produce but also because everyone is at some *unknown* future risk. Third, they demonstrate the great societal impact and implications of innovative medicine.

---

[1] The term "tragic choices" is employed by Guido Calabresi of Yale Law School to describe a group of societal decisions which he is examining in further elaboration of the work which he performed as a consultant to this project [Appendix A].

The entire heart transplant circus was no aberration; it was the tip of a massive and dangerous iceberg; it was the inevitable result of our culture's fantastic, perhaps unprecedented, fear of death; it was the symbol of our peculiar faith in machines, technology and, most basically, machismo—a faith as poignant as it is irrational.[2]

To explore these issues we have developed dual conceptual perspectives. The first examines and evaluates the authority which should be vested in each of the chief participants in the catastrophic disease process—the physician-investigator, the patient-subject and his relatives, the professions, and the state. The second perspective builds on the insight that the roles and capacities of the participants vary not only according to the basic issues they face but also according to the point in decisionmaking at which these issues arise and have to be resolved. The process of investigating and treating catastrophic diseases can thus usefully be divided into three decisionmaking stages—the formulation of policy, the administration of research and therapy, and the review of the decisions and their consequences.

We have divided this book into three parts. In Part One, which serves as an introduction, we seek to define the ambit of catastrophic diseases (Chapter One), to present the framework which we have developed for the analysis of the problems raised by catastrophic diseases (Chapter Two), to enumerate and discuss the goals and values that are served by a committed effort to investigate and treat these diseases (Chapter Three), and finally to give an account of the development of the major innovative treatments for heart and kidney diseases (Chapter Four). Our intention in Part One is not merely to convey facts but, by integrating a discussion of "facts" and "values," to point to the forces behind developments in medicine and the issues which they generated.

In Part Two we turn our attention to the principal participants in the catastrophic disease process. We describe the major pressures, conflicts, and decisions which confront the participants both individually and in their interactions with one another, in order to evaluate the extent and limits of their capacities to meet these pressures and conflicts and to make meaningful decisions. Our presentation is designed to raise searching questions about the authority that has

---

[2] Michaelson, Book Review, N. Y. Times, Apr. 1, 1973, Sec. 7 (Book Review), at 23.

traditionally been assigned to each participant and to demonstrate the need for new ways of ordering the catastrophic disease process.

Finally in Part Three we propose a number of general and specific recommendations for the regulation of the catastrophic disease process. We believe, as already indicated, that the problems which require resolution are sufficiently disparate throughout the catastrophic disease decisionmaking process that the analysis of the roles which the participants should play will be facilitated by introducing distinctions among the several stages of the process: formulation (Chapter Eight), administration (Chapter Nine), and review (Chapter Ten). Throughout this part we are particularly concerned with demonstrating the need for a variety of individuals and groups with diverse values to be involved in decisionmaking as well as the need to permit investigators to pursue their interests without undue interference. We attempt to resolve this inherent conflict by including decisionmakers from outside the biomedical establishment at the *formulation* and *review* stages of the process where they are most needed while leaving the *administration* of research and therapy largely in the hands of the professionals.

Our conclusions have been guided by a preference for open, "visible" decisionmaking. One cannot, of course, ignore the possibility that the complex and hard choices, often involving life and death, which have to be made in the catastrophic disease process have in the long run a less devastating impact on the members of society and its institutions if they are arrived at by "low visibility" rather than "high visibility" decisionmaking. We have concluded that obscuring the bases for decision can only lead to fear and misunderstanding and, most important, to abuse, particularly of those groups within society who are traditionally the objects of neglect and mistreatment. Of course, open decisionmaking is not a cure for all the problems which may plague catastrophic disease research and treatment. But on balance we believe that its benefits outweigh its drawbacks and that it should be promoted in preference to the informal and invisible—even secret—mode of decisionmaking that has characterized this area in the past.

PART ONE

Facts and Values

Too often explorations of the problems created by medical advances are undertaken with the assumption that the most clearsighted and rational decisions will be reached if the scope of the discussion is restricted to "factual" questions. At most, when the role of "values" in decisionmaking is acknowledged, it is generally treated as a separate topic and left divorced from a consideration of the facts. Since we believe that it is not possible to weigh and consider facts without value assumptions and preferences, we attempt in this introductory section to acknowledge the importance of both facts and values and to suggest the ways in which they are intertwined. By emphasizing this point at the outset, we hope to alert the reader to the need of keeping the interrelationship of facts and values clearly in mind throughout all that follows.

The tragic choices which we face in the area of catastrophic disease decisionmaking seem almost to be in a conspiracy to undercut the notion that "value-free" science is possible. For example, in the first chapter of this study certain facts about the scarcity and expense of medical resources are set forth. Only a fraction of the patients needing treatment for life-threatening kidney disease will get what they need to survive—and as greater resources are devoted to renal failure we will only become more acutely aware of other diseases which are also inadequately treated. The response to such revelations has been to call for the allocation of more money to meet the cost of treating all catastrophic illnesses. Yet this response operates on the assumption that health—or perhaps merely life—is the paramount goal in society. If the "fact" is taken to be simply that a certain amount of money is necessary to "save" everyone with a certain condition, then myriad competing values have simply been ignored. When the conclusion goes further and includes, for example, the judgment that home dialysis is the preferred treatment for kidney failure because it "costs" only about one-tenth as much as hospital dialysis, then pressures have been generated which may obscure the burdens (both economic and noneconomic) that have been placed on the families of patients in home dialysis.

By focusing on this example we do not intend at this point to reach a judgment on the merits of hemodialysis in the home compared with other treatment modalities. Rather, we have used this merely as an example (and a rather self-evident one at that) of the way in which objective decisionmaking, based on allegiance to certain values—in this instance, "health" and "economy"—can lead to the neglect (often unacknowledged) of other values.

This example also points up a challenge faced by the entire study: the difficulty in moving beyond "health" as a value to any description of "health" as an objective status. There are certain medical assumptions about what constitutes health, based largely on data about what is statistically "normal." There are also societal views about health, which seem to vary greatly among subgroups in the society. Although reconciliation of the philosophical conflicts involved would be difficult if not impossible, it is important to keep this complicating factor in mind in defining "health" (or "happiness" or "worth") for various decisionmaking purposes.

These values, and the imperatives they pose for decisionmaking, are made strikingly clear in the process of research on catastrophic diseases. For that reason, we have chosen to include in this introductory part of the book a chapter which reviews the development of some innovative treatments for heart and kidney diseases, with particular emphasis on the roles of the individual physician-investigators as well as their patients and professional colleagues. Our intention, then, in Chapter Four is not simply to convey "facts" but to suggest the moral forces behind those facts and the issues (even crises) which they precipitate.

CHAPTER ONE

Introduction to the Issues

When one examines the far-reaching social ramifications of diseases instead of being concerned only with providing therapy for them, it becomes inevitable to view disease not only as a condition which causes pain and suffering and thus requires immediate help but also as an event which creates "issues" and "problems" and thus requires analysis. The posture of analyzing misfortune—rather than treating it—is, of course, an uncomfortable one. Yet if we wish to respond in a comprehensive and intelligent fashion to the needs of people who suffer from diseases that are so crushing as to devastate them and their families, as well as to strain the resources of society, we must at some point step back and examine the means by which care is provided and also search for ways to minimize the impact of our reluctance or inability to provide it. To introduce these issues and problems, this book begins with a sketch of the major concerns faced by the participants in the catastrophic disease process and the means that the participants have devised to cope with them.

A. WHAT IS A CATASTROPHIC DISEASE?

In the past decade, the cost of medical care has risen substantially. Even relatively uncomplicated illnesses can involve considerable expense and inconvenience, and an individual, who develops a condition serious enough to require repeated medical attention, and perhaps hospitalization, faces the prospect of a heavy drain on his financial resources, even if part of the bill is borne by private or government-funded health insurance. Some of this increased expense reflects the general inflation in the economy, which has been particularly pronounced in the health sector because of higher professional fees and unionization of nonprofessional hospital employees, and some of it is attributable to the advances made in the treatment of illness. The range of therapy for most diseases has been greatly increased by new drugs and other medical devices, which place some previously incurable and inevitably fatal conditions within the power of medicine to retard, if not to control.

While all illness carries with it some threat to life and imposes some economic burdens, in certain diseases these factors are especially pronounced. These diseases, which are termed "catastrophic," more often than not represent disaster for those they strike. Fatal unless promptly treated, yet with a course of therapy so financially burdensome as to be beyond the usual resources of most persons, a catastrophic illness may radically alter a person's existence and accustomed way of life, disable him from pursuing his accustomed work and activities, and leave his private affairs and family life in disorder. Thus, as we use the term, a catastrophic disease is one for which some form of *unusually expensive* treatment must be available which can at least *sustain life* for a period of time.[1] Moreover, the availability of insurance coverage or other financial support does not remove a condition from this category; the emphasis is on the great expense of the treatment, no matter who pays for it. Both criteria must be fulfilled in order for an illness to be considered a catastrophic one. Other factors, such as the psychological and social impact of such conditions on patients and their families, though not part of this definition are, of course, important consequences of these diseases which will receive major attention in this book. Different catastrophic diseases may require somewhat different approaches than those we have developed for one group which serves as our exemplar —namely, those heart and kidney conditions which are susceptible to treatment through organ transplantation or support by artificial means. We hope, however, that the lessons to be learned from an examination of these conditions, which have been the object of recent, dramatic medical attention, will turn out to be useful for the analysis of other catastrophic diseases.

1. Heart Disease

Nearly 28 million Americans suffer from some form of cardiovascular disease, accounting for about 1,050,000 deaths annually, 300,000 of them

---

[1] Therefore, for example, fatal automobile accidents or other *sudden fatal* traumas are not catastrophic diseases for our purposes, although they may have profound effects on a family if they deprive it of its primary wage earner.

among individuals under 65 years of age. Although leaders in the field of cardiology hope that preventive measures—restrictions in diet, curtailment of cigarette smoking, better detection and treatment of rheumatic fever and hypertension—will eventually reduce this staggering toll, at present the only treatment for the patient facing imminent cardiac death is the replacement of his damaged heart with a healthy heart from a person who has just died of other causes.[2] Work is also under way to develop a totally implantable artificial pump, but success still appears to be a number of years away.[3]

At present there are practical limits to cardiac transplantation. Among persons with coronary heart disease (the largest category), the critical limitation is its sudden onset, often without prior indications, and the occurrence of death before such patients reach a hospital. Moreover, until an effective circulatory assist device for rapid, emergency use is developed, many patients for whom cardiac replacement might be indicated will die before the necessary arrangements can be made. Even the availability of such a device will not save all coronary victims; as the National Heart Institute's Ad Hoc Task Force on Cardiac Replacement observed,

on the basis of . . . relevant data, particularly pathological evidence as to the extent of myocardial destruction and the extent of coronary artery disease, it seems likely that the overall mortality rate from cardiogenic shock [now estimated at from 70 to 100 percent] will remain high despite effective temporary circulatory assistance or any other method of treatment.[4]

Upon reviewing a combined series of 183 patients[5] from the Framingham, Mass., and Tecumseh, Mich., studies, and assuming the widespread availability of a circulatory assist device, the NHI Task Force concluded that

---

[2] Various measures, such as an interaortic balloon, can be applied to support for a brief period a damaged heart which fails, for example, to start pumping following surgery but which still possesses recuperative powers; the temporary nature of such measures excludes them from our definition of catastrophic disease treatments.

[3] ARTIFICIAL HEART ASSESSMENT PANEL, NATIONAL HEART & LUNG INST., U.S. DEPT. OF HEALTH, EDUCATION & WELFARE, THE TOTALLY IMPLANTABLE ARTIFICIAL HEART: ECONOMIC, ETHICAL, LEGAL, MEDICAL, PSYCHIATRIC AND SOCIAL IMPLICATIONS 50 (1973). Replacement of damaged valves in otherwise well-functioning hearts has been a major successful and permanent surgical approach to the treatment of heart disease.

[4] AD HOC TASK FORCE ON CARDIAC REPLACEMENT, NATIONAL HEART INSTITUTE, U.S. DEPT. OF HEALTH, EDUCATION & WELFARE, CARDIAC REPLACEMENT: MEDICAL, ETHICAL, PSYCHOLOGICAL AND ECONOMIC IMPLICATIONS 5 (1969) [hereinafter cited as CARDIAC REPLACEMENT].

[5] Out of 229 deaths from all types of heart disease; this 80 percent figure is roughly equivalent to that found in national statistics on coronary heart disease in comparison with the overall cardiac causes of death.

only "30 were potential candidates for total cardiac replacement,"[6] a ratio of one in six for coronary patients.

Patients suffering from other heart conditions will probably provide an even smaller percent of potential candidates for transplantation or artificial maintenance. This results from a number of factors, primarily (1) that diseases of other organs, which compromise life, are likely to be present, and (2) that alternative medical and surgical therapies offer greater promise of success at smaller risk. For example, in rheumatic heart disease valvular replacement, rather than total heart replacement, seems to be the preferable approach, and for hypertensive patients the debilitating effects of congestive heart failure can be more conservatively treated by medication.

Thus, for some time to come few of those who suffer from heart disease will be treated by having their damaged organ replaced by a healthy one from another person or an artificial substitute. The major roadblock remains the problem of rejection, which is discussed in some detail in Chapter Four. Once that problem is solved, the number of heart replacements could rise to a level which would be an order of greater magnitude. The NHI Task Force estimated that at such a time transplantation would jump from the existing (1969) level of 100 operations per year[7] to an annual figure of about 12,000. This figure was based on an estimate that 6 percent of the approximately 200,000 persons under 65 who die from heart disease would then become candidates for heart replacement. The Task Force increased its estimate to 16 percent, or 32,000 candidates, if a satisfactory circulatory assist device and an artificial heart were also available.

Recently heart transplants at the Stanford Medical Center have cost from $30,000 to $85,000, the bulk of which goes for postoperative care. In addition, there is the expense of final care for the donor plus tissue-typing, organ removal by a separate surgical team and transportation of the organ to the waiting donor. At the moment most of this money is provided by NHI research funds, insurance, and private sources, including (in effect) contributions by the physicians and surgeons involved, who do not make the usual charges for their services. The cost of an artificial pump and its implantation would probably be about that of a transplant. Moreover, the cost of these procedures would be much higher if the beneficiaries had to amortize the investment (largely by public agencies) in their development. By way of illustration, over the past five years, NIH (through the National

---

[6] CARDIAC REPLACEMENT, note 4 *supra*, at 11.

[7] *Id.* at 16. The Task Force's estimate was on the high side even when made. While 101 transplants were performed in 1968 on a worldwide basis, only 54 were American. In 1972, the last year for which published data is available, just 14 cardiac transplants were performed in the United States. ACS-NIH Organ Transplant Registry, *Third Scientific Report,* 226 J.A.M.A. 1211, 1213 (1973).

Heart and Lung Institute and the National Institute of Allergy and Infectious Diseases) has given about $13.1 million in research grant and contract support for cardiac transplantation and immunology and about $48.4 million for the artificial heart program.

Heart disease, is, therefore, likely to remain a catastrophic disease of major proportions—killing or crippling the hundreds of thousands it strikes, imposing a heavy financial burden on those who can be treated, and creating the sometimes even heavier psychological burden of uncertainty about offering and accepting treatment for all involved, be they patients, relatives and friends, physicians or researchers.

2. Kidney Disease

As a catastrophic illness, chronic renal failure and the concomitant uremia present a somewhat different picture than heart disease. For one thing, incidence of kidney diseases is much lower. On the basis of death certificates, it is estimated that 28,000 people die each year of primary kidney diseases, including nephritis, nephrosis, kidney infections, and polycystic diseases of the kidney. Additionally, approximately 20,000 die of hypertension with arteriolar nephrosclerosis and 50,000 die of other forms of hypertension; a small portion of these can be counted as "kidney deaths," in that they would benefit from hemodialysis (treatment on an "artificial kidney" machine).

On the other hand, a second and perhaps more striking aspect of kidney disease is that the greater success rate of therapy[8] (compared with heart replacement) creates at present a much larger pool of potential candidates for treatment. Although, due largely to immunological difficulties, transplantation of the kidney continues to be far from risk-free, this procedure is much the most frequently performed type of transplantation; its frequency increases while that of heart transplantation declines.[9] One reason for its success is that since kidneys come in pairs live donors can be used, which increases the probability of finding a good immunologic "match" among a patient's immediate relatives. Moreover, hemodialysis permits patients to be maintained until they are adequately prepared for transplantation or until a suitable organ can be found. By compensating for their diseased kidney, this therapy also puts patients in a healthier state prior to

---

[8] This "success" was, of course, accomplished over the years. At an earlier date kidney transplantation was as fraught with failure as heart transplantation is at present. Other important differences, *e.g.*, availability of hemodialysis in cases of kidney transplantation failures, are noted, *infra*.

[9] Kidney transplants are currently performed at an annual rate of about 2,800 in the United States.

their surgery than is the case with cardiac recipients. Of course, some patients are maintained for long periods of time on hemodialysis, which is employed as a life-sustaining treatment in its own right.

Despite these differences, the treatments for end-stage kidney disease share with cardiac replacement two important characteristics; they are costly, and they may provoke severe psychological tension for all concerned. The cost of transplanting a kidney is less than the cost of replacing a heart, yet still better than $15,000,[10] and the patient will need further follow-up care, including dialysis or another transplant if the first kidney fails to function. Because of its continuing nature, dialysis is even more expensive. The cost for this procedure ranges from about $30,000 per year for in-hospital dialysis to about $4,500 per year for dialysis carried out in a patient's home, after an initial expenditure of $3,000 for equipment as well as the substantial expense of home alterations (plumbing, etc.).

The psychological reverberations of kidney transplantation probably exceed those of the heart operation because, in addition to a large element of uncertainty or risk, in many cases the life-saving organ will have come from another living human being, rather than from a cadaver. And even the problems inherent in such a two-way psychic debt are probably not as great as the difficulties encountered by patients undergoing chronic dialysis, who two or three times a week must spend from six to sixteen hours attached to a machine to "purify" their blood.[11] Moreover, preexisting psychopathology is often made more severe by the shifts in the dialysand's metabolic state.

B. A MATTER OF NUMBERS AND CHANCE

This brief description of the treatment of two catastrophic illnesses, end-stage renal and cardiac failure, prompts a number of questions. Prime among these is the need to explain the gap between the number of people who suffer from these conditions and the number who are being treated. The explanation for the gap in turn raises two sets of problems.

---

[10] The cost is higher if a live donor is used. Although the expense of kidney treatments (both transplantation and dialysis) have been declining over the past ten years, the figures used here are on the low side.

[11] *See generally* Calland, *Iatrogenic Problems in End-Stage Renal Failure*, 287 NEW ENG. J. MED. 334 (1972); *Renal Failure: The Agony and the Ecstasy*, 222 J.A.M.A. 829 (1972) [editorial]. Chronic dialysis is also associated with severe physiological complications. *See, e.g.*, Lindner, Charra, Sherrard & Scribner, *Accelerated Atherosclerosis in Prolonged Maintenance Hemodialysis*, 290 NEW ENG. J. MED. 697 (1974); Letters to the Editor, *Maintenance Hemodialysis and Cardiovascular Disorders*, 290 NEW ENG. J. MED. 1324-25 (1974).

1. Experimentation v. Therapy

Why does not everyone with heart disease have his heart replaced? The answer is obvious to anyone looking at the statistics on the transplants which have been performed: of the 228 persons who received transplants between December 1967 and March 1974, only 33 survived with functioning grafts.[12] While several patients have survived for more than five years after the operation, most recipients die within six months.

Such an alarming mortality rate is not, of course, unusual for a new procedure. Even procedures subjected to the most rigorous laboratory and animal testing meet such results in initial trials with human beings. Accordingly, these procedures are usually designated "clinical experimentation," although the reasons for applying this label, and the consequences which follow from it, are often not clearly articulated. A number of possibilities suggest themselves in the context of heart transplantation.

First, if a procedure is "experimental," it is generally assumed that it will be carried out only by those few physician-investigators who are specially qualified to undertake it. This relates primarily to the need for careful laboratory work and extensive experimentation with animals before the investigator tries his hand with humans. Yet heart transplantation adhered to this paradigm only to a limited degree. As Francis Moore dryly observes,

> Unlike transplantation of other organs, progressing cautiously after a slow laboratory launch, cardiac transplantation leaped into action suddenly, quickly getting off the ground, and basing its meteoric rise on remarkably brief laboratory study.[13]

Nevertheless, one explanation for the fact that fewer people get new hearts than needed them is that not every cardiac surgeon, no matter how skillful, is prepared to undertake this experimental procedure. Indeed, some leading surgeons have felt strongly that the procedure is only investigatory (and premature at that) and therefore should be carried out only on a limited scale. They dissuaded others from joining the cardiac transplantation sweepstakes of 1968-1969.[14]

Second, in classifying a procedure as "experimentation," limits are imposed on the number of persons who are selected to undergo the procedure. New medical interventions are often first tested on "normal" subjects, in order to observe their effects unobscured by the complications caused by a

---

[12] ACS-NIH ORGAN TRANSPLANT REGISTRY NEWSLETTER 4 (Spring 1974).

[13] F. D. MOORE, TRANSPLANT: THE GIVE AND TAKE OF TISSUE TRANSPLANTATION 255 (1972).

[14] The role of Dr. Dwight Harken in the Boston medical community, in particular, is discussed in Chapter Five.

disease or other abnormal condition. This is not the practice with surgical innovations, where the initial trials are uniformly performed on persons suffering from the disease in question. In selecting patient-subjects for such trials, it seems to be generally agreed that the decision to proceed turns on the probability that the surgical intervention will produce a greater improvement than can be expected from other accepted modes of treatment. In the case of experimental surgery, in which the risks (of death, injury, or lack of improvement) are speculative, investigators usually proceed only in cases which are otherwise "hopeless." As the NHI Task Force concluded, "it may reasonably be assumed that imminent death will be the basic criterion for total replacement, at least in the near future."[15]

Labelling a procedure "experimental" has other consequences besides limiting the number of times it will be performed. One important result, discussed in Part Two, concerns changes in patterns of interaction among the persons and institutions involved. According to the formal statements on "medical ethics," physicians have different obligations toward "patients" as contrasted to "subjects." It is often assumed, for example, that a subject's "informed consent" to a medical intervention must meet more exacting standards than that of a patient; various "codes" have been drafted to guide physicians in the conduct of human experimentation.[16] The physician's relationship with his colleagues, his hospital, his funding sources, and the scientific community also reflects whether his work is intended solely as therapy for his patients or is also designed to test out new procedures and yield medical knowledge.

2. Scarce Resources

Most of what has just been said about heart transplantation also applies to kidney transplantation. Although the mortality and morbidity rates are much lower than for cardiac operations,[17] only about 50 percent of the 15,000 patients (some 600 of whom have had multiple transplant operations) still had functioning grafts as of March 1, 1974, with the longest survival being a transplant between monozygotic twins performed in 1956.[18] Despite the increased sophistication of drug immunosuppression, basic

---

[15] CARDIAC REPLACEMENT, note 4 *supra*, at 2.

[16] *See, e.g., Nuremberg Code*, 2 TRIALS OF WAR CRIMINALS BEFORE THE NUREMBERG MILITARY TRIBUNALS 181 (1948); World Medical Association, *Declaration of Helsinki*, 271 NEW ENG. J. MED. 473 (1964).

[17] Additionally, there is the crucial factor that the availability of hemodialysis as "back up" protection for kidney recipients means that it makes sense to speak of "morbidity" as well as "mortality," since the failure of the transplant does not necessarily spell death for the patient, as it does in the case of heart transplants.

[18] ACS-NIH ORGAN TRANSPLANT REGISTRY NEWSLETTER 4 (Spring 1974).

problems still exist in coping with rejection, so each transplant remains to some extent an "experiment."

Yet the "experimental" aspect of kidney transplantation only partially explains the gap between those who suffer from renal disease and those who are being treated and accounts even less for the gap between the number sick and the number treated in the case of hemodialysis, which has by even more stringent criteria moved from the category of "experimentation" to that of "therapy." The major reason for the gap is rather that the allocation of needed resources falls short of the number that, for better or worse, would be utilized if they were readily available. The resources in question are of three types: medical personnel, funds, and transplantable organs. Later chapters will explore the efforts which have been made to meet these difficulties, *e.g.*, the development of home dialysis, which is less expensive and requires fewer medical professionals; the tapping of federal[19] and insurance funding sources; the easing of both the practical and legal barriers to organ donation. For the moment, it suffices to observe that the resources are still inadequate and that in the United States the 2,347 patients who received a renal transplant in 1973 and the 3,742 who began chronic dialysis during 1972[20] represent only a fraction of the more than 20,000 new patients who

---

[19] As will be seen later, the analysis of the tensions produced by the disparity between need and treatment would lead one to anticipate the provision of massive federal support, as provided for in §2991 of "H.R.1," the Social Security Amendments of 1972, Pub. L. No. 92-603, 86 Stat. 1329 (1972).

[20] Both these figures need a word of explanation. The ACS-NIH Organ Transplant Registry has records on 2,347 kidney transplants which were performed in the United States in 1973; this was an increase of 158 over the figure for 1972. While the 1973 figure may slightly overstate the number of new patients, since it includes persons who received a second, third, etc., kidney transplant, it is more likely that it *understates* the total significantly, since not all transplants are reported promptly. The ACS-NIH Registry recorded 1,863 kidney grafts for 1972 as of June 1, 1973, but the figure had been adjusted upwards to 2,189 by June 1, 1974; moreover, a number of transplants are never reported to the Registry. A more informal count kept by Dr. Donald Kayhoe of the National Institute of Allergic and Infectious Diseases shows 2,182 kidney transplants for 1971 and 2,298 already reported for 1972. In sum, it is likely that 600-800 more kidney transplants were performed in 1973 than in 1972.

The figure of 3,742 new dialysands in 1972 comes from the NIH Hemodialysis Registry; the staff estimates that this figure is 90 percent complete for the United States. At the beginning of 1972 there were 6,334 patients on longterm dialysis; during the year about 2,320 left dialysis (1,050 died; 1,200 were transplanted, 70 voluntarily discontinued, moved, or were lost to follow-up) leaving 4,014 patients who were on dialysis throughout the year. Together with the 3,742 new patients and 248 patients who were already on dialysis but who were first reported to the Registry in 1972, there were a total of 8,004 chronic dialysands as of January 1, 1973. The figure for January 1, 1974 is 9,502, but a breakdown of new patients, deaths, transplants, etc., is not yet available.

suffer from end-stage primary kidney disease each year and who will die if therapy is not available. Yet if the attempt is made to treat all "suitable candidates" for this *one* serious, chronic disorder, the cost could exceed $500 million annually.[21]

3. Blunting the Issues

Thus, the nub of the problem is that under present practices some people receive treatment and live while a larger number go untreated and die. The lack of an effective therapy or the inability to supply an effective one to all who need it results in the saving of only a portion of those in need. Of course, this is an issue throughout medicine—indeed, throughout human existence. But the matter is seldom posed as starkly as in these conditions.

Naturally, conscious and unconscious efforts are made to blunt the issue. For instance, rather than comparing the number of persons suffering from kidney disease with the number treated, health planners initially reduce the first number substantially by estimating the number of "suitable candidates" and then utilize only this smaller figure. Some of the standards for suitability are cast in physiological terms, others are psychological. The sociological criteria that underlie much of what is subsumed under "suitability" are left unspoken or at least unexamined.[22] Similarly ignored is the fact that the standards employed are far from certain or absolute; indeed, our ability to treat a larger number of patients has come to mean that we have discarded certain criteria which were used until recently as an easy excuse to exclude some categories of patients. For example, the finding of the Bureau of the Budget's Committee on Chronic Kidney Disease (the "Gottschalk Committee") that about 7,000 new cases would be eligible for dialysis in 1968 was based on a "survey of various nephrologic authorities in the United States and Europe" in which it was "estimated that, on the average, about 20 percent of all uremic patients would be suitable candidates for dialysis and are within the age range of 15-54 years."[23] The committee noted that

---

[21] *See* Friedman & Kountz, *Impact of HR-1 on the Therapy of End Stage Uremia,* 288 NEW ENG. J. MED. 1286 (1973).

[22] For example, the reasons (whether physical, psychological, sociological, or whatever) for focusing only on heart patients *under 65* were not fully articulated by the NHI Task Force. *See* text accompanying note 7 *supra.*

[23] COMMITTEE ON CHRONIC KIDNEY DISEASE, U.S. BUREAU OF THE BUDGET, REPORT 106 (1967). In addition to the 20 percent figure for primary kidney disease, the committee concluded that 2 percent of those dying of hypertension with arteriolar nephrosclerosis and 1 percent of those with other forms of hypertension "might benefit from dialysis." *Id.* at 107. The question of how selection procedures should be formulated and administered will be discussed in detail in Part Three of this book.

it had actually described the "ideal patient" as being in the 15-45 age range, but that the strictness of resulting eligibility percentage (about 16 percent) was, "in part, dictated by the relative unavailability of dialysis centers" (*i.e.,* if the capacity to dialyse were increased, as the Committee suggested, more patients would be "suitable"), so the age range was increased by ten years and the percentage of "eligibles" boosted to twenty. A similar process was employed by the NHI Task Force in arriving at its estimate of "potential candidates" for heart replacement. Clearly, both in the abstract and in particular cases, the question of "suitability" is subject to a good deal of arbitrary manipulation. Factual conclusions are adjusted, consciously or unconsciously, to relieve value conflicts.

CHAPTER TWO

Analytical Framework

In noting the incidence of heart and kidney diseases, and in highlighting the distinctions between experimentation and therapy, as well as the inadequacy of resources, it is not our purpose to suggest that these issues exhaust the problems raised by the modern treatment of catastrophic diseases. Rather, we wish to emphasize the significance of these issues and to prepare for the next step in our inquiry: Who should have the authority to make decisions about life and death? People do not "choose" to have cardiac and renal difficulties,[1] but men and women, or institutions designed by them, will have to make the decisions which by direct or indirect means permit some sick people to live and leave others without treatment. Accordingly, throughout this book, great stress will be laid on the authority which is, and ought to be, exercised by each of the participants in the process.

In order to facilitate the analysis of who should be charged with the responsibility of exercising such authority, we have developed a dual conceptual perspective. The first part grows out of an examination of the capabilities and historical roles of the major participants in research and treatment of catastrophic diseases: physician-investigators, patient-subjects and their relatives and other agents, the professions, and the state. The second grows out of our conclusion that the roles and capabilities of these

---

[1] This does not necessarily suggest that different consequences should follow if they did so choose, e.g., if it were conclusively demonstrated that cigarette smoking causes cardiac disease and persons persisted in encountering this risk by continuing to smoke.

actors will vary according to the stage of the decisionmaking process at which each basic issue arises and has to be resolved. This functional approach breaks the process of investigating and treating catastrophic diseases into three decisionmaking stages—the formulation of policy, the administration of research and therapy, and the review of the decisions and their consequences.

In Part Two of this book we examine the issues which emerge from the structural framework of physician-investigator, patient-subject, and professional and public institutions. The participants are introduced in this sequence in order first to evaluate the problems which arise if total authority were assigned to physician-investigators and to identify their special qualifications and values, then to examine the competence of patient-subjects (and their spouses or guardians) to collaborate in decisionmaking, and finally to explore the capacity of the professions and the public to play a role in the process of investigating and treating disease. All the participants have unique and conflicting constellations of motivations, capacities, and value preferences by which they chart their courses. Therefore, to analyze the tensions which arise between the participants over the objectives and conduct of research and therapy, one must not only identify each actor's values but also assess his capacity and willingness to act upon them.

Answers to the question, "What is the proper allocation of authority among these participants?" must, of course, take into account more than their capabilities and constraints. To some extent, a political judgment has to be made. For example, besides an understanding of the participants, one also needs a social theory in order to determine the limitations which should be placed on the scope of experts' control over their clients' lives or, contrarily, the degree of freedom to conduct research which should be delegated to them. This is not to say that these questions must be resolved by the political process or within government agencies, but if they are not, account must still be taken of the value assigned under our form of government to public decisionmaking about such issues as: (1) What goals should be sought by biomedical inquiry? (2) How do these goals and potential achievements compare with those which might be attained through other uses of the same resources? (3) What kinds of risk and what degree of harm are acceptable in achieving advances in the treatment of catastrophic diseases? (4) What information should be supplied to the participants and by what procedures? or (5) To what sort of review, if any, should the "voluntary" decisions of the participants in research and therapy be subjected?

Some of the "political" aspects of the allocation of authority will be dealt with in the portraits of the participants presented in Part Two, but much of it will be discussed in Part Three where we turn to a functional analysis. This complementary approach is grounded in the assumption that the authority to be assigned to each participant is not identical throughout the catastrophic disease process. For example, physician-investigators have asserted that, because of the necessary diagnostic skills they possess, the *selection* of donors and recipients for organ transplantation is a matter which should be left largely to their discretion once they have fulfilled certain obligations (of disclosure, etc.) toward the donors and recipients. Whatever the merits of this claim, it does not follow that physician-investigators should have a like degree of authority over the *formulation of standards for selecting* donors and recipients (which may raise questions of "when is a person dead?" or "who deserves to live?") or over *the review of the decisions made and their consequences.*

Our approach to the subject differs in a number of ways from those taken in the past. Previous studies were for the most part descriptive and non-comprehensive; they tended to address discrete "problems" that they believed were raised by dialysis and transplantation. Furthermore, they usually spoke in terms of "morality" or "ethics," or divided the topic into "medical," "legal," and "ethical" components. We have rejected such an approach for a number of reasons. One reason is that the compartmentalizing of the issues tends to ignore the importance of elements that run across such disciplinary lines. The customary approach also results in making unspoken assumptions about the outcome on certain important points. For instance, the suggestion that a more elaborate "code of medical ethics" is needed has been frequently advanced without acknowledging that this solution presupposes that the "problem" being dealt with is best left to self-regulation within the profession, as opposed to other forms of guidance or control. It is our hope that the structural/functional framework avoids such pitfalls, while not creating worse ones of its own.

CHAPTER THREE

The Role of Goals and Values

Cure or amelioration of one's condition may seem of such overriding concern to a person suffering from a catastrophic disease, that he or she would "give anything" to achieve it. Yet as strong as the patient's attachment to health and life may be, it is the rare individual who means this statement literally. Though the preservation of life holds a prominent, and perhaps momentarily dominant, place in a patient's scheme of values, achieving this goal may be abandoned if it is clear that the price is neglect of or injury to other important values, such as the reduction of suffering, preservation of self-respect, and protection of his or her family's well-being. Similar considerations apply to physician-investigators: Their efforts at research and therapy, for example, often involve conflict between such values as the acquisition of knowledge and the alleviation of suffering.

Although the conflict over value preferences often remains below the surface identified only in certain troublesome decisions, often long after they have been made,[1] such conflict plays an important role in decision-making about catastrophic diseases, not only for individuals' own decisions but particularly in those choices which involve more than one decision-

---

[1] Good examples of the latent value conflicts which only later come to light are found in the study of untreated syphilis conducted by the Public Health Service in Tuskegee, Ala., from 1932 to 1972, and the injection of "live cancer cells" in debilitated patients at the Jewish Chronic Disease Hospital in Brooklyn, N.Y., in 1963. *See* J. KATZ, WITH THE ASSISTANCE OF A. CAPRON & E. GLASS, EXPERIMENTATION WITH HUMAN BEINGS 9-65 (1972).

maker. One of the useful aspects of an analytic framework built around the participants in the decisionmaking process is the light it can shed on the way values and assumptions, seen separately from the vantage points of each participant, affect decisions.

In this chapter we seek to identify the values served by a commitment to research on, and treatment of, catastrophic diseases. This exploration does not, however, intend to turn the process into a mathematical one which grinds out choices based on a finely calculated resolution of value conflicts. We doubt that any such model is possible, especially since it would also have to take into account the intensity of all participants' attachment to each of these values and to other societal goals and values which may be enhanced or undermined by the choices made in the catastrophic disease sphere. The treatment and research modalities which concern us here are only one small part of health care in this country, albeit an important and highly illuminating one; the delivery of health care, in turn, is embedded in the complex of all social relationships and interactions. Instead we intend to list and discuss briefly the goals and values that are served by a committed effort to investigate and treat these diseases, so that decisionmakers can be more sensitive to the values which affect the decisions they make and which are served or neglected by those decisions.

A. PRESERVATION OF LIFE

There are many ways in which our society demonstrates that human life is a "pearl beyond price" which must be vigilantly protected. The criminal law attaches its most severe punishment to the intentional taking of life and views the criminal aspect of nonfatal conduct as aggravated when it involves a threat to life. On the civil side, the protection of life is sought through damage awards and safety regulations. Of course, the commitment to this value is often compromised, especially when the economic costs of protecting it are considered too great. The tension between the professed value assigned to protecting life and the economic restraints on implementing that value is well illustrated by the tragic history of coal miners' working conditions. Although our collective concern about loss of life manifests itself through heroic and expensive rescue measures whenever a mining disaster has trapped workers underground, adequate steps are not taken by mine owners or the government to install the safety devices which would minimize the risk of a disaster recurring.[2] Yet the anger or the twinge in the

---

[2] *See, e.g.,* Franklin, *U.S. Lags in Effort to Implement Mine Safety Law,* N.Y. Times, Mar. 23, 1970, at 15, col. 1; Franklin, *Chairmen of Two Senate Committees Urge a Federal Inquiry into Fatal Coal Mine Explosion in Kentucky,* N.Y. Times, Jan. 3, 1971, at 34, col. 1.

conscience which such undeniable reality provokes only lends further testimony to the primal nature of this value. Similarly, the current national debate about abortion law reform highlights dramatically society's concern about medical interventions which lead to the deliberate termination of life. Though the right of a woman to make decisions which affect her body has been increasingly championed and even found legislative approval in some jurisdictions, this has largely been possible because it is argued that a fetus, up to a certain stage of development, is a "non-being." At least from the time that a newborn is capable of existence independent from its mother's body, society has an interest in protecting it from all but the most compelling interventions.[3] Indeed, when an attempted abortion leads to the "delivery" of a living but premature fetus, physicians customarily devote great effort trying to save it.

If preservation of healthy life is a value to be maximized, then a thoroughgoing commitment to the treatment of and research in catastrophic diseases is required. Already hemodialysis and kidney transplantation can implement this value for those patients to whom these therapies are made available, and a major scientific breakthrough in organ transplantation immunology would greatly increase our ability to preserve life. The lengths to which physicians and patients are willing to go in maintaining life, as in other "heroic" medical treatments, require the examination of at least one underlying assumption; namely, that the *extension* of life is an aspect of preservation of life. Just as, regarding abortion, there is the need to decide when life begins, so in treating catastrophic illness in adults, particularly older people, there is a need to be clear about what constitutes meaningful human life (and the standards by which the quality of human life is to be determined) if the concept of "preserving life" is to have any meaning and deserves to be a value which we should protect.[4]

B. REDUCTION OF SUFFERING

Closely related to the preservation of life is another value which is a central tenet of physicians' professional creed: the alleviation of suffering. The historical role of the medical professional has been that of healer. Although the great increase in clinical experimentation in recent years has introduced a certain ambiguity into the doctor-patient relationship, most

---

[3] *See, e.g.,* Roe v. Wade, 410 U.S. 113 (1973).

[4] *See, e.g., Hearings on Death with Dignity, An Inquiry into Related Public Issues, Before Senate Special Comm. on Aging,* 92d Cong. 2d Sess. (1972); Capron & Kass, *A Statutory Definition of the Standards for Determining Human Death: An Appraisal and a Proposal,* 121 U. PA. L. REV. 87 (1972); D. CRANE, SOCIAL ASPECTS OF THE PROLONGATION OF LIFE (1969).

patients trust that their physicians are primarily concerned to ease the pain of disease.

The changing role of physicians suggests the question: Whose suffering should be reduced? Research or therapeutic intervention with an individual patient may be justified in an attempt to assuage his suffering. Ought it also to be employed if it will soothe the feelings of his family or be of benefit to other patients, present or future? Underlying all these concerns is a basic question about the scope of the concept of "suffering." It is usually conceived to be physical pain, yet should it not encompass mental or economic distress?

There is a point at which the alleviation of physical suffering cannot be a paramount value in our culture, for its singleminded pursuit would lead to a reign of *soma*. Indeed, certain types and degrees of suffering have been regarded as salutary for individuals. On the other hand, in the case of a terminally ill patient who is in great pain, the loss of individuality which may come from massive doses of pain killers may be seen as more humane than the loss of that individuality through unbearable suffering, even though the treatment for pain may also hasten the patient's demise.

C. PERSONAL INTEGRITY AND DIGNITY

The value placed on human life is derived not only from the importance of maintaining biological life but also from the complex implications of the word "human." In our society, with its professed respect for individual liberty and autonomy, a high place is accorded to conduct which enhances personal integrity and dignity, including the power of each individual to determine what interferences with his own mind and body he will permit or what risks he wishes to take, be they in climbing mountains or participating in research (though the latter has never been tapped as much as it might). The treatment and investigation of catastrophic diseases can serve these values by returning the individual to health and hence to a position where he can function as a full human being with control over his own life. Yet if these values are also to be respected during the process of therapeutic experimentation, certain difficult issues must be confronted.

As long as the treatment of a catastrophic disease can neither promise marked relief from suffering nor prevent the occurrence of known and unknown side-effects which impose new pains and discomfort on patients, the possibility exists that such an intervention while prolonging physical life will not extend "meaningful" human life. Thus, if an experimental treatment fails to restore better health, patient-subjects may no longer wish to continue an existence that requires a long period of unaccustomed inactivity and suffering. Respect for the dignity and personal integrity of individuals suggests that procedures be formulated which will give consideration to such requests.

Yet any resolution in favor of these values will have to contend with society's uneasiness about all procedures which permit the deliberate termination of life. These values are already recognized, however, in a number of contexts: (1) Although physicians seek to save life, even against their patients' will, if the procedure is simple, they generally recognize the right of a person to refuse hazardous treatments even though to do so may shorten life; for example, the refusal to undergo hemodialysis will generally be honored even though it may lead to death. Thus, the question can be posed: Should patients be provided with an opportunity to try out such treatments until they have determined whether this represents a satisfactory way of life? (2) The treatment of catastrophic diseases, at least in its early developmental phases, will be highly experimental with little definitive knowledge about its consequences. Patients for altruistic as well as selfish reasons may seek out and undergo such experiments to benefit themselves and science. Since no assurances can be given about success and, again, since nonparticipation would probably have led to an earlier death, should not the general rule that subjects are free to withdraw from research be applied, even though it means giving the subject an opportunity to terminate his life?

D. EQUALITY

The treatment of catastrophic diseases is expensive, and the danger is thus great that, once such an intervention promises more than "research" benefits, it will be available primarily or exclusively to persons of substantial means. Correlatively, if public or quasi-public (foundation or charity) funding is used to make a new treatment more widely available, the danger exists that it may be bestowed only on those who are considered "worthy" of help. The former method favors those whom the socioeconomic system has advantaged; the latter, unless precisely defined, is prone to favor those whose background is similar to the persons making the judgments of "worth" or "social value."

The possibility of such discrimination raises serious questions with respect to the availability of treatment because it obviously conflicts with the value attached to the equality of persons, which finds expression in the theory of "equal protection," a cornerstone of the American legal system. Many deviations from this standard are approved, or at least acquiesced in, by our society. Standard medical care itself has historically been handled by the forces of "private ordering," and this has resulted in an unequal allocation of medical care. Yet, with the growth of public support for therapy, which has led to health care being viewed as a right and not a privilege, and with research seen as a natural outgrowth of society's collective response to the "challenge" of disease, the laissez-faire attitude will not persist for long.

The concern about safeguarding equal treatment is also endangered from another side. As long as treatment of a catastrophic disease is experimental and uncertain (*e.g.*, transplantation at present), the danger is great that patient-subjects will be selected from the less educated and socially deprived classes of the population.[5] This may occur for many reasons, including their being less likely to be protected by a personal physician and more likely to be given "ward" treatment on a charitable basis in a university hospital.[6] Equality of opportunity thus dictates that procedures be devised which will preclude both omissions and exploitations resulting from biased selection procedures for therapy and research.

E. PURSUIT OF KNOWLEDGE

Research in and treatment of catastrophic diseases can, of course, make significant contributions to the acquisition of knowledge in general and to the amelioration or conquest of these diseases in particular. The pursuit of knowledge is a value cherished not only by scientists but by society as well; however, this value is increasingly called into question since it is frequently in conflict with other values, especially respect for the dignity and personal integrity of the individual. Few will disagree that the ongoing work on catastrophic diseases contributes to the acquisition of knowledge and that impediments to such research and treatment could undermine this value. But disagreement will probably arise about the kind of balancing that should take place between this and other values, about which areas of knowledge are more "worthwhile" and should therefore be pursued first given a scarcity of resources, and about who ought to play what role in this balancing. The deep commitment of the scientific community to this value is based, at least in part, on its reading of the historical record of "outside" interferences with scientists' freedom to pursue their research wherever it leads. While many of the examples cited (such as the experience of Semmelweiss) reflect more the conservatism of the scientific elite than heavy-handed government control, it is the latter which is particularly feared.

Decisions about supporting or limiting research on catastrophic diseases are more complex than similar decisions about other types of "pure re-

---

[5] *Cf.* Kelman, *The Rights of the Subject in Social Research: An Analysis in Terms of Relative Power and Legitimacy,* 27 AM. PSYCH. 989, 990-991 (1972).

[6] *See generally* R. DUFF & A. HOLLINGSHEAD, SICKNESS AND SOCIETY (1968).

search." There is a need to consider not only the possible conflict between *the knowledge* gained (and *the uses* to which it may be put) and other societal values, but also the danger that those other values will be violated or neglected *in the process* of gaining the knowledge, a process which involves human subjects as well as laboratory equipment. Any assessment of the value of pursuing knowledge will have to work through a number of issues, such as: (1) the extent to which the intervention is expected to have immediate benefits for the patient-subject; (2) the extent to which the patient-subject can be informed about the procedure, including its risks; (3) the extent to which a meaningful consent can be obtained; (4) the extent to which harm to the patient-subject can be weighed against expected benefits to science; and (5) the extent to which society actually wishes to support the acquisition of knowledge.

F. HIGH STANDARDS OF PROFESSIONALISM

The existence of diseases which lead to untimely death has always challenged the medical profession to seek daring new remedies. The value which has traditionally been placed on doing the job as well as it can be done and on persevering in the face of defeat in part explains the lengths to which some have gone in attempting to treat catastrophic illness. (It also explains in part the willingness of patients to hand over their fate—including in many cases their accustomed right to make decisions for themselves —to their physicians.) Optimal treatment of patients with catastrophic diseases requires specially trained teams of professionals from many disciplines, including internists, surgeons, immunologists, psychiatrists, nurses, social workers, and paramedical personnel. Moreover it demands sophisticated hospital and out-patient facilities, organ registries, specialized laboratories, computers, and a regional or national network of organ exchange.

The collection in one center and on a single health "team" of professionals from many disciplines may create conflicts in views, techniques and priorities, and disputes over leadership and control. Yet in the absence of such personnel or facilities the important value of professionalism can easily become eroded. To some extent this has already happened. For example, the rush of cardiac surgeons to get on the heart transplant bandwagon in 1968 resulted in a number of medical centers undertaking that procedure without adequate staff or preparation to make maximum use of the information gained or to provide the best care to their patient-subjects, particularly in combating the rejection phenomenon.[7]

---

[7] *See* R. Fox & J. Swazey, The Courage to Fail 77, 135-36 (1974).

G. RATIONALITY

Decisions about matters of life and death, to say nothing of the allocation of millions of dollars, ought to be made as rationally as possible. Yet in decisionmaking about catastrophic disease, this laudable value is often difficult to implement. Professionals disagree on the extent to which patients, their families, and the community should be apprised of the treatment and research decisions which have to be made, especially when life hangs in the balance and outcome is affected by complex and often unknown variables. There are great tensions in this area, as in many others, between rationality—by which we mean making explicit to all participants the reasons for decisions and discussing them in a thoughtful fashion—and irrationality—by which we mean decisionmaking in which some or all of the underlying reasons for decisions are not considered by the participants or in which decisions are based on factors that are unrelated to the ends being sought.

Some physicians do not inform their patients truthfully about the lack of facilities for treatment but instead give other reasons for their exclusion from therapy. The need to maintain hope—which some believe may require that a patient be kept ignorant of the gravity of his or her condition or impending death—has been invoked in support of this position. Against this is advanced the right of patient-subjects to make their own decisions; it is argued that the patients' health as well as rationality is increased by bringing to the surface and openly attempting to work through the difficult problems inherent in decisionmaking. Moreover, the difficulties, real or imagined, which are feared will arise if patients are fully informed of "the truth" are suggestive of the obstacles which lie in the way of rational decisionmaking by all of the participants. The unarticulated value preferences and deep-seated preconceptions which plague all attempts to make wise choices are sure to be increased when the topic is as emotionally charged as treatment and experimentation on fatal diseases. It is our impression from the study of existing practices that the forces of irrationality have prevailed too much in the area of catastrophic diseases in particular and medicine in general.[8] Whatever the ultimate balance, the achievement of greater rationality will require probing analysis and arduous articulation.

---

[8] This point is well illustrated by a recent newspaper analysis of the possibility that the yearly cost to the federal government of providing treatment for chronic kidney disease to all those eligible under the 1972 Social Security amendments may reach $1 billion by 1980.

The history of American medicine is such that when a new technique is discovered, it is put into practice as rapidly as possible. If the cost is high initially,

H. ECONOMY

Both individuals and society attach great weight to the husbanding of scarce resources. In modern terms, this may be expressed as the "cost/ effectiveness ratio" by which it may be determined which of a number of proposed interventions is most efficient in curing or ameliorating a particular condition at the least cost. Although the precision of such measurements may be doubted, the need to be economical, in however rational or irrational a fashion, is undeniable. Indeed, so long as the resources available for research and therapy on catastrophic disease are inadequate to meet the need, pursuit of such other values as equality and rationality demands that the benefit derived from the available resources be maximized.

I. PUBLIC INVOLVEMENT

Greater openness and participation by a wider range of people is sometimes advanced as a means of reaching sounder decisions. In a democracy, once a problem area is identified as having a significant impact on the community at large, public involvement in the decisionmaking process may be viewed as a value in and of itself. Participation by the public or its official representatives is appropriate for catastrophic diseases, since the decisions which have to be made have not only professional consequences but profound societal ones as well. Although this is true of many medical practices, little attention has been paid to sorting out which decisions are best made by the profession and which should be delegated to others. Work on catastrophic diseases, particularly heart transplantation, has evoked great public interest in professional activities and has highlighted the need for societal participation in such matters as "the definition of death"[9] and the means of organ procurement. This greater public involvement in some

---

eventually a way is found to lower it so as many patients as possible can benefit.

Accordingly, many doctors and laymen say they are horrified about the need to discuss such a basic humanitarian issue as preservation of life.

Doctors as a group are unaccustomed to thinking about the costs to society of the discoveries they make. But as the taxpayer assumes more and more of the costs for the new and more expensive therapies created by medical research, a need exists for greater public accountability. Accurate long-range budgetary predictions are essential for legislators to decide if the country can afford to finance a program like care for patients with terminal kidney diseases.

Altman, *Cost of Kidney Therapy: Two Fundamental Questions Raised*, N.Y. Times, Jan. 23, 1973, at 21, col. 1.

[9] *See* Capron & Kass, note 4 *supra*.

of the decisions has the subsidiary benefit of removing some burdens solely from the shoulders of the medical profession.

The values we have enumerated, similar to those which shape all human endeavors, conflict with one another. This reality has led some students of policymaking processes to argue that decisionmakers

> . . . must, in sum, seek a comprehensiveness and realism in focus which will encourage both a systematic, configurative examination of all the significant variables affecting decisions and the rational appraisal of the aggregate value consequences of alternatives in decision.[10]

On the other hand, some contend that:

> . . . The idea that values should be clarified, and in advance of the examination of alternative policies, is appealing. But what happens when we attempt it for complex social problems? The first difficulty is that on many critical values or objectives, citizens disagree, congressmen disagree, and public administrators disagree. . . .

> Even when an administrator resolves to follow his own values as a criterion for decisions, he often will not know how to rank them when they conflict with one another, as they usually do. . . .

> The value problem is . . . always a problem of adjustments at a margin. But there is no practicable way to state marginal objectives or values except in terms of particular policies. That one value is preferred to another in one decision situation does not mean that it will be preferred in another decision situation in which it can be had only at a great sacrifice of another value. Attempts to rank or order values in general and abstract terms so that they do not shift from decision to decision end up by ignoring the relevant marginal preferences. The significance of this . . . point thus goes very far. Even if all administrators had at hand an agreed set of values, objectives and constraints, and an agreed ranking of these values, objectives, and constraints, their marginal values in actual choice situations would be impossible to formulate.[11]

Whichever position is accepted does not eliminate the need for decisionmakers to become alert to the competing values which press for recognition and at least to identify those which are to be maximized and those to be neglected. Since value preferences shape decisions significantly, this process

---

[10] Lasswell & McDougal, *Law, Science and Policy: The Jurisprudence of a Free Society,* in J. KATZ, note 1 *supra,* at 259.

[11] Lindblom, *The Science of "Muddling Through,"* 29 PUB. ADMIN. REV. 79, 81-82 (1959).

of identification may clarify why certain decisions are reached and reveal the consequences of their implementation. Also by becoming aware of the values that are being neglected, it may become easier for decisionmakers to minimize the impact of such neglect. Even a noncomprehensive approach to decision*making* does not preclude the need for an awareness of the value consequences in decision *analysis*.

CHAPTER FOUR

The Development and Current Status of the Procedures

Before turning to an examination of the roles of the participants in the catastrophic disease process, it may be helpful to have some familiarity with the history of the research and therapy of kidney and heart ailments. What follows is a brief sketch of that history with emphasis on the medical problems which have arisen and the social and legal questions they pose.

A. HEMODIALYSIS

The artificial kidney, the backbone of the modern treatment of irreversible kidney disease, had its origins in rather inhospitable circumstances. It had been recognized since the early years of this century that uremia could be controlled if it were possible to remove the accumulating chemical wastes from the patient's blood which the diseased kidneys could no longer accomplish on their own. In 1914 a group of Johns Hopkins doctors reported that a process of "dialysis" (in which the blood of live animals was washed against a semipermeable membrane with salt water on the other side) permitted diffusible substances to be removed.[1] Further work was hampered, however, because the membranes did not work well and blood clots formed. The development and commercial manufacture of cellophane

---

[1] Abel, Rowntree, & Turner, *On the Removal of Diffusible Substances from the Circulating Blood of Living Animals by Dialysis*, 5 J. PHARMACOL. EXP. THER. 275 (1914).

tubing (intended for sausage casing) and of heparin, an anti-clotting chemical preparation, provided the means to overcome those problems.

These two innovations were first combined and put to use by Dr. Willem J. Kolff, who became interested in the treatment of nephritis when he was working in the department of medicine of the University of Groningen in Holland in the late 1930s. He was attempting unsuccessfully to construct a dialysis machine when the German army invaded the Netherlands in May 1940. After working on the establishment of blood banks, Kolff transferred his workshop to the town of Kampen where with the help of local industry, left inactive by the war, he produced the first functional artificial kidney. Kolff recently described the initial clinical application of his new device:

> From March 17, 1943, until July 27, 1944, 15 patients were treated. Of these 15 patients only one survived. . . . I sometimes wonder what would have happened to this project if I had done it, not in the Netherlands, but in some location in the United States, and if having treated 15 patients in one and one-half years I could not have claimed a single therapeutic triumph![2]

After the war, work on the development of the artificial kidney stepped up rapidly. Kolff generously donated his kidney machines (which looked like large washtubs on legs with a rotating, slatted drum inside) to various medical centers in Europe and the United States. Kolff's major publication on dialysis techniques was translated into English in 1947, and later that year he visited this country, sparking the work of a particularly active group of experimenters at the Peter Bent Brigham Hospital in Boston. There Drs. John Merrill, George Thorn, and Carl Walter, starting with the blueprints which Kolff had presented to them, led a team of internists, surgeons, and engineers in the construction of a greatly improved artificial kidney. By 1950 they could report that they had achieved excellent results in 33 dialysis procedures with 26 patients.

The artificial kidney proved highly successful in the treatment of *acute* kidney trauma and disease such as battlefield injuries and tubular necrosis (the "crush syndrome", which had been widely observed during the bombing of cities in World War II). Dialyzing such patients a half dozen times over a few weeks was usually sufficient to reverse their uremia and shock and to keep them alive while their kidneys healed. Gradually, however, the physicians began to wonder whether patients with *chronic* renal failure might not benefit from this procedure. The prevailing medical view was that chronic conditions were not suitable for hemodialysis. First it was

---

[2] F. MOORE, TRANSPLANT: THE GIVE AND TAKE OF TISSUE TRANSPLANTATION 82 (1972) [hereinafter cited as MOORE]. The reader interested in the history of research and treatment in this area will find Moore's book a valuable source, as the authors have.

believed that the need to puncture the patient's leg and arm veins and arteries repeatedly would within a few months exhaust the good sites for connecting up the dialysis tubes. Second, physicians were dissatisfied with keeping patients alive without curing them or relieving their dependence on the machine. As Dr. Francis D. Moore has written:

> If there was no likelihood that his own kidneys would heal, then the artificial kidney became merely an instrument for the merciless prolongation of a hopeless life. . . . A patient with chronic kidney failure might be kept alive for weeks, months, or years, but he had little to look forward to if his own kidneys could not be replaced.[3]

Another facet of the unending nature of dialysis raised a third objection among physicians: The spiraling demands for dialysis hours among chronic patients would make these scarce facilities unavailable for acute patients.

Early in 1960, doctors at the University Hospital in Seattle treated a near-dead comatose patient who had been referred for dialysis to reverse his acute renal failure. While the patient soon "recovered," the physicians were distressed to learn that his referring physician's original diagnosis had been mistaken: The patient's kidneys were irreversibly damaged. Shortly thereafter, saddened by having had to send that patient home to die, Dr. Belding Scribner awoke early one morning with a conception of how to save such patients. As he recalls,

> basically, it was such a simple idea—just connect the tube (cannula) in the artery to the cannula in the vein by means of a connecting tube or *shunt*, and the blood would rush through without clotting and maintain the cannulas in functional condition indefinitely. Then when an artificial kidney treatment was needed, we could simply replace the shunt temporarily with the blood circuit of the artificial kidney.[4]

Much to Scribner's amazement, his Teflon-shunted cannulas "worked right from the start." The first chronic kidney patient, Clyde Shields, was fitted with a shunt on March 9, 1960; he lived for 11 years on regular dialysis. Yet, without realizing it, the Seattle physician had opened up "a Pandora's box [of] new and difficult problems."[5] Within a few months, the hospital had to turn away patients desiring chronic dialysis, and a major problem raised most dramatically by hemodialysis—patient selection—was born.

---

[3] Moore at 85. At another point, Dr. Moore observes that even though repeated dialysis is now medically feasible, "new kidney tissue must be supplied if the patient is to be freed of the burden of frequent dialysis treatments." *Id.* at 112.

[4] Scribner, *The Problem of Patient Selection for Treatment with an Artificial Kidney* (consultant's memorandum) at 2 (1972) [Appendix J].

[5] Moore at 85.

Another major difficulty faced by Scribner was to convince his professional colleagues that chronic dialysis was an acceptable form of treatment. Scribner took the opportunity at the annual meeting of the American Society for Artificial Internal Organs in Chicago in April 1960 to announce his success with the shunted cannulas for chronic patients. Because he feared "premature" release by the press of the discovery, Scribner made his presentation at an informal closed session, at which he presented Shields and also distributed "do-it-yourself" shunt kits with which the physicians could make Teflon cannulas. Scribner recalls that Drs. Merrill, Kolff, and George Schreiner (the ASAIO President), among others, were impressed and took the kits back to their hospitals with them to try the technique out on patients.

Although the group in Seattle, which had originated chronic dialysis and was highly motivated to see it succeed, continued to have favorable results, there were no long-term survivors anywhere else in the world, except for those under the care of Dr. Stanley Shaldon who began a new center in London in 1961. Scribner told us of this "very sad" period in these words:

> None of the other investigators in this country or around the world could confirm our experience. It wasn't that the shunts failed—they didn't—but the patients all died of various complications related primarily to poor overall treatment and lack of attention to detail—so necessary in the early phase of complex research.

In searching for an explanation of his team's singular success with dialysis, Scribner notes that there was no transplant program in Seattle at this time. In other centers, where dialysis was regarded merely as a "holding operation" until the patient could be transplanted, the physicians may have been less dedicated to improving the technique and to encouraging the patient to make a "successful" accommodation to the pain and inconvenience of the dialysis regime.

Despite these difficulties in the early 1960s, regular long-term dialysis came to be recognized as a feasible, if not uniformly acceptable or lifesaving, form of innovative treatment for renal failure. Yet the new technique was not without basic problems. In addition to the dramatic problem of patient selection, already mentioned, a host of others have arisen including: What should be done for patients who cannot be taken into a dialysis program? Conversely, what should be done when a patient tires of the dialysis regime and wishes to cease treatment? Who should bear the expense of treatment, which can cost as much as $35,000 per year? New technology has provided a partial answer to these problems, primarily through the development of less expensive means of treatment which permit greater numbers of patients to be dialyzed while reducing the crushing nature of the cost for each patient. Long-term treatment is now possible at home[6] or in satellite centers,[7] at a substantial saving of both direct and indirect costs (*e.g.,* travel expenses, time, etc.). The increasing use of novel modes of care, particularly those which make use of the patient, his family, and other lay personnel, as well as the increased expenditure of funds account for the rapid growth in the number of dialysands. Only 100 Americans were being treated in 1964, and a mere 1,500 were receiving dialysis therapy as recently as September 1969, while today the number exceeds 11,000 in 450 centers. This does not mean that the lid has been closed on Pandora's box, however. Though dialysis of long-term patients probably does not prevent hospitals from having adequate facilities to treat acute renal insufficiency as well, as was originally feared, the psychological burdens of repeated dialysis, imposed on all participants, remain, as does the major stumbling block: How to select the "lucky ones," since only a portion of the *at least* 7,500 new "suitable candidates" each year are actually accepted into dialysis programs.

B. KIDNEY TRANSPLANTATION

For some doctors—particularly surgeons—the artificial kidney's greatest advantage is not its ability to maintain patients over a long period of time but to restore them to a state of relative good health preparatory to the transplantation of a new kidney. Although dialysis and transplantation are thus often interrelated, they are regarded by many physicians as separate or even competing modalities. Indeed, the first attempt at a kidney "transplant" occurred in this country before Kolff's dialysis techniques were being employed.

The experimental transplantation of kidneys in laboratory animals dates to the turn of the century. Dr. Emerich Ullmann of Vienna reported in 1902 that he had transplanted a dog's kidney to its own neck and a dog's kidney into another dog and also into a goat.[8] These initial steps were soon fol-

---

[6] The development of home dialysis techniques by Peter Bent Brigham Hospital personnel in 1963 was soon adopted on a wide scale. *See, e.g.,* Merrill, Schupak, Cameron, et al., *Hemodialysis in the Home,* 190 J.A.M.A. 468 (1964); Curtis, Cole, Fellows, et al., *Hemodialysis in the Home,* 11 TRANS. AM. SOC. ARTIF. INTERN. ORGANS 7 (1965); Shaldon, *Experience to Date with Home Hemodialysis,* PROCEEDINGS OF WORKING CONFERENCE ON CHRONIC HEMODIALYSIS 66 (1966). A current picture of home dialysis is given in Bailey, Hampers, Merrill & Paine, *The Artificial Kidney at Home: A Look Five Years Later,* 212 J.A.M.A. 1850 (1970).

[7] *See, e.g.,* Bilinsky, Morris & Klein, *Satellite Dialysis: An Economic Approach to the Delivery of Hemodialysis Care,* 218 J.A.M.A. 1809 (1971).

[8] Ullmann, *Experimentelle Nierentransplantation,* 15 WIENER KLINISCHE WOCHENSCHRIFT 1 (March 13, 1902).

lowed by the work of the noted surgeon Alexis Carrel. Both in France and, after 1904, in the United States, Carrel did extensive work in kidney transplantation with dogs and cats. His experiments and those carried out by Dr. C. S. Williamson at the Mayo Clinic in the 1920s demonstrated that the relevant surgical operations were not difficult to perform and that the transplanted organs functioned well, as shown by their almost immediate production of urine once the vessels had been sutured together and circulation was restored. They also noted, but did not investigate, the existence of a mechanism which eventually caused the recipient to "reject" the new organ.

Against this background, the first human trial of renal transplantation took place in 1947. A young, pregnant woman was admitted in severe shock to the Peter Bent Brigham Hospital. After ten days of anuria she went into deep coma, and death appeared to be imminent. Dr. Charles Hufnagel, a young surgeon who had done considerable kidney transplantation in animals and was "on the lookout for a patient in whom a kidney transplant might be needed,"[9] in consultation with Dr. Ernest Landsteiner, the urologic resident, and another young surgeon Dr. David Hume decided to give the patient a cadaver transplant "to see if she could be tided over this problem enough to get well."[10] The hospital administrators objected to the operation because of the patient's critical condition, so it was carried out, as Hufnagel recalls, "in the dark of the night . . . by the light of two small gooseneck student lamps."[11] The cadaver organ was attached to an artery and vein in the patient's arm, in which it was partially imbedded, with the tip of the ureter exposed. The transplanted organ served its purpose. Within a few days the patient's condition had improved greatly, the cadaver kidney was removed, and her own kidneys resumed normal functioning. Since just at this time the artificial kidney was being developed, no further attempts were made at short-term transplantation for acute renal insufficiency.

While the artificial kidney made transplantation unnecessary for patients with acute renal disease, it only served to increase surgeons' desire to attempt transplantation for chronic kidney disease. On March 31, 1951, Dr. James V. Scola of the Springfield (Mass.) Hospital transplanted a kidney from a patient with cancer of the ureter into Mr. A., a 37-year old man whose rapidly declining kidney function and worsening uremia had been temporarily reversed by dialysis at the Peter Bent Brigham Hospital. Although A.'s condition improved for a few days, it subsequently worsened, and he died of infection and kidney failure (through rejection) on May 7, 1951.

---

[9] A recent statement by Hufnagel, quoted in MOORE at 40.
[10] *Id.*
[11] *Id.* at 40-41.

Shortly before A. died, Hume, who had participated in the 1947 transplant, began a series of nine transplant operations at the Peter Bent Brigham Hospital which were to stretch into 1953, to be followed by Dr. Joseph E. Murray's series of six patients. Looking back at that period, Francis Moore, Brigham's Surgeon-in-Chief, recalls that

> It was hoped that the transplanted kidneys might function longer than was previously reported in animals, or that the general advances in surgery, medicine, and biology would permit some unexpected success in transplantation. There was every reason to expect something new when all the techniques of modern medicine and surgery were applied. This expectation alone justified the undertaking. . . .[12]

Despite this hope, true success was not forthcoming, and the pattern of brief recovery, followed by failure, repeated itself in patient after patient. Even the one "unexpected success," the transplantation performed on Dr. W., a young physician, on February 11, 1953, was only of fleeting duration and raised more problems than did the "failures." W.'s immediate post-operative period was turbulent, with much bleeding and no kidney output for nearly three weeks. Suddenly, the course of recovery reversed itself, and after constant improvement the patient was discharged 81 days after the operation. Nevertheless, while the new kidney behaved well, W.'s own diseased kidneys caused greatly elevated blood pressure, and he died of heart and kidney failure nearly six months after the transplant. As has so often been true in transplantation, even to this day, "[t]he explanation of precisely why this patient lived 175 days with good kidney function while none of the others had shown anything approximating such a good result must remain a mystery."[13]

At the same time, Dr. Peter Medawar and his team of researchers in England were bringing to fruition many years of study on immune reactions and rejection. Their theories had roots in the work of Dr. Emile Holman, who as early as 1924 had published his observations on the reaction of skin grafts,[14] including what Medawar later termed the "second set phenomenon"—that animals seem to become sensitized by a graft and rejected a second graft much more swiftly. These scientists discovered that an animal reacts to a graft from another animal as it does to viruses or bacteria. The graft carries with it certain antigens, proteins that excite a cellular response from the host organism which puts out other proteins, called antibodies, which with the help of another substance (the "complement") then destroy

---

[12] MOORE at 89.

[13] MOORE at 91.

[14] Holman, *Protein Sensitization in Isoskingrafting*, 38 SURG., GYNEC. & OBSTET. 100 (1924).

or bind up the invader. While simple in its conception, this process is not yet fully understood. Through the work of Medawar's group, Sir Macfarlane Burnet of Australia, and Drs. Jack Cannon and William Longmire at UCLA, much was learned in the 1940s and 1950s about the reticuloendothelial system, the tissues that are responsible for mounting the body's response to foreign protein. Burnet postulated that while this system is still developing the circulating proteins are able to destroy the cells which produce antibodies against them, leaving behind only those cells which react against other antigens not possessed by the particular animal.[15] Experiments with baby chicks demonstrated that this tolerance for new antigens persisted until birth but disappeared quickly thereafter; skin grafts in newly hatched chicks "took" uniformly, while only 1 per cent of grafts made at three days, and none at 14 days, were successful.[16] Medawar, Billingham, and Brent then demonstrated that unlike the sensitized "second set" response of mature immune systems mentioned previously, an injection of foreign protein from a donor into a fetus led to an "actively acquired tolerance" for even repeated grafts from that donor after birth.[17] In experiments on rats and then on human babies, Dr. Michael Woodruff demonstrated that at least partial tolerance could also be created by injecting cells into a newborn rather than a fetus.[18]

Yet, since this type of immunization in humans seemed impractical (and even dangerous),[19] the growing knowledge of the body's defense mecha-

---

[15] F. M. Burnett, The Clonal Selection Theory of Acquired Immunity (1959).

[16] Cannon & Longmire, *Studies of Successful Skin Homografts in the Chicken*, 135 Annals Surg. 60 (1952).

[17] Billingham, Brent & Medawar, *Actively Acquired Tolerance of Foreign Cells*, 172 Nature 603 (1953). This induced tolerance has its natural analogue in nature. Beginning with studies of cattle, Owen, *Immunogenetic Consequences of Vascular Anastomoses between Bovine Twins*, 102 Science 400 (1945), it was found that "chimerism" (the presence in one animal of genetic material from another) occasionally occurred in nonidentical human twins, apparently because the twins' blood must have cross-circulated *in utero*, Dunsford, et al., *A Human Blood-group Chimera*, 2 Brit. Med. J. 81 (1953). In 1958, Drs. Michael Woodruff and Bernard Lennox, in Scotland, grafted skin between a brother and sister with blood chimerism; as with the "actively acquired tolerance," the twins' natural tolerance for each other's antigens permitted the grafts to be accepted. Woodruff & Lennox, *Reciprocal Skin Grafts in a Pair of Twins Showing Blood Chimerism*, 2 Lancet 476 (1959).

[18] Woodruff & Simpson, *Induction of Tolerance to Skin Homografts in Rats by Injection of Cells from the Prospective Donor soon after Birth*, 36 Brit. J. Ex. Path. 494 (1955); Woodruff, *Can Tolerance in Homologous Skin be Induced in the Human Infant at Birth?* 4 Transplant. Bull. 26 (1957).

[19] Incidences were reported where this type of transplant caused a graft-versus-host reaction, sometimes termed "runt disease," that leads to weight loss and skin reactions.

nism helped to define the problems facing transplanters but did not resolve them. The publication of Medawar's work in 1953 only served to confirm the sad experience of the Brigham surgeons as they ended their series of kidney grafts that year: Transplantation would be successful only (1) if the antigens of the donor's organ did not call forth a response from the recipient (as had apparently been the case, to some degree, with Dr. W.) or (2) if the recipient's rejection mechanism could be weakened or immobilized.

1. Avoiding Antigenicity

One way of exploiting the first possibility was to perform the transplant using an organ which was genetically identical to the one replaced, *i.e.*, a graft from one identical twin to the other. It was known that skin grafts could be performed successfully between twins; like skin, a person could "spare" a kidney to help his or her ailing twin. In October 1954, the staff at the Peter Bent Brigham Hospital had the opportunity to test this theory when a young man dying of kidney disease, who had a healthy identical twin brother, was referred to them. The doctors decided that it was proper, with the healthy brother's consent, to deprive him of one kidney in the hope of restoring normal renal function in his ailing twin. Led by Dr. Joseph Murray, the Brigham surgeons placed the healthy organ in the abdominal cavity, near its normal site, attached it to the bladder, and subsequently removed the two diseased kidneys (in order to reduce the recipient's abnormal blood pressure). Within six months the young man was out of the hospital leading a normal life.[20] This success—the first true success in renal transplantation—gave the doctors a great boost "and had an immediate and far-reaching effect on the entire transplant research effort, both in this country and abroad."[21]

To some extent, of course, kidney transplantation in identical twins partakes of a "medical freak," as Moore has observed, since so many factors have to coincide, not the least of which is that "the sick twin must . . . be in the hands of a physician who will consider a transplant and seek the necessary consultations."[22] While statistically rare, twin transplants continue to be performed at a fairly even pace. Overall, 82 had been carried out worldwide by June 1, 1974[23] (equal to .5 percent of all transplants, a

---

[20] Merrill, Murray, Harrison & Guild, *Successful Homotransplantation of the Human Kidney between Identical Twins*, 160 J.A.M.A. 277 (1956).

[21] MOORE at 96.

[22] MOORE at 103.

[23] ACS-NIH ORGAN TRANSPLANT REGISTRY NEWSLETTER 2 (Spring 1972), updated by unpublished data received from the ACS-NIH Registry in June 1974; 63 percent of the 82 identical twin transplants occurred in the United States.

figure approximately the same as the rate of occurrence of twins in the population). The longest transplant survivor is a twin who received a kidney 18 years ago;[24] the average two-year survival for 1951-1966 is 85.2 percent (±5.6 percent), and in recent years it has been 100 percent.[25]

This is not to say that identical twin transplants are without problems. The major medical difficulty in patients suffering from glomerulonephritis is that the isotransplant (between identical individuals) meets with a modified rejection reaction similar to that experienced with allotransplants (between nonidentical individuals of the same species). Thus, in addition to the original twin transplant of 1954, subsequent twin recipients have experienced a reoccurrence of fatal glomerulonephritis. Consequently, some of the techniques of immunosuppression developed for nonidentical transplants are now being used in twin recipients to hold down the action of the antibody which seems to lead to glomerulonephritis.

Transplantation in identical twins has also presented the legal issue of whether the operation is permissible in children under the age of consent (recently lowered from 21 to 18 years in most jurisdictions). As far as the recipient is concerned, this presents no problem: If a minor needs a kidney transplant, permission for the operation can be given by his or her parents or guardian to whom the law gives the authority to consent to therapeutic interventions.[26] Yet when the donor is a twin, he or she will also be a minor, and the law traditionally has not given parents authority to consent to interventions that do not promise therapeutic benefit. The reasoning which courts have employed to deal with this issue is discussed in later chapters.

2. Overcoming Antibody Response

Since destructive antigenicity can be naturally avoided only in the rare circumstance of identical twinship or the still rarer unexplained "chance" case (such as Dr. W.), means have had to be found to reduce the impact of the body's natural immune responses. The first method attempted, whole

[24] ACS-NIH ORGAN TRANSPLANT REGISTRY NEWSLETTER 4 (Spring 1974) [hereinafter cited as 1974 REGISTRY NEWSLETTER].

[25] Advisory Committee to the Renal Transplant Registry, *The Tenth Report of the Human Renal Transplant Registry*, 221 J.A.M.A. 1495, 1496 (1972) [hereinafter cited as *Tenth Renal Registry Report*]. *See also* note 23 *supra.*

[26] Of the nearly 16,000 transplants performed as of December 31, 1972, 1,351 (8.6 percent) were performed on patients 15 years old or less, and another 1,770 (11.1 percent) on those 16 to 20 years of age. Although kidney disease is often traced to a severe childhood infection, it usually does not manifest itself critically until later in life. The large proportion of transplants among minors is explained by the fact that long-term hemodialysis is not recommended because of its adverse physiological and psychological effects in young, growing children.

body irradiation, proved to be too clumsy. Either too low a dose was given and the graft was rejected or the exposure was too great which destroyed the patient's ability to ward off infections and to produce platelets (necessary to prevent hemorrhages), despite transfusions of whole blood and bone marrow cells. Notwithstanding the largely unfavorable animal test results, trials of the technique were carried out on humans from 1958 to 1961 in certain "desperate situation[s]."[27] Unfortunately, the results were uniformly disappointing; it seemed that the antibody response could be suppressed only at great risk to the patient, leading to an updating of an old saying—"the graft lived but the patient died."[28]

As with the unmodified transplants of the early 1950s, however, there were rare, "freak" successes. For example, in January 1959, a kidney was transplanted between fraternal twins at the Peter Bent Brigham Hospital after the ailing brother had been exposed to doses of radiation which were below those previously used and substantially lower than the level which animal experimentation indicated was necessary to achieve immunosuppression—yet the kidney was not rejected.[29] Somehow the graft and patient "adapted" to each other. Drs. Jean Hamburger and R. Kuss of Paris followed this regime of less irradiation, first in nonidentical twins, then between close relatives.[30] This emphasis on close genetic relationship, which grew out of the French physicians' belief in and reliance on leucocyte testing[31] before it was accepted in the United States and Great Britain, prob-

---

[27] MOORE at 118.

[28] *Id.* at 109.

[29] Merrill, Murray, Harrison, Friedman, Dealy & Damin, *Successful Hemotransplantation of the Kidney Between Nonidentical Twins,* 262 NEW ENG. J. MED. 1251 (1960).

[30] *See, e.g.,* Hamburger, Vaysse, Crosnier, et al., *Transplantation d'un rein entre jumeaux non monozygotes après irradiation du receveur: Bon fonctionnement au quatrième mois.* 67 PRESSE MED. 1771 (1959); Hamburger, Vaysse, Crosnier, et al., *Renal Homotransplantation in Man after Radiation of the Recipient: Experience with Six Patients since 1959,* 32 AM. J. MED. 854 (1962); Kuss, Legraine, Mathe, et al., *Etude de quatre cas d'irradiation totale par le cobalt radioactif (A des doses respectives de 250, 400, et 600 rads.),* 10 REV. FRANC. ETUDES CLIN. BIOL. 1028 (1962).

[31] Leucocytes (white blood cells) provide a useful means of predicting graft-host compatibility for organ transplants because (a) leucocytes are easily obtained and (b) they share important transplantation antigens with organs, tissues, and lymphocytes. Beginning in the 1950s, "typing sera" from patients with antibodies of limited specificity were selected on the basis of computer analysis of their reaction with leucocyte samples from many donors. More than 20 leucocyte antigens (most of them belonging to the HL-A system, discussed *infra* at note 39) are now recognized on an international basis.

The exchange of typing sera among laboratories in different parts of the world and the holding of several international workshops in histocompatibility typing have

ably explains their success rate, which exceeded the American and British by a wide margin.

Despite the occasional successes with irradiation, a more precise means of immunosuppression was needed if transplantation was to be any more positive than Russian roulette with five chambers loaded. It had long been known that certain compounds, such as benzene, tolurene and the "nitrogen mustards" interfered with antibody production, but attempts to use this knowledge to aid transplantation were not successful until 1958. At that time, Dr. Delta Uphoff reported that amethopterin (an anti-cancer drug) prevented the "graft-versus-host" reaction ("runt disease") which occurred when bone marrow infusions were given to irradiated animals;[32] similarly, Drs. Robert Schwartz and William Dameshek described a "drug-induced tolerance" to human serum albumin in rabbits treated with 6-mercaptopurine, another anti-cancer agent.[33]

From these beginnings, there has grown up a battery of immunosuppressives—*azathioprine* (Imuran), which was found to be more effective and less toxic than mercaptopurine,[34] and *azaserine*, both of which apparently attach themselves to the DNA in the antibody producing cells and throw off normal synthesis (although the exact mode of azathioprine's action is still unclear); *actinomycin*, which binds itself onto the DNA molecule and prevents the corresponding RNA molecule from being produced; and *cortisone*, an adrenal hormone (now produced artificially) which seems to block

---

played an indispensable role in defining the reagents and the antigens, arriving at a standard nomenclature, and indicating the high degree of consistency of the results obtainable.
R. BILLINGHAM & W. SILVERS, THE IMMUNOBIOLOGY OF TRANSPLANTATION 27 (1971) [hereinafter cited as BILLINGHAM & SILVERS].

[32] Uphoff, *Alteration of Homograft Reaction by A-methopterin in Lethally Irradiated Mice Treated with Homologous Marrow,* 99 PROC. SOC. EXP. BIOL. MED. 651 (1958).

[33] Schwartz, Stack & Dameshek, *Effect of 6-mercaptopurine on Antibody Production,* 99 PROC. SOC. EXP. BIOL. MED. 164 (1958); Schwartz & Dameshek, *Drug-induced Immunological Tolerance,* 183 NATURE 1682 (1959). They subsequently demonstrated that 6-mercaptopurine would triple the survival time of skin grafts in rabbits, as well as serum injections. Schwartz, Dameshek & Donovan, *The Effects of 6-mercaptopurine on Homograft Reactions,* 39 J. CLIN. INVEST. 952 (1960). *See also* Calne, *The Rejection of Renal Homograft: Inhibition in Dogs by 6-mercaptopurine,* 1 LANCET 417 (1960); Calne & Murray, *Inhibition of the Rejection of Renal Homografts in Dogs by BW 57-322,* 12 SURG. FORUM 118 (1961).

[34] Although azathioprine is considered to be a generally "safe" drug, one transplant team recently reported a severe, irreversible liver condition which caused the death of a kidney recipient being treated with azathioprine. Zarday, Veith, Gliedman & Soberman, *Irreversible Liver Damage after Azathioprine,* 222 J.A.M.A. 690 (1972).

the antigen-antibody reaction. Not only the mechanism but the proper use of these drugs remain a matter of dispute and trial and error. While kidney transplantation is much more effective than it was just a decade ago, the unknown aspects of immunology keep it in the category of experimental therapy.

A major consequence of the availability of immunosuppressive drugs has been the increasing use of cadaver kidneys; indeed, Dr. Roy Calne, a pioneer in immunosuppression research in the early 1960s, employed organs *only* from dead donors. The results in this group are not yet as good as those with closely related donors, but they are improving. Cadavers now account for about 70 percent of all transplanted kidneys, and their survival rates are improving: Two-year graft survival[35] has gone from 27.9 percent for 1951-1966 to 46.6 percent for operations performed in 1971.[36] This improvement is due in part to increased sophistication in the use of immunosuppressives, including antilymphocyte serum (ALS) and its purified immunoglobulin (ALG) which have come into clinical use since 1966. Yet the results with cadaver kidneys remain below those for live donors: One-year graft survival is 45.4 percent for cadaver organs at last report, compared to 76.4 percent for parent donors and 74.0 percent for siblings.[37]

---

[35] Since patients whose transplant fails can be supported on hemodialysis and even given a second, third, etc. graft, the *recipient* survival rate is a good deal higher than the *graft* survival, particularly in the case of cadaver transplants.

[36] Advisory Committee to the Renal Transplant Registry, *The 11th Report of the Human Renal Transplant Registry*, 226 J.A.M.A. 1197, 1202 (1973) [hereinafter cited as *11th Renal Registry Report*]. While cadaver donors now comprise 63.4 percent of the renal grafts worldwide, the past few years have seen an increase in the number of live donors (particularly siblings) used in the United States, where cadavers constitute only 52.6 percent of the grafts. *Id.* at 1198. In Australasia 98.3 percent of the kidneys transplanted are from cadavers; the 42 percent graft survival rate at five years is considerably above the worldwide average of 29.4 percent. *Id.* at 1201-02.

[37] *Id.* In 1970 the one-year results were 56.1 percent for cadaver grafts, 74.2 percent for parental, and 82.5 percent for sibling. The data for 1967-1971 suggest that the survival rates for kidney transplants have reached a plateau. *See* Lazarus & Hampers, *Renal Transplantation—1972*, 76 ANN. INTERN. MED. 504 (1972). Moreover, the disparity between cadaver and live donors is more marked over time.

After three years, surviving recipients of related living grafts show an attrition rate that approaches zero, while that of cadaver grafts and recipients continues slowly. Since there is a trend toward increasing use of cadaver grafts, the fate of recipients of such grafts depends on improved methods to prevent rejections and greater care to insure that patients are managed properly during the pretransplant period, especially as regards avoidance of unnecessary transfusions.

Organ Transplantation, 223 J.A.M.A. 320 (1973) [editorial].

3. Combining the Techniques

Of course, the advances in immunosuppression which have been useful in cadaver transplants have also improved related-donor results.[38] But the real advantage seems to lie in the less violent rejection reaction which has to be overcome in the latter set of transplants. With increased knowledge of the molecular biology involved, "tissue-typing" of the kind originally developed by the French transplanters has played an increasingly important role in kidney grafting. Dr. Paul Terasaki of UCLA, who did his early work with Dausset and Medawar abroad, has developed an automated, routine method of typing cells from minute samples according to their antigens on the HL-A system. This antigen system is similar to the ABO system used for blood, but is much more complex. It seems to be made up of two closely connected loci, "LA" and "Four" with 13 and 26 alleles, respectively, which have been identified and labeled by Terasaki and Dr. J. J. van Rood, among others.[39] Terasaki's work and that of Dr. F. T. Rapaport have shown the need to crossmatch donor and recipient before grafting to avoid preformed antibodies which often cause immediate rejection of the new organs.[40] Even when mismatching does not lead to an immediate rejection, retrospective studies indicate that it does increase the risk of subsequent rejection. Yet knowledge of antigens is still rudimentary. As Terasaki has recently observed:

> In view of the enormous complexity of the HL-A genetic locus, which has established itself as the most complex locus known to man, it would seem naive to expect complete knowledge or immunogenicity to follow immedi-

---

[38] Drs. Murray and Wilson have also described another method of reducing lymphocyte reaction which has proven its value in transplants involving live donors. About five days before the operation the thoracic lymph duct is drained, a fairly simple procedure. Large quantities of fluid are removed, the lymph cells are centrifuged out, and the fluid returned to the patient. The result is a significant reduction in rejection crises among these kidney recipients. Murray, Wilson, Tilney, et al., *Five Years Experience in Renal Transplantation with Immunosuppressive Drugs: Survival, Functioning, Complications, and the Role of Lymphocyte Depletion by Thoracic Duct Fistula*, 168 ANNALS SURG. 416 (1968).

[39] "HL-A system" refers to the Human Leukocyte Antigen System, formerly called "Hu-1." In addition, closely linked to the HL-A loci is the MLC (for mixed lymphocyte culture) locus. For a recent review of the HL-A system, *see* Thornsby, *Human Major Histocompatibility System*, 18 TRANSPLANT. REV. 51 (1974). Although ABO blood group compatibility has recently been shown to be an important factor in transplantation of tissues, as well as in transfusion of blood, the specificities of the HL-A system have not been shown to be present on red cells. *See* BILLINGHAM & SILVERS, note 31 *supra*, at 28.

[40] Terasaki, Mickey, Singal, Mittal & Patel, *Stereotyping for Homotransplantation; XX, Selection of Recipients for Cadaver Donor Transplants*, 279 NEW ENG. J. MED. 1101 (1963); Rapaport & Dausset, *Ranks of Donor-Recipient Histocompatibility for Human Transplantation*, 167 SCIENCE 1260 (1970).

ately the serologic identification of the HL-A antigens. Overenthusiasm has led to the belief that application of histocompatibility matching to transplants from unrelated (cadaver) donors is now past the research stage and can be utilized on a strictly service basis.[41]

In sum, the present measures of histocompatibility are not yet adequate to assure that "well matched" kidneys will "take" even when employed in conjunction with advanced immunosuppressives. It is possible that certain antigen loci have yet to be identified or to be given their proper weight.[42] This is at least one explanation why some "A matches" fail while occasional "D matches" succeed.[43] Nevertheless, tissue-typing appears to be well-established today as a central part of renal transplantation. This raises important issues for physicians and the public concerning the degree to which a good match should be a prerequisite to using an organ for a particular recipient as well as problems about how kidneys should be pooled and shared among potential recipients. These questions will be explored in the chapters which follow.

Before closing this section, one additional medical difficulty should be noted. The use of immunosuppression has not been an unmixed blessing. These powerful agents not only open the patient to the danger of powerful side-effects, such as infections and psychological disturbances, but, it now appears, also create an increased likelihood of cancer. This is ironic since some of these immunosuppressives were originally developed from drugs used in even greater doses to combat cancer. A tumor may also be unwittingly transplanted along with the new kidney or it may be dwelling unnoticed within the recipient (this has been particularly true in liver transplantation); in either case, the immunosuppression permits the tumors to grow at an unusually fast rate.[44] It is not clear which drugs have what

---

[41] Terasaki, Wilkinson & McClelland, *National Transplant Communications Network*, 218 J.A.M.A. 1674, 1675 (1971).

[42] Similarly, the occurrence of some blood reactions between persons who were ABO compatible was inexplicable until the Rh-antigen was discovered. It may also turn out that important kidney antigens are not manifest in blood cells.

[43] A grading scale, from A to D, has been established by immunologists to describe the degree of histocompatibility of donor and recipient: An "A match" indicates that there is no antigenicity at any major locus.

[44] The Advisory Committee to the Renal Transplant Registry at first suggested that the incidence of malignant neoplasm following renal transplantation "is quite low." *Tenth Renal Registry Report*, note 25 *supra*, at 1051. More recent reports indicate that the rate of lymphoma following transplantation is far in excess of that for the general population, with the risk of reticulum cell sarcoma being 350 times higher than expected. *See* Hoover & Fraumeni, *Risk of Cancer in Renal Transplant Recipients*, 2 LANCET 55 (1973). *See also* Lecatsas, *Papopavirus in Urine after Renal Transplantation*, 241 NATURE 343 (1973)—virus particles typical of those with oncogenic potential found in urine of eight kidney recipients.

effect in this sorry sequence; the incidence of tumors is highest in patients on ALS, but other patients have experienced growths without ALS. Since extensive immunosuppression has come into use only recently, there is concern among physicians that the increase in tumors is only now beginning to be detected and that the incidence may be even higher than is now suspected.

These findings about tumor growth, besides being of possible help to cancer researchers, may spur transplant research into ways (such as improved matching) of avoiding heavy immunosuppression or otherwise of "enhancing" transplant acceptance. The latter possibility, which may be related to the phenomenon of "adaptation," grows out of observations on the experimental transplantation of tumors in mice. At a certain time before the transplant, a small amount of cell extract is injected into the recipient; rather than leading to a "second set" rejection, this procedure, when done at just the right time and with just the right quantity, seems to cause the donor to produce antibodies which lock into the antigen of the graft, protecting instead of destroying it, thereby "enhancing" the survival. Indeed, appropriate pretreatment with specific antisera can produce the same effect, as is shown by treatment of women delivering Rh-incompatible children.

C. HEART TRANSPLANTATION

The lack of a back-up system similar to a dialysis machine and the dependence on cadaver organs has contributed to making heart transplantation an infrequently employed experimental procedure. In contrast to the first year of heart transplantation, beginning in December 1967,[45] the present activity is a mere trickle. Nearly half of the cardiac transplants performed in the world in the six and one-half years to date were carried out during those first twelve months, as medical centers sought the public spotlight for such activities.[46] The 26 operations performed in the single month of November 1968 represent one-ninth of the total heart grafts thus far; that month also marked the beginning of the end, or at least of the present abeyance, for this dramatic procedure.[47]

---

[45] A single cardiac transplant was performed in 1964 at the University of Mississippi using a chimpanzee donor, but it turned out to be an isolated event which did not trigger the rush of followers as did Dr. Barnard's December 1967 operation in Capetown. *See* Hardy, Chavez, Kurrus, et al., *Heart Transplantation in Man,* 188 J.A.M.A. 1132 (1964).

[46] ACS-NIH Organ Transplant Registry, HUMAN HEART TRANSPLANTATION (DEC. 3, 1967—JUNE 4, 1974) at 1 (1974) [hereinafter cited as 1974 HEART REPORT]; 1974 REGISTRY NEWSLETTER, note 24 *supra,* at 4.

[47] 1974 HEART REPORT.

The public's disaffection with the procedure can probably be traced to the poor results of what was originally heralded as a great advance in life-saving *therapy* for otherwise hopeless patients. Only 15 percent of the transplanted grafts are presently surviving, the longest having just passed five and one-half years. Disenchantment in the medical community probably has the same roots, with the added fact that physicians are aware that even the grafts that last do not represent unmitigated successes. The burden of continued immunosuppressive treatment for the recipient, with all its complications, the prolonged suffering of patients who have been subjected to these operations, and transplanters' inability to determine exactly what makes some grafts work and others fail, all serve to dampen the enthusiasm with which the survival of these few heart recipients would otherwise be met.

Cardiac transplantation goes back to the animal experimentation of Drs. Norman E. Shumway and Richard R. Lower in the late 1950s and early 1960s. They demonstrated that such transplants were feasible with temporary mechanical cardiopulmonary support and were fairly simple surgically.[48] They also observed that the heart would function well even though its nerves had been severed, but that rejection (which could be monitored by electrocardiography) would, not surprisingly, remain the major problem facing cardiac surgeons and their patients.

The poor results of cardiac transplants can be traced to two factors. Under the criteria employed by all the cardiac transplanters, a patient had to be near death to be considered for this operation; the risks involved meant that the surgeons would not operate on anyone but patients with extremely limited life expectancies and no hope from conventional treatment.[49] Thus, these patients were not only very weak, with little reserve strength for the tough postoperative haul, but more importantly their period of availability as recipients was so limited that the chances of finding a compatible donor were greatly reduced. Unlike kidney recipients, heart

---

[48] *See, e.g.,* Lower, Stofer, Hurley, Doug, Cohn & Shumway, *Successful Homo-transplantation of the Canine Heart after Anoxic Preservation for Seven Hours,* 104 AM. J. SURG. 302 (1962).

[49] *See, e.g.,* EXPERIENCE WITH HUMAN HEART TRANSPLANTATION: PROCEEDINGS OF THE CAPE TOWN SYMPOSIUM, 13-16 JULY 1968, at 6 (H.A. Shapiro, ed., 1969) [hereinafter cited as CAPETOWN PROCEEDINGS]: "[A]s cardiologists have always done, we face our surgeons with the worst possible material and the worst possible cases, to begin with, on the thesis that if the surgeon can cope with the worst possible cases, in due course he will be able to deal with patients who are less ill." [Comments of Dr. V. Schire.] It has been suggested that the improved survival rates of the past few years are a consequence of a reversal of the early pattern, so that transplanters may now be biased to select healthier patients. Gail, *Does Cardiac Transplantation Prolong Life: A Reassessment,* 76 ANN. INTERN. MED. 815 (1972).

patients could not be maintained indefinitely until the "right" organ came along.

This was not the only factor lying behind the poor tissue matching which characterized the early heart grafts. The hope had existed among transplanters that the heart would prove to be a "privileged" organ with less antigenicity than the kidney,[50] but the reverse proved to be the case. More importantly, most of the transplant teams were led by doctors who were more concerned with the surgical aspects of the transplant than with its immunology. Ten of the 28 surgical teams were headed by physicians trained at two schools (Johns Hopkins and Minnesota) which had emphasized cardiac surgery, not transplant science, in the previous decade.[51] Transplants were frequently carried out before the immunological testing had been completed. For instance, Dr. Denton Cooley (known as perhaps the most driving, single-minded cardiac surgeon in a very headstrong group) has recounted how at the time of his second transplant in May 1968 he had two potential recipients and a single donor who was ABO compatible with both. He chose one patient and was relieved that the "tissue matching, which became known 24 hours after the operation," turned out to be better for the recipient selected than for the one passed over.[52] Of course, some of the cardiac transplant teams emphasized tissue typing. This was true of Dr. Shumway's group from the beginning;[53] their transplants seem to have been the best matched overall, their results are the most encouraging, and they remain today the only active heart transplant center in this country.[54] Yet most of the early heart transplants were done without regard to histocompatibility, which was seen as too primitive to be of much use. The widely held view was that the "chief limiting factor" in transplantation was "the coincidence of a recipient who needs a heart and a donor who can give a heart," and that "it would be a mistake to place a great deal of reliance" on tissue matching.[55] This is well reflected in an exchange between two leading heart surgeons:

---

[50] CAPETOWN PROCEEDINGS, note 49 *supra*, at 23 [comments of Dr. Denton Cooley], and at 24 [Dr. James Pierce].

[51] Crane & Matthews, *Heart Transplant Operations: Diffusion of a Medical Innovation* (unpub. paper, 1969).

[52] CAPETOWN PROCEEDINGS, note 49 *supra*, at 11.

[53] *Id.* at 25 [comments of Dr. Edward B. Stinson of Stanford].

[54] Seventy heart transplants were performed in the United States from January 1, 1970 to June 1, 1974; 24 of these patients were alive as of June 1. Dr. Shumway transplanted all but one of these survivors. 1974 HEART REPORT, note 46 *supra*, at 2.

[55] CAPETOWN PROCEEDINGS, note 49 *supra*, at 23 [comments of Dr. James C. Pierce]. Even those who had originally emphasized tissue typing were persuaded by the early (misleadingly positive) results of some poorly matched grafts to downplay this factor. *Id.* at 24 [comments of Dr. Donald N. Ross].

Dr. Cooley: [S]ometimes one overlooks the fact that the clinical urgency may overrule the other factors in the decision to operate. [S]uppose the surgeon has one man who is dying before his eyes with heart disease, and a donor who is ABO compatible with even a reasonable tissue cross match. To my thinking, one should not deny that recipient the possibility of even a 6-month life. So I think we are struggling too hard to find contraindications and I don't believe, in the infancy of a project, as vital to the future as cardiac transplantation, that that should be our goal. We are trying to accumulate experience so we can get more objective evidence of the limitations. Personally, I would not want my immunologist to stay my hand simply because we did not have an adequate tissue match.

Professor Barnard: Did you use tissue typing then just as a sort of research study?

Dr. Cooley: In our first 3 cases we did not have facilities for tissue typing in our hospital. We had to send our tissue typing off to Terasaki. The results of the typing were available after the transplantation had been performed.

Professor Barnard: Let me pose the problem of a patient who, you think, can still last for 6 days; he is not dying today. You have a donor with ABO compatibility and the immunologists tell you after tissue typing that he is not a good match.

Dr. Cooley: This, of course, would be an important feature. You must realize also that the donor will die within 12 to 24 hours. If the transplant is purely elective and the recipient may live for 1-2 weeks, then I think that one may hesitate to do the transplant. But none of our cases had had better than a C rating on tissue typing. I think the decision will always be difficult. . . .[56]

Thus, it is apparent that all areas of medical knowledge were not perfectly conjoined in the early days of cardiac replacement.

D. CONCLUSIONS ON FACTS AND VALUES

As we noted at the outset of this part, "facts" cannot exist in a vacuum but must imply certain value choices and conflicts. Our summary of the development of treatment for kidney failure illustrates this point repeatedly: For example, the dedication of medical scientists to persevere until "victory" is achieved was illustrated by Kolff's persistence in the face of the near total fatality rate associated with his prototype dialysis machine and by Scribner's confidence in his methods for chronic dialysis with the early Teflon "shunt" despite the lack of success in other centers. Sociological factors cannot be ignored in explaining these investigators' attitudes: Patient fatalities in a war-torn country probably seemed less crushing than they would otherwise for Kolff, and the absence of a transplant program

---

[56] *Id.* at 22-23.

in Seattle permitted Scribner's effort to gain support in its own right and not as a "second-best" adjunct to kidney grafting. Psychological factors as well as a commitment to personal and professional values of course also influenced these investigators. Similarly, the distress with the prospect of patients on long-term dialysis—which drove Moore and others on to make renal transplants work—exhibits conscious and unconscious preference for the image of human beings as dignified and independent beings.

We have also seen how medical science, driving ahead relentlessly, precipitates societal problems which were unanticipated by society's representatives but which once raised cannot be laid to rest. One example, present first in kidney disease, is the difficulty of selecting to whom rare and expensive therapy should be offered. Another is provided by the major social issue which is raised by the heart procedure, namely the definition of death. For a transplanted organ to function in its new host, it must be "alive"—that is, it must be able to make use of oxygen and other nourishment from the blood and to carry out its usual cellular activities. Even a brief period of ischemia can render an organ useless for transplantation. Thus, in kidney and liver transplantation prior to 1967, physicians had already seen the need to remove the organ from the donor promptly once "brain death" had occurred although the traditional standards (absence of heartbeat and respiration) had not yet been met. While the need for prompt removal was perhaps greater for the kidneys and liver, which are more sophisticated organs and more subject to rapid deterioration than is that simple "pump," the heart, the fact that beating was revived in the heart after transplantation from the "dead" donor caught the public's attention. Because of this apparent paradox[57] and because of the magico-religious beliefs associated with the heart, it was not surprising that in the lay mind heart transplantation was particularly startling. Society was thus presented with many problems which like those raised by the developments in kidney treatment will be discussed in subsequent chapters; prime among them is the necessity of balancing the time and care required to make certain that the donor is completely and certainly dead against the speed with which organ salvaging should occur once vital functions have ceased in order to have a healthy and useful organ to transplant.

---

[57] That is, how could a person be "dead," if death is the absence of heartbeat and his heart is still beating, albeit in another body?

PART TWO

Description of Participants— an Interactional Portrait

This part focuses separately on the major participants in the catastrophic disease process—the physician-investigator, the patient-subject, the professions, and the state. We intend to describe the major pressures, conflicts, and decisions which confront them individually and in their interactions with one another, in order to evaluate the extent and limits of their capacities to meet these pressures and conflicts and to make decisions. This approach should begin to raise questions about the authority that ought to be assigned to all participants and to suggest the need for new ways of ordering the catastrophic disease process. This in turn is the major task of Part Three of this book.

It is impossible to offer a detailed descriptive picture of the various roles played by the participants in the catastrophic disease process since extensive in-depth studies about their activities are not yet available. Such sociopsychological research is still in its infancy, though recently a number of important contributions have been made by Barber,[1] Fox,[2] Fellner,[3] Sadler,[4] and Swazey,[5] to name a few. None

---

[1] B. BARBER, J. LALLY, J. MAKARUSHKA & D. SULLIVAN, RESEARCH ON HUMAN SUBJECTS: PROBLEMS OF SOCIAL CONTROL IN MEDICAL EXPERIMENTATION (1973).

[2] R. FOX & J. SWAZEY, THE COURAGE TO FAIL (1974). Portions of their manuscript were submitted as consultants' reports to our project [Appendix B].

[3] Fellner & Marshall, *Kidney Donors: The Myth of Informed Consent*, 126 AM. J. PSYCHIATRY 1245 (1970).

[4] Sadler, Davison, Carroll & Kountz, *The Living, Genetically Unrelated Kidney Donor*, 3 SEMINARS IN PSYCHIATRY 86 (1971).

[5] Swazey & Fox, *The Clinical Moratorium: A Case Study of Mitral Valve Surgery*, in EXPERIMENTATION WITH HUMAN SUBJECTS 315 (P. Freund ed. 1969).

is, however, as detailed as Fox's pioneering participant observation **research on the activities of "Ward F-Second," a hospital unit devoted** to clinical investigation of metabolic disorders.[6] Similar studies must be undertaken to provide the factual background for any proposed reordering of the catastrophic disease process. Moreover, if on the basis of such studies changes in the authority-assignments are implemented, they will permit a subsequent assessment of the impact of this restructuring in comparison to earlier findings.

Systematic studies of the activities of and interactions between the participants of the catastrophic disease process need to be encouraged and supported. A greater number of sociologists, psychologists, and other behavioral scientists should be trained for such research and invited by the medical profession to engage in it. It is also important that they be joined by medical investigators as collaborators, for the interdisciplinary nature of such ventures will give additional depth and insights to these efforts. Moreover, medical students, under the direction and guidance of experienced investigators, should be encouraged to conduct small studies of their own in this area. This will not only make students more aware of the problems posed by investigative medicine, and thus enrich their professional training, but will also stimulate some of them to become scholars in this field.

Our encouragement of such studies makes apparent one of our major underlying assumptions, which also pervades much that we have to say throughout this book; namely, that awareness by all participants of the problems which affect the catastrophic disease process is to be preferred to ignorance. The merits of this assumption can be questioned and if rejected would significantly affect the persuasiveness of our recommendations as to how this process should be structured. This judgment we leave to others. In opting for awareness, we do not wish to suggest that there may not be exceptions to such a value preference, and indeed we shall discuss such exceptions.

Central to the discussion in the following chapters is one particular issue on which more study and attention is sorely needed: the "experiment-therapy dilemma," as it is sometimes termed.[7] In Part Three of this book, we discuss some of the policy implications of the distinction that is often drawn between "research" and "treatment," but a few

---

[6] R. Fox, Experiment Perilous (1959).

[7] Swazey & Fox, note 5 *supra*, at 335.

introductory remarks are advisable to clarify how we intend to deal with this issue. In recent years the traditional distinctions between "research" and "therapy" have been increasingly questioned. Such distinctions seem to be even less useful in analyzing the catastrophic disease process, where research and therapy remain facets of the same process for a long time; thus, one can at most speak of interventions being on a research-therapy continuum. Indeed, more generally, we wonder whether the distinctions between research and therapy serve any useful purpose, and whether instead, for all medical interventions, operational distinctions are not better based on other criteria; for example, on the degree of uncertainty about consequences, on risk-benefit equations, on risks themselves, on the quality of consent given by patient-subjects, and so forth.

While alerting the reader that we shall not dwell much on experiment-therapy distinctions, we do not intend to overlook the importance of the research aspects of catastrophic disease treatment. In fact, the "research-therapy" dichotomy is useful in the context of these chapters because it highlights a significant facet of the role definitions which concern us here. The physicians involved in innovative therapy clearly regard themselves as having a special role which sets them off from ordinary doctors and which they believe entails an overriding obligation to create and pursue new developments in medicine. Similarly, patients who are treated with research techniques may see their role as distinct from that of the ordinary patient, with a different relationship to their physician and even to their disease. To keep these special roles and obligations in mind, we speak of "physician-investigators" and "patient-subjects." These terms indicate that in the catastrophic disease process, as in all modern medicine, the dual aspects of participation—for research and therapeutic purposes—are intertwined.

CHAPTER FIVE

The Authority and Capacity of Physician-Investigators

We begin our examination of catastrophic disease decisionmaking with the role and authority of physician-investigators. At one time, this choice would have been so obvious as to be beyond comment, for

> when one examines a new area of medicine . . . the nexus of authority seems naturally to lie with the physician-investigators who have set out on the uncharted seas. While there is today widespread recognition of the need for other hands in addition to the investigator's upon the tiller, most commentators continue to take a "leave it to the investigator" stance.[1]

Even with increased attention to the potential for abuse in such unreviewed discretion,[2] the focus has largely remained on the need for more elaborate "codes of ethics"[3] in the hands of "an intelligent, informed, conscientious, compassionate, responsible investigator."[4]

---

[1] Capron, *The Law of Genetic Therapy*, in THE NEW GENETICS AND THE FUTURE OF MAN 133, 147 (M. Hamilton ed. 1972).

[2] *See, e.g.,* Beecher, *Ethics and Clinical Research*, 274 NEW ENG. J. MED. 1354 (1966); M. PAPPWORTH, HUMAN GUINEA PIGS (1967).

[3] *See, e.g.,* The Nuremberg Code, Declaration of Helsinki, and other codes, collected in J. KATZ WITH THE ASSISTANCE OF A. CAPRON & E. GLASS, EXPERIMENTATION WITH HUMAN BEINGS 305-06, 311-16, 845-46, 891-92 (1972) [hereinafter cited as KATZ]. The latest government guidelines go beyond these codes, in anticipating participation in decisionmaking by non-physicians; *see* U.S. DEP'T OF HEALTH, EDUCATION & WELFARE, THE INSTITUTIONAL GUIDE TO DHEW POLICY ON PROTECTION OF HUMAN SUBJECTS (1971) and amendments, 39 FED. REG. 18914-20 (1974). Questions about codes and other mechanisms of control are discussed in Part Three *infra*.

[4] Beecher, note 2 *supra*, at 1360.

We doubt that the physician-investigator need be accorded such a singular role or even that it accurately reflects historical fact. "Unlike theoretical scientists whose freedom to pursue their studies, though sometimes challenged, is generally accepted in contemporary society, investigators involved in human research often find their freedom encumbered by the rights and interests of their subjects."[5] Nevertheless, we turn first to an examination of physician-investigators, both for convenience's sake and in recognition of their importance in initiating the process of biomedical advance which was detailed in the previous chapter.

A. BACKGROUND CHARACTERISTICS OF PHYSICIAN-INVESTIGATORS

Though throughout this chapter we speak of "physician-investigators," we appreciate that this designation is inaccurate. The group of participants encompassed in this label includes not only M.D.'s but also Ph.D.'s from a variety of disciplines as well as nurses, social workers, psychologists, and paramedical personnel. Little attention has been paid to defining the authority and responsibility of the various members of "the team" in the catastrophic disease decisionmaking process. The traditional assumption has been that, since all of them work in medical settings, a physician or group of physicians should have ultimate authority. This assumption requires reexamination. For example, with respect to decisions involving the weight to be given to tissue typing in the selection of recipients, the question must be explored whether greater, or even primary, authority should not rest with an immunologist rather than a surgeon.

Although the professional participants in the catastrophic disease process come from a variety of professional backgrounds, two broad groupings can be identified: those with and those without prior clinical training and experience, many of the latter being graduates of basic science programs. Within both groups the extent of prior experience varies considerably. The senior persons, who head these programs, are generally professionals of long clinical experience, while the rest of the participants range from recent graduates, often of great promise,[6] to seasoned veterans. For example,

---

5 KATZ, note 3 *supra,* at 281.

6 Renée Fox, in describing the composition of the Metabolic Research Group which carried on extensive investigations with cortisone at a prominent New England medical school, noted that

The members of the Group were not only young chronologically. They were also in a relatively early phase of their professional careers. All had completed their internships and served as residents. Two members of the Group had Ph.D. degrees (one in Pharmacology, the other in Biochemistry). All had done some teaching,

when Christiaan Barnard performed the first heart transplantation he was not considered to be among the group of senior cardiac surgeons who were engaged in extensive preliminary work for the eventual performance of this operation.

Beyond the attainment of a professional degree, no formal mechanisms have been established for certifying a person competent to experiment or treat in areas, such as catastrophic disease, which are at the "frontiers of knowledge" with all the uncertainties, responsibilities, and hard choices that such work implies. In theory, any person who wishes to work in this complex and highly specialized field can do so, though, in practice, a number of informal mechanisms exist to brake rash practices, such as restrictions on access to clinical settings (for which one must first be recognized by peers and hospital boards), the fear of malpractice suits, the need for referrals of patients (which again is based on prior recognition of one's professional worth), and the like. Yet, the question remains whether standards of training and certification should be promulgated for the professionals working in innovative settings, such as catastrophic diseases, and whether the extent of their authority should not be circumscribed until such training has been obtained.

Whatever the answer to the last question, careful thought needs to be given to the kind of education which such professionals should receive, particularly because they can come to this task with varied backgrounds. Here we only wish to point to one facet of education, *i.e.,* training for professional responsibility, which has generally been neglected in all professional education and is of particular importance for those working at the frontiers of knowledge.[7]

Improvement in ethical socialization is desirable at every phase of medical training. In medical school, for example, the teachers who now instill the

---

some research (for the most part, basic rather than clinical research), and (with the exception of one physician) each had published several articles before joining the Group. (Eight members of the Group had published two articles; one had published four; and the physician with a Ph.D. in Pharmacology had published twelve articles. Only one member of the Group had spent any time in practice (one and one-half years). R. Fox, Experiment Perilous 19-20 (1959).

[7] *See generally* Katz, *The Education of the Physician-Investigator*, 98 Daedalus 480 (1969). We do not have in mind indoctrinating professionals as to what is "good" or "bad" ethical behavior. This is not only impossible but also offensive. Rather we envision opportunities for the exploration of the complex problems posed by modern medicine to increase awareness and, in turn, thoughtful analysis of these problems. At least this could lead to physician-investigators saying less often than they do now when confronted with questions about why they assumed they could proceed as they did—"I never thought about it."

value of research as they talk about their own research projects ought to address themselves in proper measure to the ethical problems that occur in such research. For it is only when medical students see that their teachers are taking research ethics as a continuing and serious concern that they will themselves come to define it in the same way.[8]

It is also necessary for educators, and physician-investigators generally, to recognize the extent to which the questions they face in the catastrophic disease treatment process force them to look for answers beyond "medical ethics," as it is traditionally conceived.

The catastrophic disease process, like other fields of clinical investigation, poses many difficult problems for the professional, commonly designated as "ethical dilemmas." Though it has often been asserted that the physicians' prior medical education or clinical experience has prepared them for these new assignments, there is little evidence that systematic exposure to the problems raised by professional responsibility has been part of their prior medical education or, if such training had been provided for their therapeutic tasks, that it is sufficient for the tasks inherent in investigative medicine. Thus it is important that such training be made available to all professionals as part of their postgraduate education. The case for such a proposal is strengthened by the particular need to educate those professionals whose major prior experience has been in basic research or other non-clinical settings.

Our concern about the training for professional responsibility has other roots as well. In the next section we shall discuss the conflicting pressures and clinical uncertainties which physician-investigators encounter in investigative medicine. To the resolution of these complex problems they bring their own unexamined biases and value preferences which always tend to exert a greater influence when conflicting intentions cannot readily be reconciled or when consequences cannot be easily ascertained. For example, some professionals have stated, without documentation so far as

---

[8] B. BARBER, J. LALLY, J. MAKARUSHKA & D. SULLIVAN, RESEARCH OF HUMAN SUBJECTS: PROBLEMS OF SOCIAL CONTROL IN MEDICAL EXPERIMENTATION 191 (1973) [hereinafter cited as BARBER]. They go on to observe: "The teaching vehicle for such courses is now, fortunately, at hand in the form of the systematic book of cases and readings on the ethics of research compiled by Dr. Jay Katz and his colleagues. Going through such a book and discussing its contents with fellow-students and an instructor would be invaluable not only for future researchers but for those many practitioners who have the ethical responsibility for patients who become research subjects. To the extent to which such explicit training is neglected, the rights of patient-subjects will continue to be violated out of simple ignorance of the relevant norms; ignorance as a source of failure to conform to the highest standards of ethical concern ought no longer to be accepted." *Id.*

we know, that unrelated persons should not be used as organ donors because their psychological motivations as volunteers are suspect.[9] Others disagree.[10] We wonder to what extent unexplored personal feelings have entered into these pronouncements and, more generally, to what extent prior systematic education for professional responsibility can bring to the surface those personal and professional beliefs and values which distort and obscure finding appropriate answers to such questions as: By what authority, under what circumstances, and in the presence of what psychopathology should offers by unrelated donors be refused?

Fox and Swazey, who have studied transplant surgeons extensively, have noted a number of crucial background factors and professional experiences which transplant surgeons have in common:

> . . . A number of them have brothers who are also physicians, to whom they are both personally and professionally close. Another family pattern a number of transplanters mention is that one or both of their parents emphasized the supreme importance of work, of striving for excellence and achievement. Two of the most prominent surgeons who have transplanted human hearts had fundamentalist religious upbringings. It is interesting that of all their colleagues, these two surgeons seem to have the most combative attitudes toward death, as well as the most zealous outlook on the present accomplishments and future prospects of cardiac transplantation. The wives of five of the surgeons we interviewed are nurses. That these men created medical families through their marriages may mean they sought and expect understanding of their day-and-night devotion to their work. Finally, the most striking similarity is that most transplant surgeons have trained in and been professionally associated with a particular constellation of medical schools and hospitals. This is what might be termed a "progenitor pattern," . . . It is also potentially important as a "social circles" phenomenon. That is, the fact that these men were trained by some of the same teachers has contributed to the attitudes and values they share and in turn transmit to younger colleagues. It also means that because they have worked together in

---

[9] Hamburger, *Protection of Donor Rights in Renal Transplantation*, in BIOMEDICAL SCIENCE AND THE DILEMMA OF HUMAN EXPERIMENTATION 44 (V. Fattorusso ed. 1967).

[10] Fellner & Schwartz, *Altruism in Dispute*, 284 NEW ENG. J. MED. 252 (1971).

The reasons for [the unrelated living donor's] rejection appear to be unscientific, emotional, and prejudicial. Furthermore, the decision to bar him appears to have been made somehow by private consensus of the medical teams involved, who do not seem to be aware that in so doing, they are grossly out of step with public opinion.

Fellner, *The Genetically Unrelated Living Kidney Donor: Unemployed and Unwanted* (consultant's memorandum) at 12 (1972) [Appendix E].

various contexts they have exerted considerable personal influence over each other.[11]

For all their similarity of background, training, and motivation,[12] the physicians involved with transplantation varied markedly in reactions to the problems raised, especially by cardiac replacement, and in their determination to persist in the face of unresolved difficulties. Indeed, Fox's description of the "types" of responses is notable for the contrasts which it highlights:

> It is interesting to note the kind of role-positions that various medical spokesmen assumed and consistently maintained in the heat of [the discussion whether to continue with heart transplantations]: the adventuresome, zealous, flamboyant, pioneering heart surgeon; the surgeon determined to be optimistic about the cardiac transplants in which he is engaged, but less histrionic and missionizing, and more publicity-shy; the transplant surgeon with a troubled conscience; the distinguished experimental surgeon, not doing heart transplants, who speaks as a judicious, historically oriented superego of the profession.[13]

This observation suggests that despite the common background factors which investigators bring to their careers, other significant individual determinants and forces shape their personal beliefs and actions in medical decisionmaking.

B. MOTIVATIONS AND GOALS

An examination of the motivations of transplanters may begin to reveal the pressures under which they operate and the reasons for the intensity as well as the variation of their response. Fox and Swazey have sketched the personal and professional drives that motivate this group of physician-investigators:

> Transplant surgeons see themselves . . . as "pioneers," "trail blazers" whose explorations carry them beyond the safely reassuring boundaries of established medical knowledge and technique. Their work, they are convinced, "mark[s] the evolution from dream to experiment and from experiment to bold human adventure." Not only do they feel that they are on the "front lines" of medicine, they are also keenly aware of the "risks" they are

---

[11] R. Fox & J. Swazey, The Courage to Fail 110-11 (1974) [hereinafter cited as Courage to Fail]. This material and that which follows from Courage to Fail is reprinted by permission of the University of Chicago Press. © 1974 by The University of Chicago.

[12] The motivations of physicians are discussed *infra* at pp. 85-94.

[13] Fox, *A Sociological Perspective on Organ Transplantation and Hemodialysis*, 169 Ann. N.Y. Acad. Sci. 406, 412 (1970).

incurring through their willingness to work "in modern acute medicine at its extreme" and to make "radical departures" from what is conventionally accepted in the field of medicine. The lives of their desperately ill patients are at stake and almost literally in their hands, they feel. In trying to create a new "beachhead," they believe that.they have as much chance of jeopardizing their professional reputations as advancing them. And the "joy of inquiry and discovery" that ideally accompanies their "frontiersman" role may be dimmed or totally eclipsed by their failure to solve the problems they have audaciously tackled.

For all these reasons the transplanters emphasize how important it is to have what they variously term "courage," "grit," or "guts.". . . "The bigger the challenge the happier I am," declares one surgeon; "stress is the spice of life," says another.[14]

In the behavior and statements of the transplanters, one senses not only exhilaration but great optimism in the face of uncertainties or even grave setbacks. Their attitudes range "from the 'cautious optimism' of a clinical investigator to the 'bellicose optimism' of a fervent missionary."[15] Moreover, the optimism of these doctors often seemed not simply to be that transplantation would prove a successful therapy but that they personally would succeed. They competed vigorously for their own individual achievements. The first year of heart transplantation exhibited this well—with the cardiac surgeons vying for public recognition of being "the first" in this or "the most" in that. "[T]hey take pride in surpassing their own accomplishments and, if possible, those of top-ranking colleagues in the same field."[16]

The "pioneer" complex of the transplanters characterizes other physician-investigators engaged in the other innovative and adventuresome aspects of catastrophic disease treatment as well. The same driving ambition to conquer death is found among the developers of hemodialysis as among the transplantation investigators. Since the original work of Willem Kolff, the physicians involved in dialysis have had to pursue their work against great odds—which involved not only seemingly inexorable natural forces but also neglect or opposition from colleagues.[17] Those who eventually established the success of dialysis treatment manifested great faith in the ultimate value of the new therapy and confidence in the face of uncertainty. Their optimism was often reinforced by a need for them to reassure and encourage their patients to continue with the arduous treatment regimen.

The significance of the physician-investigator's personal commitment to

---

[14] COURAGE TO FAIL, note 11 *supra*, at 111 (citations omitted).

[15] *Id.* at 112.

[16] *Id.* at 117.

[17] Fox, note 13 *supra*, at 410-411.

his work became starkly evident in the controversy surrounding long-term dialysis in the early 1960s. The introduction of the new technique, based on the shunted cannulas which obviated the need for repeated venepuncture, was met with skepticism, especially in those kidney centers which were dedicated to improving transplantation and which viewed dialysis as merely a "holding" procedure to maintain the patient until a donor could be found. Dr. Belding Scribner, the shunts' inventor and major proponent, was almost alone in reporting success with dialysis. Since his team in Seattle regarded chronic dialysis as "our baby," they were untiring in pushing on with the procedure despite the criticism of their fellows. Indeed, competition played an important part in their efforts.[18] As Scribner very insightfully told us, in recalling the Seattle group's driving ambition and motivation,

> This factor was pin-pointed by [Dr. George] Schreiner at a private meeting in about 1963 when he accused me in front of my peers of making dialysis work just to satisfy my ego. I was resentful and embarrassed at the time, but probably I should have been pleased.

Scribner's pleasure in Schreiner's criticism reflects again the enthusiasm and "courage" which typify physician-investigators and which may be necessary to sustain them through periods of uncertainty and adversity in the development of new means of treatment. Similarly, transplanters appear incredibly dedicated to their work despite the great risks of failure and criticism. "A few of the transplanters are even more ardent; their conviction borders on zealotry. They see themselves as "defending the cause" of transplantation or, as one surgeon put it, "spreading the gospel."[19]

Transplant and dialysis physicians' driving ambition to succeed against death and their colleagues reflect background factors that are apparently common to all innovators. George Sarton expresses it well:

> Curiosity, one of the deepest of human traits, indeed far more ancient than mankind itself, was perhaps the mainspring of scientific knowledge in the

---

[18] There is an edge of bitterness and frustration, as well as competition, in one of Scribner's comments to us concerning the poor results in most of the early dialysis programs:

In many centers this situation actually went from bad to worse because the dialysis program was run by some "underling" who was considered a flunky of the transplant surgeon. . . . The net effect of all this was disastrous both for dialysis patients and transplant patients. In many centers the patient mortality following transplantation was enormous mainly because the surgeon had no interest in the quality of his dialysis program and hence operated on patients who were severely ill and even near death. And those patients who did survive provided an enormous boost to the surgeon's ego because he had rescued them from a fate worse than death—namely chronic dialysis.

[19] COURAGE TO FAIL, note 11 *supra*, at 115.

past as it still is today. Necessity has been called the mother of invention . . . but curiosity was the mother of science. The motives of primitive scientists . . . were perhaps not very different from those of our contemporaries; they varied considerably from man to man and time to time and then as now covered the whole gamut from complete selflessness, reckless curiosity, and spirit of adventure down to personal ambition, vainglory and covetousness.[20]

From the vantage point of a psychoanalyst, Anna Freud has probed the origin of these traits among persons who choose a medical career:

According to our experience, there are three different ways which urge a young person to choose the medical career. One, and a very good one, is curiosity. The wish to know . . . arises very early in the human individual. Already at the age of two, three and four, certainly later also in the school ages, you can distinguish the curious children from those who have no special interest in the mysteries, in the riddles of their surroundings. But the curious ones want to know everything. Parents and teachers are plagued by the continual "why" of the young child—a "why" that they are not always able to counter with the proper answer. And very often when parents and teachers do their best to answer the child as fully as they can, the "why" continues, because it springs from rather deep sources. . . . But also at these early ages you can find something else. In every nursery school, the nursery school teacher is prepared that . . . a hospital will be established, and this hospital will be usually for insects, frogs or lizards or any other small animals that can be found. And these small animals will be tended carefully in boxes, fed and looked after and, as the child says, cured. Sometimes, especially when it is an insect, legs will be pulled off beforehand so that a patient is produced, and the patient is cured afterwards. Which means that the child's wish to help and to cure is still very close to the wish to hurt and to maim. The younger the child, the more dangerous he is to smaller children or to animals, the stronger his wish to hurt. The older and more socially adapted he becomes, the more this aggressive wish can be submerged under a strong urge to help. Both wishes can lead the growing individual straight into medicine. . . . There's a third source—a very respectable one, too—the wish to become a doctor. I remember very vividly when I was a child myself, of being impressed by those fairy tales usually placed somewhere in the middle ages, where an unusually trained or gifted medical man took up straightforwardly the battle with death, and proved that he could conquer death at any time and save his patients. Death was his enemy. He was the savior and the hero. And this image behind the medical profession that they are the heroes strong enough and wise enough to conquer death or at least to put off and postpone death is certainly an idea which is attractive to many people. . . .[21]

---

[20] G. Sarton, A History of Science 16 (1952).
[21] A. Freud, *The Doctor-Patient Relationship*, in Katz, note 3 *supra*, at 642-43.

The pressures operating on and within physician-investigators who work in the catastrophic disease process are great. By definition, they are working in an area which constantly forces them to confront death and the lack of knowledge and of adequate resources to combat it effectively. Fox and Swazey found a "counterphobic dimension" in the way several of the cardiac surgeons they studied threw themselves into daily confrontation with what the surgeons "considered the most fearsome, with the need to challenge and win out over it every time."[22] In many ways the physician-investigators of catastrophic diseases are like top athletes driven by forces deep within themselves, intensely competitive, and forever pressing on to "victory" in the face of adverse odds, fatigue, and pain. But their behavior goes beyond that of the athletes. By throwing themselves into the battle they seemingly attempt to deny the innate human horror at the radical nature of their interventions and instead to take on the mythic status of superhuman heroes who are "not afraid," in the words of one heart surgeon, "of blood, or death, or the heart, or any structure of the body."[23]

Because they are, by definition, operating in a field where medical science and technique are not yet fully adequate, physician-investigators must cope with dual motivations—to save lives and to accumulate knowledge. Though the two motivations may complement one another, they do not do so necessarily—for example, there may be conflict in the process of selecting donors among healthy volunteers or of determining when a donor is sufficiently close to death to justify the removal of an organ.

> Dr. Cooley recalls, "Well I was worried because I was taking the heart out of the donor while it was still beating and putting it over here, and that meant the cadaver over there was completely wiped out. No question of life or death! I satisfied myself completely that death was in the process at the time we removed the heart and I didn't worry about those things. I didn't worry whether the donor was dead or alive. . . . My concern was primarily with the recipient and everyone . . .—the public, most physicians—were more concerned with protecting the rights of the donor. Well, to me the donor was dead. . . . Therefore, we wanted to see that [the recipient] got the best chance to live and there are ways one could jeopardize his chances by, say . . . trying to satisfy everyone that this donor was completely wiped out and waiting until the heart was almost at the point of cessation entirely. Then you say, okay, now we'll take it out and put it over here. So you are giving the recipient a badly abused organ, which is not fair to the recipient." Dr. Hallman described similar feelings even more starkly, ". . . it gives you the impression that you have . . . influence over life and death. . . . When . . . [we] take the heart out of a donor, we've gone through the medico-legal

---

[22] COURAGE TO FAIL, note 11 *supra*, at 115.
[23] *Id.*

procedures that . . . [say that] the patient is legally dead when the brain is dead, but yet you are the one who makes the final blow and takes out the heart and this is a peculiar feeling the first time you do it . . . I guess just like an executioner who has to pull the switch on the electric chair because it's his job. It bothers him the first time, but the more times he does it, the less it bothers him. . . . This was upsetting to me personally the first time I did it, but the more I did it the easier it became. . . . But the first time you do it you have the feeling as if you are killing the patient. The only justification that one can have for doing [it] is that the patient is for all practical purposes . . . dead and that everybody has agreed to this. . . ."[24]

Furthermore, the motivation to safeguard life may come up short against the need to make choices among recipients all of whom might benefit to various extents from receiving a transplant.

> Dr. A: So, at our center, we are looking very definitely in the direction now of the younger age recipients of a heart [transplant].
>
> Dr. B: On the other hand, I think we must remember that with our present sort of limitations and expectation of not a very long survival, a year in an old patient means more than a year in a young patient.
>
> Dr. C: I don't know about that. To redefine that, a year in a younger person is a lot longer than a year in an older person.
>
> Dr B: I think if you give a child of six years an extra year of his life it is about a sixtieth of his life expectancy whereas if you give a man of sixty an extra year of life, you have given him a twentieth of what he has lived.
>
> Dr. X: Metabolically it is a shorter period.[25]

In addition, choices may also have to be made between the saving of certain lives and the acquisition of knowledge, *i.e.,* selecting patient-subjects on the basis of the contributions they can make to science, so that others can benefit from it eventually. Moreover, in the quest to pierce ignorance, procedures may have to be tried which actually could shorten life if expected and unexpected complications cannot be controlled. On the other hand, the desire to gain knowledge may be impaired by the traditional posture to expose only moribund patients to new and unknown procedures. Such patients are not necessarily the best subjects for research, since the failure of the intervention could in part rest on their already debilitated state rather than on the procedure itself. And investigations with moribund patient-subjects confront investigators with the dilemma of having "at once

---

[24] Castelnuovo-Tedesco, *Cardiac Surgeons Look at Transplantation—Interviews with Drs. Cleveland, Cooley, DeBakey, Hallman and Rochelle,* 3 SEMINARS IN PSYCHIATRY 5, 13 (1971).

[25] 1ST ANN. JOHN F. KENNEDY SYMPOSIUM ON RECENT SIGNIFICANT DEVELOPMENTS IN MEDICINE & SURGERY (1968), quoted in Fox, note 13 *supra,* at 419.

to prolong life, alleviate suffering, and respect the right of patients to die mercifully and with dignity."[26]

More generally, as Swazey and Fox have pointed out within the ethics of human experimentation, the physician-investigator "incurs the obligation to conduct research with patients. His goal is to advance medical science and practice in ways that he hopes will benefit his subjects and other patients with similar or related medical problems."[27] This sense of obligation may be particularly strong when the physician-investigator is searching for a therapeutic breakthrough to hold off a patient-subject's death. Thus, the argument is often made that the "heroic" treatment which physicians provide in such life-threatening circumstances not only demonstrates their commitment to the individual patient but also justifies the special privileges held by experimental medicine and reaffirms the primacy of human life as a value in our culture.

Though increasingly stressed, the conflicting implications of personal ambitions for success and fame on physician-investigators' activities have not been sufficiently acknowledged or explored. The myth of the dedicated and unselfish physician-scientist is still all too uncritically asserted, notwithstanding the institutional pressures for those working in more academic settings to succeed and to publish in order to be promoted, secure research grants, and so forth. As Dr. Szent-Gyorgi forcefully observed: "Research wants egotists, damn egotists, who seek their own pleasure and satisfaction, but find it in solving the puzzles of nature."[28] While it is hard, if not impossible, to differentiate between personal ambition, the striving for excellence, or the quest for knowledge, it should at least be acknowledged that personal motivations are an ever-present and inevitable concomitant of advances in science.[29] Such desires may lead physician-investigators to underestimate the importance of self-interest in their decisions and to overvalue the significance they assign to more socially acceptable altruistic motivations.

Investigators, depending on the relative weight they consciously and unconsciously assign to their obligations to research, to their patients or to their need for recognition, will make different personal choices. Thus the question arises: To what extent should this balancing be left to individual decisionmakers, especially since they may not notice or be inclined to probe into their conflicting motivations? There is a need to subject these individual attitudes to more rigorous analysis so that the catastrophic dis-

---

[26] Fox, note 13 *supra*, at 406.

[27] Swazey & Fox, *The Clinical Moratorium: A Case Study of Mitral Valve Surgery*, in EXPERIMENTATION WITH HUMAN SUBJECTS 315, 348 (P. Freund ed. 1969).

[28] Quoted in *From a Correspondent*, 1 THE LANCET 1394 (1961).

[29] *See* BARBER, note 8 *supra*, at 59-60.

ease process will not be unquestioningly shaped by personal preferences. Since, for example, the decision of surgeons to proceed with or to put a halt to transplantations seems to be motivated also by powerful conscious and unconscious determinants, questions arise about the kinds of mechanisms which would reduce idiosyncratic decisionmaking. Hence it will be profitable to inquire whether such controls as the sharing of authority with other members of the team besides the transplant surgeon, the participation of patients in decisionmaking, peer consultation and review, and regulation by the profession and state will prove to be useful safeguards. We shall return to these issues in Part Three of this book.

C. LIMITATIONS AND RESTRAINTS

To note that physician-investigators may not be ideally suited to make decisions about catastrophic diseases alone is not to suggest, however, that at present they have a free hand to do so. There are a number of restraints, formal and informal, on a physician's freedom to do as he chooses. Prime among these, especially in a research area such as the development of treatment for catastrophic diseases, is the uncertainty of outcome of his choices. This was initially recognized as a major problem for physicians by Talcott Parsons,[30] and Renée C. Fox has written extensively on this theme:

> Some of these [uncertainties] result from limitations in current medical understanding and technique; others from the physician's own incomplete mastery of available medical knowledge and skills; and still others grow out of difficulties in distinguishing between personal ignorance or ineptitude and the imperfect state of medical science, technology, and art.[31]

Uncertainty reinforces the drive for knowledge, for only knowledge and experience can defeat uncertainty. But uncertainty also brakes this motivation, for it engenders personal anxieties about the impact of a new procedure on the patient-subject and social anxieties about the liabilities which the physician-investigator and science might incur if a new intervention proves more detrimental than non-intervention would have. Thus valuable leads may not be followed up because the investigator doubts his authority to proceed.

Similarly, the extent of the physician-investigator's authority to proceed at his own initiative is put in question by the problem of scarce resources. Who should decide

> [H]ow much time, energy, skill, and money ideally ought to be invested in fields like hemodialysis and organ transplantation? In a personal statement

---

[30] *See* T. Parsons, The Social System 447-454 (1951).
[31] Fox, note 13 *supra*, at 406-07.

concerning why he has desisted from doing cardiac transplantations, Dr. Dwight E. Harken has presented some of the reasons he feels it is not urgent for additional medical teams to carry out this procedure. From his point of view, it is more important to care for a larger number of less hopelessly ill patients and to engage in less audacious forms of clinical research [quoting Dr. Harken]:

"Heart transplantation in an early experimental prototype form is here. Each man who contemplates entry into the field of cardiac transplants must arrive at his own decision by balancing the use of the considerable resources for a few transplants, against his obligation to treat ailing people and extend heart surgery techniques in other ways. So far, I have elected the rehabilitation of a fair number of people while attempting to improve prosthetic valves, coronary circulation, and mechanically assisted circulation. I reserve the right to change tomorrow but today I am proud of our restraint in not performing heart transplants yesterday."[32]

In addition to these largely internal restraints, the major external restraints on research are imposed by codes of ethics, peers, hospitals, institutional review committees, and the law generally. Beginning with the "basic principles" set forth by the Nuremberg judges, numerous attempts have recently been made to propose "improved" codes of ethics to guide medical research.[33] The proliferation of such codes testifies to the difficulty of promulgating a set of rules which do not immediately raise more questions than they answer. By necessity these codes have to be succinctly worded and, being devoid of commentary, their meaning is subject to a variety of interpretations. Moreover, since they generally aspire to ideal practices, they invite judicious and injudicious neglect. Consequently, as long as they remain unelaborated tablets of exhortation, codes will at best have limited usefulness in guiding the daily behavior of investigators.

Many commentators, particularly from medicine, have championed the safeguards provided by professional training, peer consultations, and group pressure as well as by internal hospital regulations. These have recently taken on more structural form under the mandate of the United States Public Health Service and, of late, the Food and Drug Administration and the overall aegis of the Department of Health, Education and Welfare (HEW) that research conducted in institutions be approved by a "peer group review committee." Though all these mechanisms provide opportunities for voluntary and involuntary consultation and review and may

---

[32] *Id.* at 418.

[33] "The need to identify and develop acceptable standards of care as an aid to the courts . . . began to receive limited but respectable support in the clinical research community in the late 1950's and early 1960's." Curran, *Governmental Regulation of the Use of Human Subjects in Medical Research,* 98 DAEDALUS 542, 545-46 (1969).

thus modify individual idiosyncratic practices,[34] they share a major fault already noted with respect to codes. In most instances neither an investigator's peers nor even those who serve as members of review committees have given systematic thought to the problems raised by investigative medicine and thus at times, particularly when decisions are difficult, their approvals or injunctions may be as questionable as the activities of individual investigators acting on their own.[35]

Law, though generally an important external restraint, has had little to say about medical research except through HEW regulations. Judges in malpractice settings have made pronouncements about informed consent and the right to self-determination, and these doctrines will most likely be applied to the research setting when such litigation comes before courts.[36] However, the problems raised by research medicine are not necessarily similar to those in therapeutic practice, and thus the question must be explored whether a sustained dialogue between law and medicine would help to define, independently of the existing law for malpractice situations, the ambit of the authority of physician-investigators in human research.

At present no constituted body exists to which an investigator can turn to obtain such authority. At the heart of the matter is the problem of making decisions about risktaking, with and without subject consent, in the quest of advancing knowledge. In Chapter Seven we shall discuss at greater length the problems raised by the lack of definition of harm in the Public Health Service regulations which delegated to institutional review committees the task of evaluating risks. On the one hand, these regulations (and the bureaucracy behind them) pose a definite, formal restraint on investigators; yet, on the other hand, the imprecise nature of the rules and guidelines create additional problems for investigators who, before proceeding, are thrown back on their own interpretations of the regulations. To guide investigators properly, such regulations should define categories of harm "to which research may expose subjects and society and then . . . identify additional elements of experimental design and objectives (*e.g.,* the subject's awareness of participating in an experiment, the subject's under-

---

[34] Previously, it had been "the posture of both the FDA and NIH to allow and to encourage clinical investigators to use a high level of imagination and freedom in the pursuit of their research objectives. They were to be guided by their own professional judgment and controlled by their own ethical standards as well as those of their institution." *Id.* at 549.

[35] *See generally* BARBER, note 8 *supra*, at 145-67, and TUSKEGEE SYPHILIS STUDY AD HOC ADVISORY PANEL, U.S. DEP'T OF HEALTH, EDUCATION & WELFARE, FINAL REPORT 29-37 (1973).

[36] *See, e.g.,* Halushka v. University of Saskatchewan, 53 W.W.R. 608 (Sask. C.A. 1965) and Kaimowitz v. Department of Mental Health for the State of Michigan, Civil Action No. 73-19434-AW (Cir. Ct. Wayne County, 1973).

standing of its risks, or the benefits of the investigation to subject, science, and society) which may aggravate or mitigate an experiment's harmful consequences. Both the nature of harm and the conditions under which it may arise must be examined in any attempt to define the proper scope of an investigator's authority. . . ."[37] Answers have to be found to such questions as:

1. What constitutes a harmful intervention?
2. To what extent should the degree or type of harm to the individual or society affect the authority of decisionmakers?
3. To what extent is the harm of an intervention mitigated by what immediate or long-range, certain or uncertain benefits, and to whom should benefits accrue?
4. To what extent is the harm of an intervention aggravated or mitigated by an explanation of the risks and benefits involved?
5. To what extent should knowledge or lack of knowledge about harm affect the authority of decisionmakers?
6. Under what circumstances should the balancing of risks and benefits be left to the persons affected and when, if ever, should other decisionmakers impose limits on risktaking?

Moreover, investigators need to become better informed about the ambit of their authority to pursue investigations whenever their studies may be contrary to existing mores or laws. This problem is dramatically illustrated by an example from a scientific field unrelated to catastrophic diseases. A scientist interested in interspecies hybridization believes that important knowledge may be gained from studying the genetic mix resulting from breeding human beings and the higher apes. He is aware of the possible social, legal, and ethical problems arising from such investigations, yet wonders whether they may not be outweighed by the resulting knowledge. Yet he has no one to consult to learn whether society might not wish to approve his work.[38]

The restraints upon physician-investigators suggest that for a variety of reasons the drive for developing new treatment modalities for catastrophic disease may be impeded. Many, particularly the dedicated investigators, regard this as an unfortunate consequence. Others, like Hans Jonas have argued that the advancement of knowledge should not be the primary objective:

> Let us not forget that progress is an optional goal, not an unconditional commitment, and that its tempo in particular, compulsive as it may become,

---

[37] KATZ, note 3 *supra,* at 202.

[38] *See* Remington, *An Experimental Study of Man's Genetic Relationship to Great Apes, By Means of Interspecific Hybridization,* in *id.* at 461.

has nothing sacred about it. Let us also remember that a slower progress in the conquest of disease would not threaten society, grievous as it is to those who have to deplore that their particular disease be not yet conquered, but that society would indeed be threatened by the erosion of those moral values whose loss, possibly caused by too ruthless a pursuit of scientific progress, would make its most dazzling triumphs not worth having. . . .[39]

Scientists have paid insufficient attention to the question of whether some of their internal restraints may not conflict with the wishes of society to pursue research more relentlessly. Procedures need to be formulated which will facilitate public discussion of the needs of science, and institutions will have to be created that can approve investigations which are beyond the authority of physician-investigators to decide on their own.[40] For example, this is already an existing problem for experimentation with children in general and the use of healthy children as organ donors in particular. Though championed by some and condemned by others, there exist today no mechanisms for arriving at a professional and public consensus as to permissible limits to which investigators may go in experimentation with children.[41]

D. MORATORIA AND THE AUTHORITY OF PHYSICIAN-INVESTIGATORS

Recently Swazey and Fox have called attention to the phenomenon of "the clinical moratorium," which they consider "generic to the process of therapeutic innovation."[42] They define it "to mean a *suspension* of the use of a still experimental procedure on patients, a suspension which may last for weeks, months, or years depending on the particular case."[43] It represents a period of "reflection, re-evaluation, and study for the research physicians formerly conducting clinical trials. During this time, they often return to laboratory experiments in an attempt to solve certain of the problems that led them temporarily to cease human trials."[44] Swazey and Fox

---

[39] Jonas, *Philosophical Reflections on Experimenting with Human Subjects*, 98 DAEDALUS 219, 245 (1969).

[40] *See* 118 *Congressional Record* S16335-37 (September 11, 1973) debating H. R. 7724, which was adopted in 1974 as the National Research Act and which established a broadly constituted commission for the regulation of human experimentation. Its membership includes representatives from the public at large.

[41] Draft regulations prepared by the National Institutes of Health to govern research with children and other "incompetent" subjects appeared at 38 FED. REG. 31738 (1973).

[42] *See* SWAZEY & FOX, note 27 *supra*, at 315.

[43] *Id.* at 316.

[44] *Id.* at 345.

also state that such moratoria can result by virtue of "internal" or "external" pressures. The internal pressures originate within "the research physician who feels that he ought to discontinue clinical trials," while the external pressures "are generated by the opinions of colleagues or lay persons that trials should not proceed, and by the actions they may take to implement their judgment."[45] Moreover, these pressures may be invoked formally, (for example, by withdrawing operating privileges from individual surgeons or halting a procedure altogether) or informally (for example, by colleagues' pleas that the reputation of surgery would be damaged if trials were continued).

Swazey and Fox give a very broad definition to the clinical moratorium which encompasses any individually or group-sponsored, externally or internally motivated, formally or informally imposed or declared, temporary or more permanent cessation of research activity. They stress the frequency of such events in the process of therapeutic innovation, though it seems that "moratoria" constantly occur in medical practice whenever sufficient doubts arise about the efficiency or risks of a procedure, however well established it had been until that time. Thus the concept of clinical moratorium, as defined by them, merely points to the variety of potential mechanisms existing in clinical and investigative medicine to pause and reflect about the current state of a particular intervention. From the vantage point of hindsight, the informal mechanisms reveal all their capricious weaknesses. They allowed, for example, the erroneous views of one of the world's most prominent cardiologists, Sir James MacKenzie, to exert undue influence over the progress of cardiac surgery, and the ingrained beliefs of referring physicians to halt the pioneering work on mitral valve surgery initiated by the English surgeon Souttar. To be sure, informal mechanisms do not necessarily impede progress; for example, it was only the encouragement of a leading cardiologist that kept surgeon Dwight E. Harken from calling off his pioneering work on mitral vavuloplasty:

> At this point [in the winter of 1948-1949] I went home depressed and said "I quit." Some people suggested I should try my techniques on better-risk patients, in order to help me get better results, so I wouldn't "ruin the reputation of cardiac surgery." But I wouldn't do that. After I lost my sixth patient, I had a call from Dr. Laurence Ellis [then President of the New England Cardiovascular Society]. I told him I wouldn't kill any more patients [through mitral valve surgery], and that no respectable referring physician would send me any more patients anyhow. Ellis asked me what I meant: didn't I realize that these patients surely would die if I didn't operate? He said he would still refer patients to me, and didn't I think he was a good

---

[45] *Id.* at 346.

cardiologist? This talk with Ellis was a turning point. I went back and operated and my patients suddenly started doing better. But I almost called a moratorium.[46]

Even when a halt in clinical trials results, this may still benefit science; the personal moratorium declared by Drs. Cutler and Beck in 1929, in the light of the staggering operative mortality rate of mitral valve surgery, led to a return to the laboratory for much needed additional animal experimentation.[47]

The problems created by informal mechanisms are that they tend to function inconspicuously and thereby preclude a public review of the merits of maintaining a moratorium. The same weaknesses are inherent in the more formal moratorium mechanisms. The discouraging results of Dr. Charles P. Bailey's initial efforts to reintroduce mitral valve surgery led three different hospitals in the Philadelphia area to terminate his privileges to perform intracardiac surgery at their institutions. Similar discouraging results with heart transplantations led the Directors of the Montreal Heart Institute to impose a "moratorium" on further operations in January 1969. The impact which a moratorium has on physician-investigators of course will vary with the procedures used to implement it. Similarly, the effect on patient-subjects and medical progress will depend on whether moratoria are formally or informally invoked; if the latter, the prestige of the invoker may have far-reaching consequences for at least a considerable period of time. Beyond the imposition of such prohibitions no further thought has been given to such questions (to which we shall return in Part Three) as: Who should have the authority to make such decisions, when and by whom should they be modified, and to whom can they be appealed?

Finally, Swazey and Fox's description of "moratoria" illustrates again two characteristics of medical practice generally: (1) the influence of personal beliefs and attitudes on decisionmaking which have major consequences because of the absence of procedural mechanisms for challenging these beliefs and attitudes, and (2) the reluctance of the profession to impose more formal procedures of self-regulation. The merits of self-regulation deserve greater scrutiny, if only to avoid more cumbersome and unnecessary controls by nonprofessional institutions.

Physician-investigators have been left too much to their own devices in coping with the problems posed by investigative medicine. Though many informal mechanisms exist which place constraints on their authority, it is not at all clear whether they have worked to their benefit or to that of

---

[46] Dr. D.E. Harken, quoted in *id.* at 331.

[47] For a detailed account of the history of mitral valve surgery, *see* Swazey & Fox, note 27 *supra*, and KATZ, note 3 *supra*, at 793-817.

patient-subjects, science, and society. Indeed it is more than likely that the informal mechanisms have also impeded progress. Physician-investigators have contributed to this state of affairs by their concern that any encroachment on their freedom by insiders and outsiders alike would only restrict their activities. The extent, if any, to which such fears are justified remains an open question. In fact, it is conceivable that if the authority of physician-investigators and of others became more clearly defined, greater research options would open up. Be that as it may, the concern over interferences has also contributed to the lack of careful scrutiny of the extent and limits of the participants' proper authority, and this raises questions to which we shall return in Part Three.

CHAPTER SIX

The Authority and Capacity of Patient-Subjects

In this chapter we are concerned primarily with those persons who are the "beneficiaries" of the new treatments for catastrophic diseases and who at the same time are also the "means" through which necessary testing to develop these new treatments is performed. In addition to the values and choices of these patient-subjects, attention will also be focused on their relationships to relatives and physician-investigators.

We begin our evaluation of the capacity of patient-subjects to participate in decisionmaking about catastrophic diseases by exploring the rapidly developing doctrine of "informed consent." We shall present an "informed consent model" of decisionmaking as a means of illustrating and examining the extent and limits of patient-subjects' authority and capabilities. The model attempts to incorporate a realistic view of the limitations and constraints that psychological forces and personal interrelationships place on informed and voluntary decisionmaking, and it lays a basis for some of the recommendations made in Chapter Eight.

A. THE "INFORMED CONSENT" MODEL

1. Genesis of the Requirement

In the spring of 1955, after a mastectomy, Irma Natanson was referred by her surgeon to Dr. John R. Kline, a radiologist, for cobalt therapy in order to reduce the risk that her breast cancer would recur or spread.

Thereafter Mrs. Natanson suffered injuries which she believed to have been caused by the radiation treatment. She sued Kline and the hospital where she had been treated, claiming *inter alia* that Kline had failed to advise her of the nature of the proposed treatment and of its hazards. The appellate rulings on her contention, in articulating a requirement that physicians obtain the "informed consent" of their patients before undertaking any medical intervention, proved to be seminal decisions in the law of malpractice. The trial court had declined to instruct the jury on this issue, but the Kansas Supreme Court reversed and announced a new duty for physicians:

> the obligation . . . to disclose and explain to the patient in language as simple as necessary the nature of the ailment, the nature of the proposed treatment, the probability of success or of alternatives, and perhaps the risks of unfortunate results and unforeseen conditions within the body. . . .[1]

The last dozen years have seen a flood of "informed consent" cases pour forth across the country in the wake of *Natanson*. Not that the case created any wholly new legal concepts or was without precedent. Indeed, the Kansas court drew upon a number of prior opinions in other jurisdictions which had brought this issue to a similar resolution.[2] The basic premise from which the *Natanson* court operated—that everyone has the right to decide for himself what shall be done to his person—is a fundamental tenet of English and American common law. The importance of volition in the medical context was forcefully stated by Judge Cardozo in *Schloendorff v. Society of New York Hospital:*

> Every human being of adult years and sound mind has a right to determine what shall be done with his own body; and a surgeon who performs an operation without his patient's consent commits an assault for which he is liable in damages.[3]

But the Kansas court did plow new ground. It moved the legal concept of consent beyond simple assault and battery law; it recognized that for the right to self-determination to be meaningful for the patient, it must be conjoined with a right to the information one needs to formulate an intelligent opinion. *Natanson* and its progeny thus carried the law beyond merely giving body to "the wish on the part of the individual to be his master . . .

---

[1] Natanson v. Kline, 186 Kan. 393, 410, 350 P.2d 1093, 1106 (1960), *clarified*, 187 Kan. 186, 354 P.2d 670 (1960).

[2] Most particularly, Salgo v. Leland Stanford, etc. Bd. of Trustees, 154 Cal. App.2d 560, 317 P.2d 170 (1957).

[3] 211 N.Y. 125, 129, 105 N.E. 92, 93 (1914).

to be a subject, not an object"[4] to include the rational processes involved in the desire

> to be moved by reasons, by conscious purposes which are my own, not by causes which affect me, as it were, from outside. I wish, above all, to be conscious of myself as a thinking, willing, active being, bearing responsibility for his choices and able to explain them by reference to his own ideas and purposes. . . .[5]

In the past dozen years the courts have developed a number of ways of applying the doctrine of informed consent. The legal points still at issue—whether the wrong involved is properly regarded as an assault and battery without consent (where full disclosure is absent) or as malpractice (the failure to inform being seen as professional negligence),[6] or whether the extent of disclosure required ought to be judged by standards set by a physician's fellow practitioners or by what lay jurors would want to know in similar circumstances[7]—remain unresolved. The requirement of informed consent in itself, however, is of major importance in examining the

---

[4] I. BERLIN, TWO CONCEPTS OF LIBERTY 16 (1958).

[5] *Id.*

[6] Traditionally, when a physician did something to a patient for which he had not obtained permission, he was liable in an action for battery. *See, e.g.,* Moore v. Webb, 345 S.W.2d 239 (Mo. App. 1961)—sixteen teeth extracted while patient, who had agreed to removal of two, was under sodium pentathol; Bang v. Charles T. Miller Hospital, 251 Minn. 427, 88 N.W. 2d 186 (1958)—as part of prostate operation spermatic cords were tied off without patient's prior knowledge or consent; Corn v. French, 71 Nev. 280, 289 P.2d 173 (1955)—mastectomy performed when patient had limited consent to a biopsy; Hively v. Higgs, 120 Ore. 588, 253 P. 363 (1927)—tonsils removed during course of minor operation on patient's nose. The battery theory has been carried forward in some of the modern "informed consent" cases. *See, e.g.,* Dow v. Kaiser Foundation, 12 Cal. App.3d 488, 90 Cal. Rptr. 747 (1970)—held, physician's willful and unreasonable withholding of material information constitutes battery. On the other hand, the majority of courts, following Natanson v. Kline, 186 Kan. 393, 350 P.2d 1093 (1960), have characterized failure to obtain "informed consent" as giving rise to a cause of action based in negligence. *See,* Plant, *An Analysis of "Informed Consent,"* 36 FORDHAM L. REV. 639, 648-55 (1968).

[7] In most jurisdictions, "expert testimony of medical witnesses is required to establish whether [the physician's] disclosures are in accordance with those which a reasonable medical practitioner would make under the same or similar circumstances," as the Kansas Supreme Court declared in its rehearing of Natanson v. Kline, 187 Kan. 186, 354 P.2d 670 (1960). Recently that viewpoint has been squarely repudiated in three forceful decisions. Canterbury v. Spence, 464 F.2d 772 (D.C. Cir. 1972); Cobbs v. Grant, 502 P.2d 1 (Cal. 1972); Wilkinson v. Vesey, 295 A.2d 676 (R.I. 1972). It seems likely that these opinions will prove influential and attract further courts to this position. *See also* Glass, *Restructuring Informed Consent: Legal Therapy for the Doctor-Patient Relationship,* 79 YALE L.J. 1533, 1559-1562 (1970).

duties and obligations which physician-investigators and patient-subjects have toward one another in the treatment of catastrophic diseases—treatment which involves highly specialized care, usually provided by persons other than the patient's primary physician and often carrying unknown risks. To evaluate particularly the authority which can and should be wielded by patient-subjects in this process, it becomes important to discuss the functions and limitations of informed consent.

2. The Functions of Informed Consent

a. To Promote Individual Autonomy. The requirement of informed consent has two parts, both of which must be met before a medical intervention is permissible: (1) that sufficient information is disclosed to the patient so that he can arrive at an intelligent opinion, and (2) that the patient agrees to the intervention being performed. The latter facet in particular reflects the concern, traditional in Western societies, that the autonomy of each person be respected. This principle is embodied in two great branches of the law: contracts and torts. Protection of the patient's autonomy is accomplished by means of a treatment contract between the physician and patient. Even though the terms of such contract are often not reduced to writing, its existence is a prerequisite for therapy. In addition to using the flexibility of contract law (which supplies a basic relationship for the parties while permitting them to vary its specifics according to their needs), the courts have also relied upon tort law to regulate the doctor-patient relationship. In sum,

> the free citizen's first and greatest right, which underlies all others—the right to the inviolability of his person, in other words, his right to himself—is the subject of universal acquiescence, and this right necessarily forbids a physician or surgeon, however skillful or eminent, who has been asked to examine, diagnose, advise, and prescribe . . . to violate without permission the bodily integrity of his patient by a major or capital operation, placing him under an anaesthetic for that purpose and operating on him without his consent or knowledge. . . .[8]

b. To Protect the Patient-Subject's Status as a Human Being. The "inviolability of [one's] person" is clearly reflective of a deep-seated feeling about what it means to be "human." This concept is a complex but very important one, and it partakes of remarkably contradictory connotations. On the pejorative side, the human aspect is disapproved at both extremes: "To err is human, to forgive divine," and "Untouched by human hands."

---

[8] Pratt v. Davis, 118 Ill. App. 161, 165 (1905), affirmed, 224 Ill. 30, 79 N.E. 562 (1906).

Contrarily, the term "human" is applied to suggest the sanctity of conduct, event, or rule, most particularly in the prohibitions against killing (which protect, in the normal course, humans but not other animals or machines) and in the condemnation of conduct such as that of the Nazis in the concentration camps who failed even to accord their prisoners the status of human beings.

While part of the concern for human beings contained in our culture relates to protecting men physically, part also relates to the respect which is deemed proper for "nonphysical" aspects of man, such as his power of thought. This mental component of the concept of "humanness" is expressed through the first facet of the informed consent rule: the "information" requirement. By emphasizing the importance of involving the patient in decisionmaking in a genuine fashion, this facet of the rule gives further recognition to his status as a human being. As Margaret Mead has perceptively commented,

> To fail to acquaint a subject of observation or experiment with what is happening—as fully as is possible within the limits of the communication system —is to that extent to denigrate him as a full human being and reduce him to the category of dependency in which he is not permitted to judge for himself.[9]

Paul Ramsey has observed that informed consent is an important example of the faithfulness among men that is normative for all moral interaction. "The principle of an informed consent is the *canon of loyalty* joining men together in medical practice and investigation."[10] He goes on to explain:

> Consent as a canon of loyalty can best be exhibited by a paraphrase of Reinhold Niebuhr's celebrated defense of democracy on both positive and negative grounds: "Man's capacity for justice makes democracy possible: man's propensity to injustice makes democracy necessary." Man's capacity to become joint adventurers in a common cause makes the consensual relation possible; man's propensity to overreach his joint adventurer even in a good cause makes consent necessary. In medical experimentation the common cause of the consensual relation is the advancement of medicine and benefit to others. In therapy and in diagnostic or therapeutic investigations, the common cause is some benefit to the patient himself; but this is still a joint venture in which patient and physician can say and ideally should both say, "I cure."[11]

---

[9] Mead, *Research with Human Beings: A Model Derived from Anthropological Field Practice*, 98 DAEDALUS 361, 375 (1969).

[10] P. RAMSEY, THE PATIENT AS PERSON 5 (1970).

[11] *Id.* at 5-6.

For informed consent to create a true "joint enterprise"[12] or partnership between physician-investigator and patient-subject, the latter's right to full information and to give or withhold assent must be scrupulously respected.[13] The danger always exists that a physician's belief in the potential benefits of a new medical procedure, such as heart transplantation, will subtly erode his willingness to regard his patient as a full partner in the undertaking. This is especially true as medical procedures become increasingly complicated, such as the modern treatments of catastrophic diseases which involve not a lone physician treating the patient but a corps of specialists. The physician, often a surgeon, who is in command of this veritable army undeniably has the upper hand in the doctor-patient relationship.[14] Indeed, he may be the originator of a new technique which offers a desperate patient a chance for cure which he cannot get from any other practitioner.[15] Yet if the patient's authority is seen as being at an end once he takes the step of initiating the relationship, if he is presumed to have given a blanket consent to all steps directed by the physician-investigator, not only will his status as a human being be diminished but rational decisionmaking will have been seriously undermined.

Having the patient place himself entirely within the physician's hands has been an accepted part of medical ideology, justified by the physician's concern for the patient's well-being and his alleged need for complete freedom to undertake whatever steps are believed necessary to promote it. But

---

[12] Similarly, Talcott Parsons suggests that although research subjects cannot stand on an equal footing with the investigators they still participate in an "associational collectivity." Parsons, *Research with Human Subjects and the "Professional Complex,"* 98 DAEDALUS 325, 344 (1969).

[13] This posture, of course, does not preclude a patient-subject explicitly instructing his physician not to tell him. He may do so for many reasons, including complete faith in his physician's actions. *See* Putensen v. Clay Adams, Inc., 12 Cal. App. 3d 1062, 91 Cal. Rptr. 319 (1970).

[14] Among the members of the transplant team, only one or two—the surgeon and, perhaps on a more sustained basis, the immunologist who must supervise the difficult postoperative period and administer the immunosuppressive drugs to fight tissue rejection—will have personal contact with the patient; even this contact will probably be more fleeting than that of the patient with his referring physician or "family doctor."

[15] This was dramatically illustrated in the only implantation of a mechanical heart substitute to date. In that case, the patient had experienced severe heart troubles for ten years and was near death when he went to Houston to be treated by Dr. Denton Cooley, who was then the only surgeon willing to attempt an "artificial heart" operation. The patient signed a consent for the temporary use of a mechanical heart replacement in case an attempt to reconstruct his own heart (ventriculoplasty) was unsuccessful. *See* Karp v. Cooley, 349 F. Supp. 827 (S.D. Tex. 1972).

the risk is great, especially in experimental medicine, that the patient's abdication of his decisionmaking authority will convert him from an end in himself to a means that can be employed along with others at the physician's command to serve the goal of the procedure, as defined by the physician and his peers. One need not even observe that in clinical research an experiment may succeed without restoring the patient-subject to health to conclude that the requirement of an ongoing collaboration among the participants, expressed through a process of renewed "informed consents," is needed to protect the human status of all.

   c. To Avoid Fraud and Duress. In addition to these more philosophical aspects of informed consent, the requirement serves practical functions as well. One consequence of truly informed consent is to remove, or at least to avoid, the danger of fraud and duress. The legal model of the doctor-patient relationship should, of course, recognize the very real limitations on rationality which serve to undermine the practical force of the informed consent rule; these are discussed more fully later in this chapter. Yet the model constructed by the law of informed consent still has validity: To the extent that the physician-investigator engages the patient-subject in a comprehensive and comprehensible discussion of the proposed treatment, he reduces the likelihood of misleading or overbearing the patient-subject. The danger that the physician will neglect this duty is probably greater in the case of standard therapy than it is for the major interventions which concern us here. Nevertheless, physician-investigators' desire to avoid discussing difficult and painful matters and incurring the risk of upsetting the patient-subject, as well as the pressures of time and economics which operate in the catastrophic disease context, may tend to undermine careful adherence to the letter of the law.

   Moreover, the idea that the treatment contract is bargained out between equals is considered as somewhat naive; indeed, the patient usually finds himself faced with an agreement which is *à prendre ou à laisser.*[16] In such cases, two remedies present themselves: The law can either remove the choice from the hands of the weaker party (in this instance, the patient-subject), or it can attempt to buttress his ability to exercise choice by erecting certain formal requirements of disclosure. Since the former would represent such an abandonment of the basic principles of individual freedom, resort to it is usually limited to situations in which a repeated pattern has demonstrated that "as a matter of law" agreements of the type in question are unconscionable, *e.g.,* they do not result from the unfettered exercise

---

[16] *Cf.* Kessler, *Contracts of Adhesion: Some Thoughts about Freedom of Contract,* 43 COLUM. L. REV. 629 (1943).

of rational choice.[17] In the doctor-patient context, the trend seems to be toward the second alternative, the establishment of rules of disclosure. While this process has not become formalized in *Miranda*-style[18] requirements, most medical centers have their own "informed consent" forms for patients, and the federal government has issued a "guide" for the protection of human subjects which sets forth the elements of informed consent:

1. A fair explanation of the procedures to be followed, and their purposes, including identification of any procedures which are experimental;
2. A description of any attendant discomforts and risks reasonably to be expected;
3. A description of any benefits reasonably to be expected;
4. A disclosure of any appropriate alternative procedures that might be advantageous for the subject;
5. An offer to answer any inquiries concerning the procedures; and
6. An instruction that the person is free to withdraw his consent and to discontinue participation in the project or activity at any time without prejudice to the subject.

• • •

No such informed consent, oral or written, . . . shall include any exculpatory language through which the subject is made to waive, or to appear to waive, any of his legal rights, including any release of the organization or its agents from liability for negligence.[19]

---

[17] *See, e.g.,* 25 U.S.C. §§174 *et seq.* (1964)—limitations on Indians' right to contract; N.Y. GEN. OBLIG. L. §5-321 (1964)—contract exempting lessor from liability for negligence void as against public policy; Williams v. Walker-Thomas Furniture Co., 350 F.2d 445 (D.C. Cir. 1965). The same provision may be valid as to one group and invalid as to another; cognovit clauses (confession of judgment) have been upheld where a debtor effectively waives his rights, D. H. Overmyer Co. v. Frick Co., 405 U.S. 174 (1972), but declared unconstitutional when applied to debtors with incomes below $10,000, Swarb v. Lennox, 314 F.2d 1091 (E.D. Pa. 1970), *affd.* 405 U.S. 191 (1972).

[18] Miranda v. Arizona, 384 U.S. 436 (1966). This case established strict procedures for what has to be told to persons who are subjected to custodial police interrogation. *Cf.* Glass, note 7 *supra,* at 1561-62 (suggesting "formal rules of disclosure").

Midway between these two approaches is one perhaps best exemplified by the federal government's approach to cigarette smoking. Rather than banning it outright in light of the practice's demonstrably deleterious effects on users' health (which would be a deprivation of the right to contract) or requiring that certain information be conveyed (which was the approach taken initially by the FCC in requiring "equal time" for anti-smoking advertisements), Congress finally banned cigarette commercials from the air waves, counting on the beneficial effects of a *lack* of "information" (*i.e.*, advertising) while also requiring a health warning to be placed on each cigarette package.

[19] U.S. DEP'T OF HEALTH, EDUCATION & WELFARE, THE INSTITUTIONAL GUIDE TO DHEW POLICY ON PROTECTION OF HUMAN SUBJECTS 7 (1971) [hereinafter cited as INSTITUTIONAL GUIDE], as amended by 39 FED. REG. 18914 (1974). *Cf.* 21 C.F.R. Sec. 130.37 (1972)—FDA policy on informed consent.

Thus, by detailing the obligation of physician-investigators to warn their patient-subjects fully about their rights, such statements increase the likelihood that the informed consent rule will help to avoid intentional and unintentional fraud and duress.

d. To Encourage Self-scrutiny by the Physician-Investigator. The requirement of disclosure contained in the informed consent rule raises some perplexing problems for a physician working on the frontiers of catastrophic disease treatment. Perhaps foremost among these is the question: How can one disclose the risks and benefits of new and often untried techniques? A partial response to this query is that one can at least be candid with the patient about the unknown nature and experimental status of the treatment offered as well as about the existence of other established methods, inadequate as they may be. Beyond this, however, the physician-investigator has the additional duty of discovering as much as possible about the new techniques he proposes to employ. At a minimum this would include making a thorough inventory of the risks of such techniques which have been described in the literature by other investigators. In most situations it would also encompass the duty to explore this matter through animal experimentation and the like; this duty is reflected in the scientific principle, independent of the law of informed consent, that human trials ought to be undertaken only after a medical innovation has been shown in animal tests to be relatively risk-free (compared with its potential benefits).

Although some risks will still remain "unknown," a candid physician-investigator can still involve his subjects in a valid informed consent process. This would be encouraged if consent to "unknown risks" is taken to include only those "unknown risks" of which the subject is made aware. Such a position does not involve a contradiction in terms, for there *are* risks of unknown probability and degree (of which the patient can certainly be informed), and there are others which he cannot be said to have accepted since neither he nor the investigator had any way of anticipating them; on a strict view of this requirement, it may reasonably be assumed that in most cases the latter category would be very small. A distinction also exists between risks to which it was reasonable to expose a patient-subject and those which were unreasonable. A physician-investigator who proceeded in the latter instance would, of course, not be able to assert "consent" as a defense to a claim of negligence.[20]

The need to obtain the patient-subject's informed consent also serves to enhance the scientific validity and the safety of the trials of new medical procedures in man. This derives from the "reflexive effect [of the obligation

---

[20] *See* Waltz & Scheunemann, *Informed Consent to Therapy*, 64 N.W.U.L. Rev. 628, 635 (1969).

to obtain consent] on the management of the experiment itself," as Paul
Freund has pointed out.

> To analyze an experiment in terms of risks and benefits to particular groups
> by way of presentation for consent is a salutary procedure for self-scrutiny
> by the investigator—like the preparation of a registration statement by a
> corporation issuing securities.[21]

If, for example, the surgeons engaged in the initial heart transplants had
felt they had to give a full explanation of the risks of graft rejection to the
proposed cardiac recipients, they might have proceeded more slowly in the
light of the rather disheartening results which were then reported in animal
trials and in human kidney transplants at that time (when immunosuppression was still in its infancy).

As useful as the informed consent requirement may be in encouraging
professional self-scrutiny and thereby avoiding thoughtless disrespect of
patient-subjects, there is no reason to believe that the end result is assured.
Indeed, rather than undertake this process, physician-investigators may
instead raise arguments over whether their subjects have the capacity to
understand what they are told. Yet this is "a displacement from the real
issue, which is the dread of an open and searching dialogue between the
investigator and his subject. This displacement is caused by the unacknowledged anxiety over making the invitation in the first place."[22] The rules
constructed by the law for medical practice and research may thus force
the profession to confront this underlying anxiety, or they may themselves
be rendered ineffective by these undeniable yet unspoken psychological
forces.

e. To Encourage Rational Decisionmaking. Thus far we have emphasized
the role of informed consent in protecting patients' autonomy. The preceding section, however, has suggested that reliance on consent can also help
physician-investigators to perform their functions more satisfactorily. The
beneficial effects of informed consent in terms of rationality in the process
of decisionmaking about catastrophic disease treatment and research go
beyond influencing the investigator. The requirement of informed consent
symbolizes a commitment to making the process of developing new therapies a joint enterprise as proposed by Ramsey. By actively including the
patient-subject in the process, informed consent serves to place him on a
plane with the physician-investigator and to involve him as a person in
the work and not merely as an object on which it is being performed. For

---

[21] Freund, *Legal Frameworks for Human Experimentation,* 98 DAEDALUS 315, 323
(1969).

[22] Katz, *The Regulation of Human Research—Reflections and Proposals,* 21 CLIN.
RES. 787 (1973).

the participants to remain on the same plane requires a commitment that they view each other not only as equally important individuals but also as joint participants in decisionmaking. Accomplishing this will require, beyond a change in attitude, learning how to communicate to patient-subjects those aspects of the proposed research which will allow them to make decisions at least as rationally as they have made others about their lives.[23] If the basic elements of information and agreement (as suggested in this chapter and in documents such as the HEW guidelines) are faithfully adhered to, patient-subjects can help to promote rational decisionmaking.

A rule of informed consent congenial to the model of catastrophic disease decisionmaking elaborated here would view patient-subjects as exercising a major influence on the plans of physician-investigators. Thus, they can also become guarantors of their own rights to autonomy and dignity, by exercising a check over the judgment of physicians who all too often may be biased by their strong desire to "conquer disease."

Moreover, there is no objective, "medical" way to determine the proper treatment for an individual, since disease itself is not an objective concept but depends upon the degree of dysfunction experienced under given conditions by each individual. Thus rationality in resource allocation is possible only when the individuals who bear the costs and receive the benefits from the allocation determine the value of the outcomes. The determination whether a particular project will yield returns to science and society in excess of its costs is best made by biomedical researchers and representatives of the collectivity (to the extent that such an issue is capable of resolution at all). But who, other than the patient-subjects, can determine whether the benefits of a procedure, conventional or experimental, outweigh the burdens that will be imposed on them? If responsibility follows choice in a system of voluntary interactions, the costs of the system will be minimized when responsibility (with the consequent incentive to avoid harm) also determines who shall have authority to exercise choice.[24]

Some physicians have always been acutely aware of the value of the old adage "two heads are better than one." Their commitment to informing and consulting with their patient-subjects has been based on a recognition of the value of intelligent and dedicated partners, be they patients or fellow scientists. A well-informed patient, after all, is more alert to facts about his own condition that may be of great significance to the investigator, and he also feels freer about reporting what he experiences to his physician, without fear of upsetting him or losing his support. Similarly, a "patient-partner"

---

[23] The difficulties with which "rational decisionmaking" must contend are discussed on pp. 121-32 *infra.*

[24] Cf. G. CALABRESI, THE COST OF ACCIDENTS (1969).

is better able to endure the often arduous period of recuperation. Many physician-investigators recognize the value of such dedication and take the opportunity of medical publication or meetings to give credit and thanks to their "co-adventurers."[25]

f. To Involve the Public. A final function of informed consent looks beyond the physician-patient setting to an involvement of the larger society, a topic which will be discussed at greater length in the next chapter. Primarily, the obtaining of consent can be important for the public relations of a physician or a medical center. The reverse is certainly true: A physician who develops the reputation of using his patients as guinea pigs for his studies or medical innovations without their informed consent will be avoided by those who know that reputation.[26]

Informed consent may also function beyond the area of public reputation and serve to increase society's awareness about human research. This phenomenon is particularly noticeable in the area of organ transplantation. The need to obtain consent from large numbers of potential donors for the removal of their kidneys after death has led to an extensive program of information about renal transplant programs. While the motivation for this information campaign was to recruit individual donors, it also enlightens the public at large about a new development in medicine. Thereby, the general public becomes an informed decisionmaker, able through legislative actions, and so forth, to accelerate, halt, or alter transplant efforts should the details which are disclosed meet with unfavorable public reaction.

3. The Limitations of Consent

For the "informed consent" model of decisionmaking sketched above to be useful, it must take account of the limitations on patient-subjects' capacity to make intelligent and insightful choices. Some of these constraints are inherent in the intellectual faculties, psychological forces, and social pressures affecting the participants, while others result from individual and societal judgments about the scope of the authority which patient-subjects should be allowed to exercise. An awareness of these problems on the part of all the participants should aid in overcoming the failures of communications, understanding, and intelligent decisionmaking that now distort the process; in any event, we believe that a review of the limitations is crucial for the construction of a useful model.

---

[25] *See* Fox, *Some Social and Cultural Factors in American Society Conducive to Medical Research on Human Subjects*, 1 CLIN. PHARM. & THERAP. 423, 432-441 (1960).

[26] *See* Kidd, *Limits of the Right of a Person to Consent to Experimentation on Himself*, 117 SCIENCE 211, 212 (1953).

a. The Impact of the Inner World. In contemporary society the importance of unconscious forces on personal conduct is increasingly acknowledged, though recognition of the extensive scope and pervasive effect of these influences is often still resisted. To note the existence of such unconscious forces does not, of course, deny the role in decisionmaking played by the conscious mind, which is likewise the product of environmental influences and hereditary preconditions. Yet the impact of unconscious drives and feelings is even greater when it comes to the pressing issues which are involved in catastrophic disease treatment: life and death, giving and receiving, mutilation and restoration.

A revealing study by Drs. Carl H. Fellner and John R. Marshall[27] illustrates this point. They interviewed a group of live kidney donors after (and in a few cases, before) surgery, concerning the reasons for their decision to donate a kidney to a close relative and the process by which the decision was reached. They had assumed that the donors would make up their minds at the end of the lengthy process during which they were first told of the need for a kidney, then subjected to medical examinations, and finally informed of the transplant team's conclusions about their suitability and of the risks of giving up a kidney. Fellner and Marshall were surprised to discover that the decisions of the donors were apparently made long before there had been an opportunity for adequate information-gathering and considered balancing of pros and cons:

> . . . Not one of the donors weighed alternatives and rationally decided. Fourteen of the 20 donors and nine of the ten donors waiting for surgery stated that they had made their decision immediately when the subject of the kidney transplant was first mentioned over the telephone, "in a split-second," "instantaneously," and "right away." Five said they just went along with the tests hoping it would be someone else. They could not recall ever really having made a clear decision, yet they never considered refusing to go along either. As it became clear to each of them toward the end of the selection process that he was going to be the person most suited to be the donor, each had finally committed himself to the act. However, this decision too occurred before the sessions with the team doctors in which all the relevant information and statistics were put before these individuals and they were finally asked to decide.
>
> Of all the subjects who made their initial decision on the telephone upon first hearing of the possibility of the kidney transplant, none had consulted his or her spouse. When questioned about this particular circumstance, each explained that the spouse later on had either been neutral or reinforced the decision. To the hypothetical question of "What would you have done if your

---

[27] Fellner & Marshall, *Kidney Donors: The Myth of Informed Consent,* 126 Am. J. Psychiatry 1245 (1970).

spouse had said no?" each answered, "I would have gone ahead and done it anyway. . . ."[28]

Similarly, the few relatives who failed to show up for the initial blood test (ABO compatibility was used as the preliminary screening device) also had made their decision instantaneously and only later developed the "necessary" reasons to support their action.

The phenomenon observed by Fellner and Marshall may not establish, as they believe, that the kidney donors failed to decide "rationally." While it is possible to articulate all the elements and processes of formal, rational decisionmaking,[29] too little is known about actual human thought processes to preclude from the realm of the rational decisions arrived at "instantaneously." Yet the fact that a decision, once reached, seems not to be subject to reconsideration as additional, arguably material information is supplied raises questions about whether optimum choices are being made. At the least, the phenomenon observed by Fellner and Marshall (which one may safely assume is not restricted to decisionmaking about renal transplants) would suggest that to be effective, the model of the informed decisionmaker propounded depends upon a collaborative give-and-take beginning with the earliest contact of physician-investigator and patient-subject. At a minimum the latter should be made aware, as early as possible, of an outline or sketch of the project on which he is being asked to embark, even if some of the potential steps are still far in the distance. There will, of course, be a need to review each step as it materializes, but the practice of waiting, as is the prevailing practice, until the very point of the intervention (for example, the night before major surgery, after the patient has already checked into the hospital) seriously undermines the patient's comprehension and voluntariness which are supposedly embodied in his "informed consent."[30]

The results of the Fellner-Marshall study raise the additional issue whether, given the not inconsiderable risks and the suddenness of the decision, the donors were in any way mentally unbalanced; they conclude not. Dr. Harrison Sadler and his colleagues found strikingly similar results among genetically unrelated kidney donors, although they clearly believed that the donations were proper and were made for "healthy" reasons. Sadler and the San Francisco transplant team found no indications that their donors manifested psychopathology, character disorders, or infantile impulses which would undercut the altruism of their acts; the "primary motive" of these unrelated donors "was not in the drives but in the very

---

[28] *Id.* at 1247.

[29] *See e.g.,* NOMOS VII—RATIONAL DECISION (C. Friedrich ed. 1964); H. LASSWELL, THE DECISION PROCESS (1956).

[30] *See* Schonberg, *Informed Consent,* 230 J.A.M.A. 38 (1974).

personal area of self-identity, a self-ideal quite unconscious to them at the time."[31] Still, they concluded that the donors' decisionmaking seemed to have been dominated by nonrational forces, yet forces which seem to be an integral part of their overall personality structure:

> The most remarkable and universal quality of this group was their aura of sureness which pervaded the whole transplant encounter. They "knew" they would respond to the appeal. They spoke of an "inner quickening" as though an already programmed circuit had been aroused. They "knew" their response was wholesome and they "felt sure" that they would match and be chosen and that the operation and post-operative period would be successful and uncomplicated.[32]

The donors of kidneys are not the only ones in whom the decisional process is deeply affected by "inner forces" which do not comport with the "model" of conscious and careful choice. The burden of disease also alters kidney transplant recipients' thinking, because of both the physiological changes and psychological problems they experience. As with other life-threatening conditions, the physician's disclosure to the patient that he has end-stage renal disease usually brings on depression,[33] followed by "denial" which "functions as a buffer after unexpected shocking news, allows the patient to collect himself and, with time, mobilize other, less radical defenses."[34] For terminal patients, denial of their condition and its gravity may thus have certain adaptive value, and this psychological process is exhibited by most patients at some point.[35] This defense may, however, seriously interfere with the patient's ability to make realistic decisions, especially since he is also probably suffering from feelings of helplessness, dependency, and further depression.

> Those factors . . . repressed by the denial alter the orderly processing of data, and decisions made at this level are processed by mechanisms which

---

[31] Sadler, *Summary Notes on a Clinical Decision-Making Model* (consultant's memorandum) at 1 (1972) [Appendix H].

[32] Sadler, Davison, Carroll & Kountz, *The Living, Genetically Unrelated, Kidney Donor*, 3 SEMINARS IN PSYCH. 86, 89 (1971).

[33] B. GLASSER & A. STRAUSS, AWARENESS OF DYING 122 (1965).

[34] E. KÜBLER-ROSS, ON DEATH AND DYING 35 (1969).

[35] Although differing somewhat about the sequence, the in-depth psychological studies of patients with terminal illnesses portray patients as passing through a number of "stages" of attitude, behavior, and feeling after they learn of their condition. *See, e.g.,* GLASER & STRAUSS, note 33 *supra*, and KÜBLER-ROSS, note 34 *supra*. While these studies thus contradict the accepted medical folklore about the way patients react to "the truth" (*see* pp. 132-39 *infra.*), they also indicate that patients' ability to work their way through the stages beyond denial and depression is highly dependent on their having candid, trusting relations with their physician and other hospital personnel.

fail to account completely for reality factors and give them symbolic quality in keeping with the dominant wish.[36]

Taken together, the startling evidence about kidney donors' and recipients' decisionmaking illustrates and confirms the importance of internal and often unperceived influences on decisionmaking about kidney transplantation. One has every reason to suppose that these same forces also play a major role in patient-subjects' decisions to accept or reject other catastrophic disease treatments, such as hemodialysis and heart transplantation.

  b. The Impact of the Outer World. More readily apparent, but not much easier to quantify, are the environmental influences on patients.

> A family member is dying of renal disease, and his best chance for survival with a tolerable life is to be the recipient of a kidney from a relative whose tissue-type closely matches his own. No matter how scrupulously low-keyed and sensitive the medical team's process of screening candidates may be, the fact remains that . . . prospective donors are under very great inner and outer pressure to give an organ to their suffering relative who, in turn, is under extraordinary pressure to receive one.[37]

Fellner and Marshall found that while families did not necessarily decide who would be the donor, they often determined who would be excluded from consideration, either to protect that person or because he or she was believed to be unsuitable in terms of intrafamilial relations. The opinions of family and friends did not need to be expressed overtly to be influential. The pronounced effect of environmental stimuli on the decision to volunteer has been well recognized.[38] It strains credibility to think, for example, that the teenage children who were asked to give up a kidney for their ailing twin had any difficulty in perceiving the response expected from them even when they were told that the choice was entirely "up to you." Whatever they really thought of their fate, once their parents had had them tested in the hospital and had petitioned for permission to authorize surgery, it is not surprising that they uniformly told judges and psychiatrists that they desired to donate their kidney.[39]

Heavy psychological burdens that can seriously distort any process of informed and rational decisionmaking are not restricted to organ donors and recipients but affect patients on hemodialysis as well. In those centers

---

[36] Sadler, note 31 *supra*, at 6.

[37] Parsons, Fox & Lidz, *The "Gift of Life" and Its Reciprocation,* 39 Soc. RESEARCH 367, 413 (1972).

[38] Rosenbaum, *The Effect of Stimulus and Background Factors on the Volunteering Response,* 53 J. ABNORMAL & SOC. PSYCH. 118 (1956).

[39] *See* Curran, *A Problem of Consent: Kidney Transplantation in Minors,* 34 N.Y.U.L. REV. 891 (1959).

in which dialysis was viewed as a stopgap until the patients could have their kidneys replaced, the spirits of the patients would rise with the approach of each long holiday weekend, for they knew that there would be a large number of automobile accidents, which would heighten their chances to receive a kidney from an accident victim. This macabre "holiday syndrome," as it was labeled by Dr. Patrick McKegney,[40] had an equally sinister backlash; if the weekend passed without a suitable donor becoming available, deep depression would spread through the dialysis units. Such a state of mind is clearly not conducive to a sound or lucid decisional process especially on whether to persevere with the arduous dialysis regimen.

Similarly, some families feel pressured to provide dialysis at home because of many physicians' preference for its lower cost (over treatment in a kidney center) and such other advantages as fewer medical complications, flexible scheduling, and reduction of cross-infections between dialysands. Despite some reports of "psychologic improvement, family unity and a feeling of self-confidence and accomplishment," it must be recognized that not all families truly want or are really able to take on the burden of caring for kidney failure at home.[41]

Finally, a patient-subject's concern for his family's economic and emotional well-being may weigh heavily on his decision to embark on a lengthy course of dialysis or undergo a risky and costly transplant operation. These factors even affect decisions in circumstances where the family professes indifference to their possible financial suffering or where other funding sources are available to defray most of the expense.

c. The Impact of the Relationship. Families do not exert the only "outside" influence on patient-subjects' decisionmaking. Indeed, in many respects the relationship of physician-investigator to patient-subject may have greater impact. A great deal has been written on doctor-patient interaction, especially concerning the "transferences" and "countertransferences" which are the hallmark of this process. The childlike expectations on the patient's part, encompassed in the transference concept, and the physician's reciprocal feelings, are nowhere more evident than in the treatment of life-threat-

---

[40] McKegney's observations about, and name for, this phenomenon among dialysis patients were reported to us by one of our consultants, Dr. Belding Scribner.

[41] *See* Friedman & Kountz, *Impact of HR-1 on the Therapy of End-Stage Uremia,* 288 NEW ENG. J. MED. 1286 (1974)—concluding that problems of home dialysis "are only now emerging in perspective," making it too early to set a limit on extent of center dialysis; Blagg, Hickman et al., *Home Hemodialysis: Six Years' Experience,* 283 NEW ENG. J. MED. 1126 (1970)—continued severe stress with maladjustment found in 19 percent of home dialysands; DePalmer, *Open Forum: Home Dialysis,* 2 DIAL. TRANSPLANT 10 (1973)—home dialysis not suitable in approximately 80 percent of cases.

ening diseases. Any illness may undermine a person's normal ego strength; a crippling disease which puts a patient in a sickbed without prospect of recovery can call forth ultimate dependence, cooperation, and devotion to the all-powerful physician who possesses the magical means of curing him. This combination of infantile regression and projection of a parental image onto the physician has often been observed in treatment and research settings, particularly when the patient has sought out the physician as a specialist, especially "*the* outstanding specialist" in his field.

The impact of these reciprocal and largely unconscious feelings and ideas is well illustrated by a few rather illuminating passages from Dr. Philip Blaiberg's account of his transplantation experience:

> The day after my admission to Ward D 1, I was lying in bed with eyes closed, feeling drowsy and thoroughly miserable when I sensed someone at the head of my bed. I opened my eyes and saw a man. He was tall, young, good-looking with features that reminded me a lot of General Jan Christian Smuts in his later years. His hands were beautiful; the hands of the born surgeon.
>
> "Don't you know me?" he asked.
>
> "No," I said with little interest, "I don't."
>
> "I'm Professor Chris Barnard," he said.
>
> "I'm sorry, Professor," I replied, "but I didn't recognize you. I have never seen you in person, and you look so different from your photographs in the Press."
>
> He spoke earnestly. "Dr. Blaiberg, how do you feel about the prospect of a heart transplant operation? You probably know, don't you, that I am prepared to do you next?"
>
> "The sooner the better," I said fervently, "and I promise you my full cooperation at all times."
>
> Though our conversation was brief and he stayed only a few minutes, I was immediately impressed with the stature of the man and his air of buoyant optimism. He inspired me with the greatest confidence, an invaluable asset in the relations between a surgeon and his patient.
>
> I felt somewhat better. Here was a man to whom I would willingly entrust my life. I came to know him well in the weeks and months that followed. He is a vital, determined, somewhat mercurial, personality, utterly dedicated to his profession.
>
> • • •
>
> On the morning of December 21, 1967, I was surprised to see my wife walk into my ward at about 9:30. Her visits had always been in the afternoon because of her morning job.
>
> "Aren't you working today?" I asked.
>
> "No," she said. "I just felt I wanted to see you."
>
> "The nurses have told me that Professor Barnard is also coming to see me this morning," I said.

It seemed strange and unusual, but I did not give the matter further thought. I accepted Eileen's explanation and believed Professor Barnard's visit would be mere routine. Soon afterward he walked in. Eileen rose to excuse herself.

"No, don't go," Professor Barnard said to her. "I want to speak to you together." I looked more closely at him. He was haggard and drawn as though he had not slept all night. He no longer resembled the handsome Smuts, to whom I had compared him, but more a martyred Christ. I felt a twinge of pity for him when I noticed the pain in his face and eyes. Something, I was sure had happened to dampen the gaiety and boundless optimism I had seen before.

. . .

Professor Barnard spoke in low tones. "I feel like a pilot who has just crashed," he said. "Now I want you, Dr. Blaiberg, to help me by taking up another plane as soon as possible to get back my confidence."

Still I did not know what he was driving at. "Professor," I said, puzzled, "why are you telling me this? You know I am prepared to undergo a heart transplant operation at any time you wish."

"But don't you know that Louis Washkansky is dead?" he asked. "He died this morning, of pneumonia."

It dawned on me why Eileen and Professor Barnard had paid me this unexpected visit. Now I knew the reason for his distress and agitation.

"Professor Barnard," I said at once, "I want to go through with it now more than ever—not only for my sake but for you and your team who put so much into your effort to save Louis Washkansky."

. . .

"Don't worry," he said a little more cheerfully now, "everything is going to be fine."[42]

This description by Blaiberg vividly depicts the strong dependencies and expectations running both ways between physician and patient which affect, and even play havoc with, the rational decisionmaking that was part of our preliminary "informed consent" model. Similarly, countertransference phenomena probably also lie behind the policy of a number of physician-investigators, as described in the previous chapter, not to permit kidney donations by nonrelated living donors.[43] Where the doctor-patient relationship leads the transplanter to a degree of identification with the donor he may find it distressing to contemplate a donation "for no reason" (*i.e.*, without the pull of family obligation) which poses a threat to the physician's highly-

---

[42] P. BLAIBERG, LOOKING AT MY HEART 65-70 (1968). Copyright © 1968 by Philip Blaiberg. Reprinted with permission of Stein and Day/Publishers.

[43] *See* pp. 62-63 *supra;* Fellner & Schwartz, *Altruism in Disrepute,* 284 NEW ENG. J. MED. 282 (1971).

valued bodily integrity.[44] When a genetically unrelated but willing person is excluded from being a kidney donor, the transplant surgeon is, in effect, withholding *his* "informed consent" to the procedure.[45]

Additional complications are added when, as is often the case, the professional and his patient are of different, and even markedly separate, social classes.[46] Besides their effect on the transference and countertransference reactions, such educational and class differences have an even more palpable effect on the degree of communication and comprehension which can be expected in the relationship. Furthermore, any number of factors can conspire to interfere with doctor-patient communication: for example, the doctor's preoccupation with other matters, particularly when he has a heavy caseload as the leading physicians do; the natural desire of the hospital staff to "routinize" procedures, in order not to burden the patient with anxiety or themselves with the added chore of coping with that anxiety; and the inclination of physicians not to complicate patients' decisionmaking by reviewing with them the alternatives to the proposed treatment on the assumption (probably faulty) that these questions had been gone over by someone else earlier in the process.

If experience in other areas provides any indication, even when physicians attempt to adhere scrupulously to the model of informed consent, patients may fail to absorb their cautions.[47] In fact, the danger that physician-investigators will overreach their patient-subjects is probably greater in therapeutic settings than in experimentation outside the context of therapy, since a patient is very poorly situated to arrive at a disinterested weighing of the risks and benefits of the proposed new treatment or to turn it down if it seems to be favored by the physician to whom he probably already owed such great emotional (and perhaps financial) debts for his

---

[44] Fellner and Marshall tell of a resident physician whose blood was used as a control in a leukocyte test and proved to be compatible with the proposed kidney recipient. When told of this finding, he immediately refused to be a donor without even being asked. Fellner & Marshall, note 27 *supra*, at 1247. This reaction contrasts with that which Fellner and Schwartz found among non-physicians.

[45] *See* Fellner, *The Genetically Unrelated Living Kidney Donor: Unemployed and Unwanted* (consultant's memorandum) at 5 (1972) [Appendix E].

[46] *See, e.g.,* A. B. HOLLINGSHEAD & F. REDLICH, SOCIAL CLASS AND MENTAL ILLNESS (1958); R. S. DUFF & A. B. HOLLINGSHEAD, SICKNESS AND SOCIETY (1968).

[47] A study of highly educated young men who were interrogated by FBI agents after they had turned in their draft cards (in protest against the war in Vietnam) indicated that despite clearly delivered *Miranda* warnings (*see* note 18 *supra*) they nevertheless gave the agents statements (which could be used in court against them) although they had for the most part not intended or "wanted" to do so. Griffiths & Ayres, *A Postscript to the Miranda Project: Interrogation of Draft Protestors*, 77 YALE L.J. 300 (1967).

past care and on whom he is dependent for his future well-being. Moreover, a new, untried technique is probably offered despite its unknown qualities only because more conventional modalities have proven ineffective. As Francis Moore has observed:

> People in this country have been weaned on newspaper accounts of exciting new cures. Particularly in the field of organ transplantation, patients are pressing their doctors to be the subject of innovation.[48]

Thus, in the context of the doctor-patient relationship there are many impediments to the patient's being able to exercise rational judgment about whether to undergo a new and experimental treatment proposed by his physician.

d. The Role of "Faith." As the previous chapter suggested, none of the forces that tend to undermine rationality is likely to be mitigated by the traditional training or orientation of clinical researchers. If anything, prevailing attitudes among physicians only serve to increase the impact of those influences.

First, as a matter of communication and comprehension, most physicians doubt that their patients can be told simple, unvarnished information about their disease and the prospects for treatment. "[I]t is meaningless to speak of telling the truth, the whole truth, and nothing but the truth to a patient. It is meaningless because it is impossible—a sheer impossibility."[49] Physicians are particularly likely to withhold information relating to diagnosis or prognosis, as opposed to the nature of a proposed intervention, not only on the grounds suggested (that there is no such thing as "the truth" which can be conveyed) but also because they believe they have a "therapeutic privilege" to do so.[50] Yet there are good reasons why such medical discretion should be narrowly confined. For one thing, a broadly defined privilege "would afford a perfect shield to cover the negligence of many [physicians] who were unable to reach a timely or accurate diagnosis of the true illness."[51] Moreover, serious questions have been raised about the validity of the premise underlying therapeutic privilege—that it is beneficial to the

---

[48] PROCEEDINGS OF THE CONFERENCE ON THE ETHICAL ASPECTS OF EXPERIMENTATION ON HUMAN SUBJECTS (Daedalus-National Institutes of Health) 31 (1967).

[49] Henderson, *Physician and Patient as a Social System,* 212 NEW ENG. J. MED. 819, 822 (1935).

[50] *See, e.g.,* Bolam v. Friern Hospital Comm., [1952] 2 All E.R. 118—defendant physicians found not negligent in failing to warn where it might interfere with treatment; Note, *Physician's Duty to Warn,* 75 HARV. L. REV. 1445 (1962)—duty should be based on patient's needs, not physician's practice; Canterbury v. Spence, 464 F.2d 772, 789 (D. C. Cir. 1972).

[51] H. W. Smith, *Therapeutic Privilege to Withhold Specific Diagnosis from Patient Sick with Serious or Fatal Illness,* 19 TENN. L. REV. 349, 350 (1946).

patient's course of treatment that he be protected from learning bad news about his condition. Irving Janis marshalled observational and psycho-analytic data which led him to conclude that it is vital for patients to engage in "the work of worrying" if they are to be able to cope with their disease and treatment, among other stressful experiences. Particularly germane to a model of informed consent in surgery or dialysis for catastrophic illness is Janis' conclusion that

> the arousal of some degree of anticipatory fear may be one of the necessary conditions for developing inner defense of the type that can function effec-tively when the external dangers materialize. In many of the individual case studies we have examined, the patient had received very little information about the suffering that he would undergo and, in some cases, this lack of information seems to have been a major factor in determining the relative absence of anticipatory fear. One surmises that most people ignore proble-matical dangers of the future unless they receive specific warnings or predic-tions from respected authorities. The unpleasant task of mental rehearsal, which appears to be essential for developing effective danger-contingent re-assurances, is apt to be shirked, even when a person knows that he is going to be exposed to some form of suffering or deprivation.[52]

Consequently, it appears that for transference and other reasons, the patient is likely to expect the physician to protect him from all harm, so that it is only the physician who can impart to his patient a more realistic view of what may develop during the illness and proposed treatment.

While ignorance may not be bliss, physician-investigators are prone to rely on it not only to exploit the curative potential of patients' "faith" in the ordinary course of treatment but also to avoid what they regard as the even more worrisome consequences of disclosure where a life-threatening illness is involved. For example, 90 percent of physicians are reported to follow the policy of withholding the information that a patient has cancer, although they typically tell the patient's relative, so to avoid legal liability as well as to share the burden that the knowledge had placed on them and to enlist the family's cooperation in keeping the patient on the desired treatment regime.[53] Physicians seek by this course of conduct to maintain their patients' "hope" and to avoid the risk that a patient, knowing the end is near, will attempt to take his own life. As was suggested in the preceding chapter, the medical practice of withholding information seems to be based largely on personal predilection, supported by a shared value system among

---

[52] I. L. JANIS, PSYCHOLOGICAL STRESS: PSYCHOANALYTIC AND BEHAVIORAL STUDIES OF SURGICAL PATIENTS 352 (1958).

[53] Oken, *What to Tell Cancer Patients: A Study of Medical Attitudes*, 175 J.A.M.A. 1120 (1961).

physicians, even though nearly all the doctors surveyed reported that "clinical experience" was the major factor in determining their policy on disclosure. Only a small percentage, however, had ever tried any policy different from their current one.

> It was the exception when a physician could report known examples of the unfavorable consequences of an approach which differed from his own. It was more common to get reports of instances in which different approaches had turned out satisfactorily. Most of the instances in which unhappy results were reported to follow a differing policy turned out to be vague accounts from which no reliable inference could be drawn.[54]

While most physicians apparently believe that knowledge of a life-threatening disease is "the cruelest thing in the world,"[55] they take a less emotional and paternalistic view of how they would like to be treated were their own physician to discover that they have cancer; most indicated that they would want to know the diagnosis.[56] This double standard demonstrates the physicians' unresolved conflicts about disclosure and interestingly enough puts them in line with what laymen state to be their own wishes regarding disclosure, which, according to one study, is desired by 77 to 89 percent.[57]

The implications of this evidence for the informed consent model of catastrophic disease decisionmaking are twofold. On the one hand, the present attitude of physician-investigators, which may seriously detract from the possibility of establishing a mutually informed joint working relationship, will probably be difficult to overcome. Though it is a limitation on informed consent which is imposed by some of the participants (*e.g.*, the physician-investigators), its roots obviously run deep into the inherent barriers to informed consent which were discussed in the previous sections. Consequently, it is unlikely that formal regulations on disclosure or mutuality of decisionmaking could have much effect in the short-run. On the other hand, if there is a genuine commitment to informed consent, it should

---

[54] *Id.* at 1124.

[55] A representative comment from interviews with physicians, who also used such terms as "a death sentence," "torture," and "hitting the patient with a baseball bat." *Id.* at 1125.

[56] "The explanation usually given was that 'I am one of those who can take it' or 'I have responsibilities.'" *Id.* This difference in some physicians' attitude toward what they themselves wanted to know had no effect (or an inverse effect) on their policy toward other doctor-patients.

[57] Feifel, *The Function of Attitudes toward Death,* in DEATH AND DYING: ATTITUDES OF PATIENT AND DOCTOR (G.A.P. Symposium #11) 632, 635 (1965). This statistical result is fully supported by the impression gained through in-depth psychological studies. *See, e.g.,* KÜBLER-ROSS, note 34 *supra.*

be possible, as part of the curricular revision suggested in Chapter Five, to bring about a change in physician-investigators' attitudes and practices. While the present policies have important psychological aspects, they could probably be overcome if medical instructors in both the classroom and clinic were to demonstrate the feasibility and desirability of giving patient-subjects a meaningful role in making choices about their own treatment or nontreatment by providing them with "the truth" about their conditions and potential alternative therapies.

Such an approach has the advantage of taking realistic account of the state of knowledge that most patients achieve anyway, their physicians notwithstanding.[58] Present medical practice carries the danger that when patients find out their real condition or the actual benefits and risks of their treatment they may lose confidence in the physician who "lied" to them or at least withheld important facts from them. Of course, a policy of informed patient decisionmaking does not require that the "cruel truth" be unloaded on the patient in a single interview.

> The central question is not whether or not to tell a patient about his dim outlook, but *who* shall tell, *how much* to tell, *what* to tell, *how* to tell, *when* to tell, and *how often* to tell.[59]

This formulation suggests that the central duty of professionals is to devise means of bringing the patient-subject into the decisionmaking process rather than creating excuses for keeping him out "in his own best interests." If the physician spends sufficient time with the patient it should be possible to convey the necessary data to him in a comprehensible form.

> Initially, most patients should be advised of the doctor's findings *and the treatment planned.* Frankness does not mean hopelessness. At the beginning, the patient need not be told more than the facts of the illness. His doctor's directness should convey a more important, non-verbal message that he will not be abandoned. Gratuitous reassurances, overly precise predictions, and philosophical precepts are to be avoided.[60]

A final advantage of the adoption of such a policy would be to decrease the possible exploitation of patient-subjects' too eager consent to research procedures. If physician-investigators adopt the new policy suggested here to guide their actions, they are less likely to misuse the undeniably great

---

[58] "As at least three-quarters of the patients here studied became aware that they were probably dying, the question 'Should the doctor tell?' loses much of its force." Hinton, *The Physical and Mental Distress of the Dying*, 32 Q. J. MED. 1, 19 (1963).

[59] Weisman, *The Patient with a Fatal Illness: To Tell or not to Tell?* 201 J.A.M.A. 153 (1967).

[60] *Id.*

impact which a sudden disclosure of impending death can have on a patient, converting him from a rational, if ailing, person into a pliant subject who will consent to any experimental intervention "since he has no hope anyway." The abandonment of the physician's supposed blanket privilege to withhold information in the patient's "best interests" does not mean that the physician should be permitted to overpower his patient with a needlessly harsh or ill-timed presentation.[61] Nor do we mean to suggest that "faith"— that is, a less than fully realistic belief in the physician and hope that the treatment will succeed—is out of place in the treatment of catastrophic illnesses.[62]

There is certainly a place in medical innovation for the brave subject who, realizing that his life is near its end, decides selflessly to participate in research so that more can be learned about the disease that is killing him or about new possibilities of treating it;[63] indeed such subjects are probably crucial to "medical progress." But their participation should be based on an unpressured weighing of alternatives and not on a dejected view of their own worth or a desperate bid to maintain the friendship and support of a physician who, by the manner in which he informed them of their condition and the possibilities of treatment, has left them with the impression that he will abandon them if they fail to cooperate in his project.

e. Societal Constraints. The final limitations on informed consent are those imposed by society, which on occasion either refuses to sanction the choice made by a patient-subject or insists that he consent to a medical procedure which he does not want. Needless to say, these two situations are often hard to distinguish: If "no treatment" were the procedure chosen by a patient who needed treatment to preserve his life and the state declines to sanction his decision, this might also be framed as the state insisting on his undergoing an intervention which he opposes.

Formal challenges are seldom made in the first situation, in which the

---

[61] [T]he 'best interests' doctrine is acceptable to the extent it mirrors the physician's Hippocratic duty to 'do no harm' but . . . it should be abandoned to the extent it would permit a physician to substitute his judgment for his patient's. Thus, this modified 'best interests' would place a floor under the standard of acceptable conduct by physicians, by refusing to excuse intentional or reckless harm to patients, without allowing this protection against potential harm to swallow up the patient's whole right to information and consent.

Capron, *Legal Rights and Moral Rights,* in ETHICAL ISSUES IN HUMAN GENETICS 221, 241 n.22 (Hilton, et al. eds. 1973).

[62] For example, the faith and hope developed in patients by the self-described "zeal and enthusiasm" of Dr. Belding Scribner was probably responsible for his extraordinary success with hemodialysis in the early years of long-term treatment. *See* pp. 38-39 *supra.*

[63] *See also* pp. 114-15 *infra.*

state overrides a patient's willingness to participate in a medical procedure. Edmond Cahn argues, however, that a patient-subject's consent should be passed upon by someone (the state?) when the procedure involves substantial risks and that in instances where the risk of permanent physical or psychic mutilation is "serious . . . the consent should not be accepted."[64]

> For example, a consent would be unacceptable if the experiment involved a serious risk of converting a subject who is mentally normal into a psychotic. On the other hand, as every physician knows, there are psychiatric conditions grievous or critical enough to warrant even the risk of psychic mutilation, but in such conditions the justification for taking the risk must be found in the possible benefit to the ailing subject, not alone in his consent or in the possible increment of scientific knowledge.[65]

Were the intervention a criminal act, the consent of the patient-subject could, of course, be disregarded by the state, either in attempting to prevent the event from occurring or in prosecuting the physician-investigator subsequently.[66] Yet we have seen no indication in the literature that the acts to which catastrophic disease patients have submitted come within the category of crimes.

More pertinent to our topic is the second category of state interference with informed consent: the insistence that a person submit to an undesired medical procedure. Outside the context of life-threatening illness, this issue arose in the early years of compulsory vaccination for contagious diseases. The objections of persons not wanting to be inoculated were found to be outweighed by the public interest in preserving the health of other citizens.[67] Where refusal of lifesaving treatment is at issue, the state's primary interest moves away from protecting others[68] to a paternalistic concern to safeguard

---

[64] Cahn, *Drug Experiments and the Public Conscience,* in DRUGS IN OUR SOCIETY 255, 264 (P. Talalay ed. 1964).

[65] *Id.* at 264-65.

[66] If the patient-subject's agreement to the intervention were found to be voluntary and informed, he would probably be unsuccessful in suing the physician-investigator for the intervention, albeit that it was criminal. For example, in Spead v. Tomlinson, 73 N.H. 46, 59 A. 376 (1904), the court assumed that a statute on the unauthorized practice of medicine made treatment by a Christian Science practitioner illegal, and that this statute was passed to benefit those such as the plaintiff who had been injured as a result of a violation of the statute. Nevertheless, the court held that the plaintiff could not recover, because she had submitted to the treatment of her own choice, but it also noted that this act on her part would not have relieved the defendant of criminal liability, had he been so charged by the state.

[67] *See, e.g.,* Jacobson v. Massachusetts, 197 U.S. 11 (1904).

[68] In some of the cases discussed *infra, e.g.,* Application of President and Directors of Georgetown College, 331 F.2d 1000 (D. C. Cir. 1964), the patient had a young child who might have been adversely affected by the loss of a parent; this factor does

the individual from his own unwise decision, a ritualistic desire to uphold "the sanctity of life," and a collective interest in preserving each person's productivity for society's benefit.[69]

In recent years the notable litigation has been the so-called Jehovah's Witnesses cases, as well as other cases which do not involve the complicating religious factor but present the same issue: Does a person have the right to refuse lifesaving medical treatment? The judiciary is divided on this issue. In *Application of President and Directors of Georgetown College,*[70] Judge J. Skelly Wright presented two lines of reasoning for his decision that the hospital could administer a transfusion over the Jehovah's Witness' objections. First, he concluded that the patient, a Mrs. Jones, had yielded to the hospital some or all of her authority to make a decision by coming to it for treatment in the first place; he distinguished her situation from that of the patient who "has refused to seek medical attention."[71] The more important part of his argument was that Mrs. Jones may have wanted to adhere to her religious beliefs and refuse to "drink blood," but she did *not* desire the consequences of that choice, that is, she did not want to commit suicide. Thus, Judge Wright concluded that his decision comported with her real, though not with her expressed, wishes.[72] In a similar case, [73] Chief Justice Weintraub of New Jersey confronted the issue of suicide more directly. He, too, concluded that the state has the authority to override a

---

not play a prominent role in the cases as a whole, however. *Cf.* Raleigh Fitkin-Paul Morgan Memorial Hospital v. Anderson, 42 N.J. 421, 201 A.2d 537, *cert. denied,* 377 U.S. 985 (1964)—transfusion ordered for woman 32 weeks pregnant.

[69] *See* Cantor, *A Patient's Decision to Decline Life-Saving Medical Treatment,* 26 RUTGERS L. REV. 228, 242-54 (1973).

[70] 331 F.2d 1000 (D. C. Cir.), *cert. denied,* 377 U.S. 978 (1964).

[71] There was no indication, however, that the patient knew upon entering the hospital that the treatment on which the doctors would insist would include whole blood transfusions. Furthermore, while Judge Wright acknowledged the "normal principle" that a patient has a right to decide the treatment to which he will consent, he wondered "where a patient would derive her authority to command her doctor to treat her under limitations which would produce death." *Id.* at 1009. Of course, this really stands the issue on its head—the real question is the source of the physician's or state's authority to insist on certain treatment over a patient's objections; seemingly recognizing this problem, Judge Wright did not push this question of "martyrdom" but at this point in the opinion reverted to his second argument, discussed in the text, that Mrs. Jones did not want to die.

[72] Judge Wright also stated that he was able to avoid violating Mrs. Jones's religious beliefs, since he understood her to say that she could not request any blood but that it could be given to her "against [her] will." *Accord* Powell v. Columbia Presbyterian Medical Center, 49 Misc. 215, 216, 267 N.Y.S.2d 450, 452 (Sup. Ct. 1965): "This woman wanted to live. I could not let her die!"

[73] John F. Kennedy Hospital v. Heston, 58 N.J. 576, 279 A.2d 670 (1971).

patient's refusal to accept a treatment necessary to save his life, just as it may prohibit suicide. He dismissed the distinction advanced by the patient "between passively submitting to death and actively seeking it," but he acknowledged that an exception does occur when "the medical opinion itself is laden with the risk of death or of serious infirmity."[74] Yet such a standard is fraught with difficulties—if, as Justice Weintraub seems to assume, blood transfusions lie at one end of the spectrum (despite the risk of transfusion hepatitis), where on the continuum of risk do hemodialysis, kidney transplantation, and heart transplantation fall? The potential confusion is not helped by the court's expansive view of the role of the medical profession:

> Hospitals exist to aid the sick and the injured. The medical and nursing professions are consecrated to preserving life. That is their professional creed. To them, a failure to use a simple, established procedure in the circumstances of this case would be malpractice, however, the law may characterize that failure because of the patient's private convictions. . . .[75]

In other jurisdictions, courts have arrived at the opposite conclusion. The Supreme Court of Illinois faced with an appeal from a probate judge's order appointing a guardian, to consent to a transfusion on a Jehovah's Witness, held that:

> Knowing full well the hazards involved, she has firmly opposed acceptance of transfusions, notifying the doctor and hospital of her convictions and desires, and executing documents releasing both the doctor and hospitals from any civil liability which might be thought to result from a failure on the part of either to administer such transfusions. . . . Even though we may consider appellant's beliefs unwise, foolish or ridiculous, in the absence of an overriding danger to society we may not permit interference therewith in the form of a conservatorship established in the waning hours of her life for the sole purpose of compelling her to accept medical treatment forbidden by her religious principles and previously refused by her with full knowledge of the probable consequences. . . .[76]

---

[74] *Id.* at 581-82, 279 A.2d at 672-73.

[75] *Id.* at 582, 279 A.2d at 673. Particularly puzzling is the court's use of the term "malpractice," by which it apparently means a medical view of misconduct, eschewing the legal view of "malpractice," to which the term usually refers. It is hard to know if the court is being critical when it notes that the viewpoint of the law may be determined by "the patient's private convictions" about whether he wishes to be treated. A major tenet of our legal system has traditionally been its respect for each person's choices about his own body and the interferences with it he will permit.

[76] *In re* Brooks Estate, 32 Ill.2d 361, 372-73, 205 N.E.2d 435, 442 (1965). The Illinois Court placed heavy emphasis on the religious basis of Mrs. Brooks's objections; the case is thus primarily a First Amendment "free exercise" decision.

Similar reasoning was applied in the New York opinion *Erickson v. Dilgard*[77] in which the judge concluded, contrary to the *Georgetown* and *Heston* courts, that the refusal to accept medical treatment when made by a competent adult, irrespective of religious reasons, did not fall under the criminal law's prohibition on suicide.

[I]t is the individual who is the subject of a medical decision who has the final say and . . . this must necessarily be so in a system of government which gives the greatest possible protection to the individual in the furtherance of his own desires.[78]

In the last few years a number of cases have reached the courts involving treatments besides blood transfusions and patients other than Jehovah's Witnesses. A particularly dramatic case related to the area of catastrophic disease treatment arose recently in New York when a physician sought court approval for the reenergizing of a 79-year-old man's cardiac pacemaker. The patient, a Mr. Bettman, was found to be unaware of his condition and incapable of making the decision himself; his wife refused permission for the operation "because, she said, her husband 'is turning into a vegetable.' "[79] The physician—in the apparent belief that he was taking a value-neutral and nonjudgmental position—argued that "As a physician I cannot take it into my hands to play God. If there is any step I can take to save life, I am committed to do it."[80] The judge agreed, and permission was granted for the hospital to proceed.

In contrast to the *Bettman* decision, a Florida court in 1971 permitted a daughter, who had been appointed guardian for her 72-year-old mother, to decline further treatment; Mrs. Martinez died the following day of hemolytic anemia.[81] Similarly, in Wisconsin a judge upheld the objections of a Mrs. Raasch to further amputations of her leg; he determined that although her condition prevented her from communicating verbally, she was "not incompetent" and her wishes (as expressed nonverbally) should be respected.[82]

Although the common law does not point in any single direction,[83] it

---

[77] 44 Misc.2d 27, 252 N.Y.S.2d 705 (Sup. Ct. 1962).

[78] *Id.* at 28, 252 N.Y.S.2d at 706.

[79] Crafton, *Doc: Ethics Made Me Save Heart Man*, Daily News (N.Y.), Jan. 29, 1972, at 5, col. 1.

[80] *Id.*

[81] Palm Springs General Hospital v. Martinez, No. 71-12687 (Fla. Cir. Ct., filed July 1, 1971).

[82] D. HENDIN, DEATH AS A FACT OF LIFE 67-69 (1973).

[83] This is, if anything, a great understatement; seemingly any attempt to bring order to the cases will fail to explain some exceptions. Initially, the distinction between competent and incompetent patients seems most attractive; such a distinction

seems to us that cases such as *Erickson* and *Raasch* state the better rule, both as a matter of legal and social philosophy and as a practical matter. Almost insuperable problems of administration would be presented if physician-investigators were free to second-guess the informed decisions made by patient-subjects. This problem is not more acute only because the manner in which physicians now control the process of information-giving and decisionmaking seldom places them in irreconcilable opposition to the choices made by their patients. If adherence to the informed consent model increases these instances, physicians might in fact not welcome the power explicitly to override their patients' wishes in the name of society and of their professional commitment to maintaining life at all costs, as seems to be suggested by the decisions of Judge Wright and Justice Weintraub.

B. THE SPECIAL PROBLEMS OF "CONSENT" FOR THE LEGALLY INCOMPETENT

As was recognized in Chapter Four, "consent" for a procedure will have to come from someone besides the patient whenever the latter is legally incompetent. If the patient is the primary beneficiary of the procedure, this presents some problems but not particularly taxing ones. For example,

---

would explain the contrary results in the two New York cases, *Erickson* (where a competent patient's refusal of treatment was upheld) and *Bettman* (where the wife of an incompetent was not permitted to refuse treatment for her husband). Unfortunately, the distinction runs into trouble from both sides. On the one hand, in a third New York case, a justice of the Supreme Court rendered a decision inconsistent with the distinction by refusing to grant the petition of Beth Israel Hospital for permission to amputate the leg of a 80-year-old woman; although incompetent, she apparently did not want the operation performed, and one of her three sons refused to agree with the others to consent to it. Petition of Nemser, 51 Misc.2d 616, 273 N.Y.S.2d 624 (Sup. Ct. 1966). Similarly, the Florida Circuit Court was willing in the *Martinez* case (discussed in the text accompanying note 77 *supra*) to permit the guardian to refuse treatment for an incompetent. Conversely, in the *George* case Judge Zampano granted a temporary restraining order permitting a hospital to administer necessary blood transfusions to a Jehovah's Witness who was "coherent and rational." United States v. George, 239 F.Supp. 752, 754 (D. Conn. 1965). Moreover, even if theoretically sustainable, the distinction would probably break down in practice, since courts which wish to permit the physicians to operate seem inclined simply to find that the patient's weakened condition renders him "incompetent." In *Nemser*, Justice Markowitz went so far as to suggest that the physicians should avoid seeking judicial review of their plans at all; they should instead wait until the patient's condition became an "emergency" and then proceed to exercise "sound medical judgment with respect to necessary treatment" without being deterred by the "threat of possible legal action"—a fear which the judge apparently thought to be unfounded and even unseemly. 51 Misc.2d at 622, 273 N.Y.S.2d at 629. *See generally* Cantor, note 65 *supra*, at 229-30, n.6 (cataloging extensive legal commentary on refusal of lifesaving treatment).

when a patient is admitted to an emergency room, his condition may be such (due to cardiac arrest or acute renal failure) that he is unable to participate in the deliberations about his treatment, and the decision must then be made instead by a member of his family; this was the situation with the first heart transplant in man, in which the recipient's sister gave permission for the operation.[84] As a theoretical matter, difficulties certainly arise when any person is given power over another, and these may be exacerbated rather than reduced (as is assumed by the law) when the persons involved are members of the same family. Yet there are reasons of sentiment, convenience, and even good sense for this allocation of authority,[85] and it is a practice which is so well known in society at large that any individual who finds the prospect particularly odious has ample warning to make other arrangements better suited to protecting his own ends or interests.

More troublesome problems are raised when consent is sought for an intervention which is not for the patient's benefit. It is generally assumed, though not authoritatively established, that a guardian lacks the authority to give consent in such circumstances. This issue has been raised in a number of the kidney transplants involving identical twins[86] and bone marrow transplants between siblings.[87] Where the potential donor is a

---

[84] *See* Hardy & Chavez, *The First Heart Transplant in Man: Historical Reexamination of the 1964 Case in the Light of Current Clinical Experience*, 1 TRANSPLANT PROC. 717, 721 (1969) [consent form signed by sister].

[85] There are any number of explanations for this societal allocation of authority [in the case of parental consent for interventions in their children]: respect for the family and a desire to foster the diversity it brings; the fitness of giving the power to decide to the same people who created the child and have the duty to support and protect him; the belief that a child cannot be much harmed by parental choices which fall within the range permitted by society and a willingness to bear the risks of harm this allocation entails or a belief that in most cases 'harm' would be hard for society to distill and measure anyway; or simply the conclusion that the administrative costs of giving authority to anyone but the parents outweigh the risks for children and for society unless the parents are shown [in a particular case] to be unable to exercise their authority adequately. Capron, *Legal Considerations Affecting Clinical Pharmacological Studies in Children*, 21 CLIN. RES. 141, 146 (1973).

[86] Hart v. Brown, 29 Conn. Super. 368, 289 A.2d 386 (1972); Strunk v. Strunk, 445 S.W.2d 145 (Ky. 1969); Foster v. Harrison, Eq. No. 68674 (Mass. Sup. Ct., filed Nov. 20, 1957); Huskey v. Harrison, Eq. No. 68666 (Mass. Sup. Ct., filed August 30, 1957); Masden v. Harrison, Eq. No. 68651 (Mass. Sup. Ct., filed June 12, 1957).

[87] During 1971 and 1972, the National Institutes of Health received permission from the Maryland Circuit Court for Montgomery County to undertake bone marrow transplants from minor donors to their ailing siblings in a series of five cases: Smith v. Smith, Eq. No. 43-919; *In re* Wayne Landry, Eq. No. 44-338; *In re* John Sharp, Eq. No. 44-478; *In re* Michael Jones, Eq. No. 44-601; *In re* Cynthia & Russell Martin, Eq. No. 44-602.

minor, the apparent rule that a parent cannot consent to a nonbeneficial operation has been sidestepped by the courts' finding that the healthy child *would* benefit from the operation because "the risk of emotional disturbance [would] be reduced." The decisions in the first cases, involving kidney transplants in teenage twins at the Peter Bent Brigham Hospital in Boston, have proven very influential with subsequent courts faced with similar issues. Therefore, it is particularly significant that in one of those cases the court went so far as to rule—after shifting the ultimate decision as to risks and benefits back to the physicians, "if [they] decide to perform the operation"—that the operation was not merely permissible but "necessary to [the well twin's] future welfare and happiness."[88]

This rather unsatisfactory handling of the issue invites a number of responses. First, one might simply conclude, with David Daube, that "children should on no account be donors, and there should be no cheating by maintaining, for example, that the child would suffer a trauma if he were not allowed to give his twin a kidney or whatever it might be."[89] Yet a prohibition on being a kidney donor is not enough, as was made clear by the case of Mrs. L., an early kidney recipient who was given massive radiation treatments and then injections of bone marrow from 11 donors to restore health to her system and (it was hoped) to achieve "cross-acceptance" of the eventual kidney graft. Then a questionable step was taken:

> As the days went by, it appeared inadvisable to take a kidney from a healthy normal donor. There were too many uncertainties and unknown variables in the plan. Therefore, a kidney that had to be removed from a young child having the hydrocephalus operation was placed in the patient's right thigh by Dr. Murray. . . . Although the abdominal cavity is the preferred position for a kidney transplant, this patient had received such severe radiation dosage that it was deemed wiser to put the graft in the thigh where it could be done very simply and easily.
>
> Just before the kidney graft, the patient received another 170 million bone marrow cells from the same donor who gave the kidney. Thus, by adding this procedure, the identity of donor for both marrow and kidney was achieved.[90]

---

[88] Unreported decision, Foster v. Harrison, Mass. Sup. Jud. Ct., Suffolk, Eq. No. 68674 (Nov. 20, 1957). When attempting to make a rule about a guardian's power to consent to nonbeneficial interventions, those drawing on the Massachusetts cases and their progeny seldom acknowledge the particular problems involved in such a situation where the guardian (parent) had a conflict of interest between helping the sick twin and protecting the well one, although this factor probably at least in part explains why the cases were litigated in the first place.

[89] Daube, *Transplantation: Acceptability of Procedures and the Required Legal Sanctions,* in ETHICS IN MEDICAL PROGRESS: WITH SPECIAL REFERENCE TO TRANSPLANTATION 198 (G. E. W. Wolstenholme & E. M. O'Connor eds. 1966).

[90] F. MOORE, TRANSPLANT: THE GIVE AND TAKE OF TISSUE TRANSPLANTATION 115 (1972).

Moore goes on after this passage to recount how the four-week survival of the kidney graft in Mrs. L. (who died of bleeding since the bone marrow injections were unsuccessful in restoring her platelet level) was a key event in the history of transplantation, because it showed that if the immunological barrier were sufficiently incapacitated a transplanted organ could survive. No mention is made of the problematic nature of taking 170 million bone marrow cells from the infant kidney donor (with the permission of his parents one supposes). Moore mentioned earlier that marrow donation "does not harm the donor at all," yet like all medical procedures it does carry some risk, pain, and inconvenience.[91]

Diametrically opposed to Daube's complete disapproval of child donors (and, one assumes, other legally incompetent persons) is the position taken by Beecher and Curran who argue that American statutes, medical codes, and cases permit parents to give consent for medical interventions of *no direct* and, in some instances, *no indirect* benefit to their child.[92] This is one reading of the leading case in this area, *Bonner v. Moran*.[93] The trial court had told the jury in *Bonner* that it could find that no parental approval was necessary for the 15-year-old plaintiff to have given valid consent to donate a skin graft to his cousin if he was "capable of appreciating the nature, extent, and consequences of the invasion" (as phrased by the *Restatement of Torts*). The jury found for the doctor-defendant, and on appeal the court reversed. It held that the consent of an "immature colored boy" was not sufficient for an operation on himself that was not for his benefit and that was "so involved in its technique as to require a mature mind to understand precisely what the donor was offering to give."[94] The case was returned to the lower court for a retrial in which the jury was to be instructed that the surgeon was liable unless the boy's mother had given her consent, directly or by implication.

Beecher and Curran argue that

> the case does *not* hold that medical procedures cannot be performed on minors where there is no direct benefit to them. On the contrary, it holds that such procedures *can* be legally permitted as long as the parents (or other guardians) consent to the procedure.[95]

This casts more weight onto the opinion than it can bear. The actual ground for the decision appears to be that the boy was simply too immature to give

---

91 Indeed, as suggested above, the National Institutes of Health have sought judicial approval before aspirating bone marrow from minors for transplantation to their siblings. *See* cases cited in note 83 *supra*.

92 Curran & Beecher, *Experimentation in Children*, 210 J.A.M.A. 77 (1969).

93 126 F.2d 121 (D.C. Cir. 1941).

94 *Id.* at 123.

95 Curran & Beecher, note 92 *supra*, at 79.

discomforts, and benefits of the proposed procedure and of alternative procedures. In addition to the points set out by HEW, others of primary importance in the context of the research and treatment of catastrophic diseases include: (1) the experimental or established nature of the proposed treatments, particularly if the proposed intervention represents an initial trial of a new procedure on a human being, and (2) the physician-investigator's degree of personal experience with the proposed procedure. The doctor should also share with patients in research settings his opinion on the degree of uncertainty which surrounds the new technique and the extent to which its use on the patient may help in resolving that uncertainty. If the patient is to be a partner in this enterprise, it will require him to be aware of the scientific as well as the personal purposes and objectives involved so that he can be alert for any important developments. It should be possible to discuss this information with him in such a way as not to increase the probability that his observations will be improperly colored by what he expects to find, any more than the physician-investigator's are by what *he* expects.[100]

3. The Nature of the Patient's Participation

While a full and frank partnership between physician-investigator and patient-subject is the aim of the informed consent model, the model also recognizes that patients' decisional processes may not always operate in a rational and unfettered manner. Dying patients, especially, may be led, often in an unconscious fashion, to offer their cooperation in return for some special favor from those who are caring for them. Dr. Kübler-Ross sees in such bargaining "an attempt to postpone" something (such as an operation) that reminds the patient of how imperiled his life is; in exchange, he may promise his "good behavior," perhaps in the form of an offer to let himself be used for scientific work that may lead to life-extending knowledge.[101]

Our suggestions have been intended, in light of the undeniable "inner" and "outer" pressures felt by patient-subjects, to place the parties as nearly as possible on comparable footing in the seeking and granting of informed consent for the treatment of a life-endangering condition. We see "informed consent" not as a single act but as a process of contracting, negotiating, and recontracting. In the treatment of, and research on, catastrophic diseases, this model of informed consent is the only realistic one, since the treatment process requires constant physical and psychic rededication over time by

---

[100] Special rules and procedures must be promulgated to govern instances in which double-blind studies are called for scientifically.

[101] KÜBLER-ROSS, note 34 *supra*, at 73-74.

patient and physician alike. Dr. Harrison Sadler even suggests that "a basic requirement is a patient who is intelligent enough to negotiate" an "honor able and dignified working partnership and alliance."[102] An honest recognition of the "bargaining" nature of the doctor-patient relationship is particularly important when the physician-investigator is seeking to enroll the patient-subject in a procedure which is not solely for the latter's benefit.

[102] Sadler, note 31 *supra*, at 5.

CHAPTER SEVEN

The Authority and Capacity of Professional and Public Institutions

The interaction between physician-investigators and patient-subjects, on the one hand, and professional and public institutions, on the other, has always been an uneasy one, characterized less by friendly collaboration than by avoidance, suspicion, criticism, and hostility. This is due, in part, to deep-seated convictions among physician-investigators that their authority should not be circumscribed since they alone have the expertise to make decisions, are the guarantors of their patient-subjects' best interests, and can be relied upon to make joint decisions with patient-subjects whenever this proves necessary. These convictions tend to be reinforced by a lack of appreciation of the complex issues that arise in the catastrophic disease process which cannot be resolved by physicians alone or between them and their patients. Some of these problems, such as the selection of hemodialysis recipients or the lack of adequate resources, involve not only medical but also social judgments and require the active support of professional and public institutions. Thus, there is insufficient awareness that participation by professional and public institutions in decisionmaking may indeed lighten the burdens placed on physician-investigators.

In this chapter, as a prelude to what is to follow in Part Three, we shall describe and evaluate the strengths and weaknesses of the decisionmaking processes currently utilized by professional groups (*i.e.,* medical schools, specialty boards, editorial boards of journals, peer review committees), public bodies (*i.e.,* presidential and congressional commissions, regulatory and administrative agencies, courts), and quasi-public groups (*i.e.,* private foundations, newspapers, litigants and attorneys).

A. PROFESSIONAL GROUPS

1. Medical Schools, Specialty Boards, Hospitals, and Professional Organizations

The authority of professional groups is most formally structured and fully applied at the time when future members of the profession seek admission for training, during the period of graduate and postgraduate education, and prior to the conferring of final certification. During this prolonged training period, the profession has its greatest opportunity and authority to influence future colleagues. The function of medical schools, according to Robert K. Merton, is to transmit and advance "the culture of medicine,"[1] including the values basic to the effective practice of medicine.

> It is their task to shape the novice into the effective practitioner of medicine, to give him the best available knowledge and skills, and to provide him with a professional identity so that he comes to think, act, and feel like a physician.[2]

On the whole, medical educators have done a competent job preparing students for the technical tasks required by medical practice. We have already pointed out, however, some deficiencies in training for professional responsibility. As centers for biomedical research, medical schools inculcate their students with the importance of conducting experiments to improve treatment capabilities. But they seem "to be more effective at the present time in socializing their students who become clinical investigators into the value of research than into the ethics of the use of human subjects in the research that is so highly valued."[3] Bernard Barber and his colleagues found in their sociological study of clinical investigators that even at the *end* of their medical school training more than 40 percent were unaware of the ethical problems in using human subjects.

> Even work with humans . . . does not necessarily socialize medical students into the ethical problems of research. Nineteen per cent of the respondents reported that they had conducted some research with human subjects while they were in medical school, but of these 59 respondents, only 31 reported that ethical issues had ever been considered in the course of such research.[4]

---

[1] Merton, *Some Preliminaries to a Sociology of Medical Education*, in THE STUDENT PHYSICIAN 7 (R. Merton, G. Reader & P. Kendall eds. 1957).

[2] *Id.*

[3] B. BARBER, J. LALLY, J. MAKARUSHKA & D. SULLIVAN, RESEARCH ON HUMAN SUBJECTS: PROBLEMS OF SOCIAL CONTROL IN MEDICAL EXPERIMENTATION 174 (1973) [hereinafter cited as BARBER].

[4] *Id.* at 101-02.

Beyond the period of training, the prevailing relationship between individual physicians and the profession is based primarily on informal methods of control. This relationship has been implicitly and explicitly designed to maximize individual autonomy and to permit any restraints to operate through peer pressure, expressed, for example, in practice through referrals and non-referrals of patients, in academic settings through promotions, or in hospital settings through facilitating or impeding the comfort and working conditions of practitioners. Though these restraints have at times been unfair and burdensome to some, they have not become sufficiently stringent to disturb the general climate of freedom of professional conduct.

In the catastrophic disease process the problems raised by the informal nature of professional decisionmaking are considerable, and they are not eased by the few official pronouncements that are available for consultation. For example, the *Principles of Medical Ethics* promulgated by the American Medical Association—of limited value to practitioners because of their all too general nature—are even less useful to investigators. For example, Section 10 states that

> The honored ideals of the medical profession imply that the responsibilities of the physician extend *not only to the individual, but also to society* where the responsibilities deserve his interest and participation in activities which have the *purpose of improving* both the health and the well-being of *the individual and the community.*[5]

In catastrophic diseases the issues which must be confronted if one wishes to balance the responsibilities to one's patients, to future patients, and to the needs of society loom large but little guidance is provided by the general promulgations contained in this code or its accompanying commentary.

Codes of investigative ethics suffer from similar deficiencies. For example, the framers of the *Declaration of Helsinki* have promulgated separate principles for "clinical research combined with professional care" and for "non-therapeutic research."[6] In the catastrophic disease process, it is often not at all clear which set of principles to consult or, even when that is possible, how to determine "therapeutic value" as the physician-investigator is instructed to do by such statements as "[t]he doctor can combine clinical research with professional care, the objective being the acquisition of new medical knowledge, only to the extent that clinical research is justified by its therapeutic value for the patient."[7] Like the famous medical dictum

---

[5] *Principles of Medical Ethics*, in AMERICAN MEDICAL ASSOCIATION, OPINIONS AND REPORTS OF THE JUDICIAL COUNCIL vii (1969) (emphasis supplied) [hereinafter cited as AMA OPINIONS].

[6] World Medical Association, *Declaration of Helsinki*, 271 NEW ENG. J. MED. 473 (1964).

[7] *Id.*

primum non nocere, the *Principles of Medical Ethics* and the variety of extant ethical codes provide physician-investigators with abstract moral imperatives to guide their professional life, but in daily decisionmaking they at best serve only as reminders or warnings which are prone to being overwhelmed by more immediate and personal needs and pressures.

In the discussion of moratoria we noted two specific control mechanisms which on occasion the profession imposes on individual physicians: withdrawal of operative privileges, as was imposed on Dr. Charles Bailey of Philadelphia, and the formal declaration of a heart transplant moratorium, as was promulgated by the Montreal Heart Institute. In both instances the decision was based in part on concern over the surgical mortality rate and in part on the belief that further investigative work was necessary before exposing additional patients to these procedures. As far as we know, these decisions were *ad hoc* ones, based neither on already existing criteria of the permissible limits of investigative procedures with patients nor on prospective criteria to govern future professional conduct. The Montreal Heart Institute declared an absolute halt, though other centers continued with heart transplantation. While this suggests a healthy pluralism, it also points up the disagreement within the profession as to the risks to which patient-subjects may be exposed with or without their consent. Whatever agreement is eventually reached emerges through consensus arrived at informally, as demonstrated by the current decline in the number of heart transplants or through limited formal restraints which may not extend beyond individual medical centers.

The more broadly based formal rules and procedures for administering medical practice and research, such as the institutional review of research projects or the requirement for obtaining "informed consent," have been largely instigated by pressure from outside the profession. A notable exception is the Ad Hoc Committee of the Harvard Medical School, under the chairmanship of Dr. Henry K. Beecher, which formulated a "Definition of Irreversible Coma."[8] The Ad Hoc Committee was convened in response to the felt need for a new definition of death in the light of the improvements in resuscitative and supportive measures which allow a person to "live" even though his brain is irreversibly damaged and of the anticipated controversy over obtaining organs for transplantation stemming from obsolete criteria for determining death. Perhaps the most noteworthy aspect of this effort and the resulting document is that such projects occur so infrequently. Members of the medical profession rarely take the initiative in anticipating problems already close at hand or in proposing rules and pro-

---

[8] Ad Hoc Committee of the Harvard Medical School to Examine the Definition of Brain Death, *A Definition of Irreversible Coma,* 205 J.A.M.A. 85 (1968).

cedures for dealing with these problems; more often such problems are sidestepped and left for action by groups from outside the profession. If such attempts at formulating policy, like the one initiated by the Harvard Ad Hoc Committee, have merit and should be encouraged, a number of questions must be considered. For example, what kind of procedures will facilitate the convening of such a group when needed? Who should be represented on such a committee—should its composition be local, regional, or national, be restricted to physicians or encompass other professions as well as representatives of the public? What weight should be given to their recommendations? What consequences should follow from nonadherence to their promulgations?

Professional organizations, like the American Medical Association and its affiliated state and county societies, as well as the various specialty associations, provide important benefits to their members through their medical journals, scientific conventions, and educational postgraduate programs. These activities create considerable consensus among physicians with respect to acceptable medical practices, which are also useful in judicial proceedings or legislative deliberations whenever prevailing standards of practice are in issue. However, their influence does not extend to a significant degree to research settings, particularly because professional organizations have shied away from addressing themselves in depth to the complex problems raised by investigative medicine.[9] Research physicians also have the weakest ties to these organizations and tend to respond more to the approbation or disapproval of colleagues engaged in similar pursuits. Moreover, professional organizations function more like "political" bodies when faced with such complicated ethical and social issues as those raised by catastrophic diseases. In hammering out position statements, the push is more toward accommodation of a variety of views, and thus toward more

---

[9] For example, the Judicial Council of the American Medical Association believed the following brief opinion sufficed to cover "Experimentation: New Drugs or Procedures":

In order to conform to the ethics of the American Medical Association, three requirements must be satisfied in connection with the use of experimental drugs or procedures:

(1) the voluntary consent of the person on whom the experiment is to be performed should be obtained;

(2) the danger of each experiment must be previously investigated by animal experimentation; and

(3) the experiment must be performed under proper medical protection and management.

AMA OPINIONS, note 5 *supra*, at 9 (1969). This opinion was not revised or extended from 1946 when it was issued until 1966 when the "Ethical Guidelines for Clinical Investigation" were promulgated.

general pronouncements about controversial issues, rather than incisive presentation of problems and their resolution. Consequently, it seems that the task of thinking through these problems can better be performed through individual scholarship in medical school settings and from there filter down to professional organizations.

2. Journals

In recent years increasing attention has been given to the responsibilities which biomedical journals and their editors should exercise in the research process. The debate has centered primarily around the question whether data unethically obtained should be published. Some have argued that

> While the loss to medicine might be great, it is never as great in any reasonably conceivable circumstances as the moral loss sustained by medicine when unethically obtained data are published. Suppression of unethically obtained data will do much to curb the enthusiasm of the careless or occasional unscrupulous investigator to carry on unacceptable practices.[10]

Others have felt the opposite:

> [I]t would be unfortunate if data "improperly obtained" were not published. Such an editorial policy would maintain the low visibility of unethical experimentation and preclude not only review but also careful and constant appraisal of the conflicting values inherent in experimentation.[11]

Exactly how and by what standards journals should exercise nonscientific review of the research submitted for publication is not clear. An editor of *The Lancet* declared that his journal does "not *want* to publish information which, according to professional ethics, has been wrongly obtained; [we] believe that no use should ever be made of such information."[12] To avoid such a possibility *The Lancet* editors feel entitled to ask questions "which must sometimes be more than a little irritating."[13] Moreover, they believe that an explanation of the voluntary participation of the subjects should be sufficient. "[W]here criticism may arise, an author should avert it by explaining," according to *The Lancet*, "that the people on whom he experi-

---

[10] THE MASSACHUSETTS GENERAL HOSPITAL, HUMAN STUDIES: GUIDING PRINCIPLES AND PROCEDURES 10 (1970). [Hereinafter cited as MGH GUIDE.]

[11] Katz, *Human Experimentation*, 275 NEW ENG. J. MED. 790 (1966). *See also* Levine, *Ethical Considerations in the Publication of the Results of Research Involving Human Subjects*, 21 CLIN. RES. 763 (1973), which argues that it is wrong to withhold publication since to do so may cause more subjects to be exposed to the risk of the same experiment in the future.

[12] Fox, *The Ethics of Clinical Trials*, 28 MEDICO-LEGAL J. 132, 139 (1960).

[13] *Id.*

mented were true volunteers; or that valid consent was given on their behalf."[14] The references to "professional ethics" and "valid consent" seem to presuppose that a clear standard exists and is generally accepted by clinical researchers and medical journals alike. The Committee on Editorial Policy of the Council of Biology Editors has recently recommended a far more comprehensive set of procedures, which were endorsed by the Council's Board of Directors:

> (1) As a regular policy, the editor should require that the published report of any research on human beings should contain a statement that the institution's committee on ethics (or other responsible person or group) approved the description of the proposed research on a certain date. The author should be asked to supply with the manuscript submitted for publication, a photocopy of the comment of prior institutional approval. (2) If, despite such a statement of prior institutional approval, the research reported seems to the editors or reviewers not to have been conducted in accordance with ethical principles, the editor should inform the author that a question of ethical propriety has arisen, and should request a copy of the original proposal of research approved by the institutional committee, along with a copy of the ethical guidelines formally adopted by the institution. (3) If, after having received the information specified in step 2, the editor or his advisors remain in doubt about the propriety of the research as carried out, the editor should request from the present chairman of the responsible institutional committee on ethics a signed statement to the effect that he has personally reviewed the actual research and has found it to be ethically proper. If that committee chairman is dissatisfied, he will undoubtedly take steps to prevent any future unethical experimentation in that institution. (4) If the research has been carried out under circumstances in which formal certification of the ethical propriety of proposed research is not required or no mechanism exists for such certification, the author should be asked to state how the ethical aspects of the investigation were evaluated, and the editor should feel obliged to form his own judgment on the basis of this information.[15]

A policy of this sort may seem to abrogate the responsibility of a journal editor to form his own independent opinion on the ethics of the research reported just as he does on its scientific merits and accuracy. Yet serious problems arise when scientific and medical journals attempt to exercise moral or ethical censorship. A journal's publication of data which may have been "unethically obtained" should not be taken as an indication that the editors approve or condone such experimentation. The real need is for

---

[14] *Id.*

[15] Woodford, *Ethical Experimentation and the Editor*, 286 NEW ENG. J. MED. 892 (1972). *But see* Katz, *Editorial Rewritten*, 21 CLIN. RES. 10, 11 (1974), holding that the CBE procedures "are unworkable, dangerous and counterproductive."

professional groups which are closer to the scene (such as peer review committees or state medical societies) to exercise before-the-fact scrutiny over medical research; having journal editors assume this function not only puts the shoe on the wrong foot but threatens to create confusion, contradiction, and duplication of effort.

Whatever the merits of delegating policing functions to editors of journals, the current debate reflects an appreciation of the important role which journals might play in opening up discussion of the catastrophic disease treatment process. Thus, journal editors could properly require authors to provide detailed explanations of how subjects were informed, what risks were considered, what benefits were expected, and so forth. Debate could be encouraged through publication of "letters to the editor," editorial comments, and invitations to scholars of many disciplines to discuss particularly troublesome investigations. Thus conceived, journals would exert their authority primarily at the stage of review and not at the stage of formulating policy, although policies will be significantly affected by this review process.

3. Institutional Review Committees[16]

Although medical school training, professional certification, and journal publication provide some means for formal control by biomedical professionals outside of a physician-investigator's own circle of colleagues, these means are—as we have seen—only partially effective. Moreover, more extensive or formal types of regulation are resisted by physician-investigators almost as an article of faith. Indeed, while it is possible to speak, as Barber does, of "the medical profession at large and the biomedical profession in particular" making "strong claims to autonomy and self-regulation on the grounds that only they have sufficient knowledge, skill, and moral trustworthiness" to regulate their members' activities,[17] the concepts of autonomy and self-regulation are really conceived of as fundamentally being *personal* attributes and not simply those of the profession. The physician is most likely to look to his immediate colleagues or "peers" for advice and to expect that they will be the ones, if anyone, to tell him when he errs.[18]

---

[16] Though conceptually the discussion of institutional review committees, established pursuant to a governmental rule, belong in the next section—Public Bodies—we place it here since in practice the composition of these committees has been largely drawn from the medical profession.

[17] BARBER, note 3 *supra*, at 173.

[18] Indeed, it is only recently that the courts have begun to abandon the "locality rule," which limited testimony in malpractice cases to evidence concerning the standards set by other physicians in the defendant's community (or, at most, in "similar" ones). *See, e.g.*, Naccarato v. Grob, 384 Mich. 248, 180 N.W.2d 788 (1970); Brune v. Belinkoff, 354 Mass. 102, 235 N.E.2d 793 (1968); Pederson v. Dumouchel, 72

Moreover, it is also a strongly held value in the medical profession that, as far as possible, controls should be *informal* colleague controls. Such controls are much preferred to either local-institution or professional *formal* controls. Formal controls are seen as unnecessarily restrictive and involving bureaucratic red tape and distant authorities who are not as competent to judge an individual professional's work as are his local peers.[19]

Although the development of federal controls has, of necessity, compromised this medical attitude to some extent, it is striking how greatly these medical values influenced the design of the system of reviewing investigations into catastrophic and other diseases, in marked contrast to ways in which the government claims to supervise other risk-producing activities.

While some attention was focused on the need for greater scrutiny of medical experimentation by Senator Estes Kefauver's hearings from 1959 to 1962 and the resulting amendments to the Food, Drug, and Cosmetic Act,[20] the first major development came in 1966 when the Surgeon General of the United States Public Health Service promulgated the following policy statement:

No new, renewal, or continuation research or research training grant in support of clinical research and investigation involving human beings shall be awarded by the Public Health Service unless the grantee has indicated in the application the manner in which the grantee institution will provide prior review of the judgment of the principal investigator or program director by a committee of his institutional associates. This review should assure an independent determination: (1) of the rights and welfare of the individual or individuals involved, (2) of the appropriateness of the methods used to secure informed consent, and (3) of the risks and potential medical benefits of the investigation. A description of the committee of the associates who will provide the review shall be included in the application.[21]

Initially this review only applied to research and research training grants but it was soon extended to all PHS grants which involved research with human beings. Three years later the PHS policies were revised,[22] requiring

---

Wash.2d 73, 431 P.2d 973 (1967). *See generally* W. PROSSER, HANDBOOK OF THE LAW OF TORTS 164 (1971).

[19] BARBER, note 3 *supra*, at 173.

[20] Act of Oct. 10, 1962, Pub. L. No. 87-781; *see* 21 U.S.C. §355 (1964).

[21] W.H. Stewart (Surgeon General), *Memorandum to Heads of Institutions Conducting Research with Public Health Grants* (8 February 1966). This memorandum was the first official response to the judicial extension of "informed consent" to experimental interventions which had occurred the previous year in Canada, in Halushka v. Univ. of Saskatchewan 52 W.W.R. 608 (Sask. C.A. 1965).

[22] PUBLIC HEALTH SERVICE, U.S. DEP'T OF HEALTH, EDUCATION & WELFARE, PROTECTION OF THE INDIVIDUAL AS A RESEARCH SUBJECT (1969) [hereinafter cited as PROTECTION OF THE SUBJECT].

now that (1) research be given not only initial but also continuing review;
(2) the institution adopt an already existing statement of principles (*e.g.,*
the Nuremberg Code) or develop its own statement; (3) the committee be
composed of sufficient members with varying backgrounds to assure complete and adequate review of the research; (4) the committee determine
independently possible hazards to subjects, the precautions taken, the relative weight of the risks and benefits of the procedures to the subjects, and,
if the subject is a volunteer, his motivation in accepting risks in the interest
of humanity; and (5) the committee find that the risks to the individual
are outweighed by the potential benefit to him or by the importance of the
knowledge to be gained.

Spurred on by the Surgeon General's promulgations most research institutions established review committees,[23] and many now are charged with
reviewing not only projects supported by HEW but all human research
carried on within their institution.[24]

An example of an ambitious structure for the evaluation of research
proposals is that established under the Trustees' Advisory Committee on
Research and the Individual at the Massachusetts General Hospital. In
addition to a set of guidelines for clinical research with various categories
of patients,[25] the Mass General document also specifies that the Advisory
Committee is (1) to render opinions to the hospital's General Director and
trustees whenever questions or controversy develop over a particular
project, and (2) to "conduct at least an annual review of Research and the
Individual at the M.G.H."[26] The composition of this Committee is not
limited to physicians but includes faculty members from many disciplines

---

[23] Two studies conducted in the early 1960s indicated that few medical schools
had committees to review human research, although a larger number favored such
bodies and some reported that they planned to draw up the relevant procedural documents and establish committees. See Welt, *Reflections on the Problems of Human
Experimentation,* 25 CONN. MED. 75 (1961); Curran, *Governmental Regulation of
the Use of Human Subjects in Medical Research,* 98 DAEDALUS 542 (1969). Barber's
responses indicate that 70 percent of the biomedical research institutions had a review
procedure prior to the PHS requirements. Therefore he concludes, "it would seem
that there had been a gradual increase in the non-required review procedures and
committees from 1960 to 1966." BARBER, note 3 *supra,* at 148.

[24] Although 85 percent of research institutions report that "all clinical research" is
reviewed, this may not cover nearly all human research since medical schools (which
do a great deal of human experimentation) are heavily represented in the group in
which *not* all protocols are reviewed. "It is clear then that a perhaps significant
volume of human research is still not subject to review by a peer review committee."
BARBER, note 3 *supra,* at 149. Moreover, a sizeable number of research projects are
carried out on an *ad hoc* basis without review.

[25] *See* MGH GUIDE, note 10 *supra.*

[26] *Id.* at 14.

who are affiliated with Harvard University. These procedures were designed to share decisionmaking authority in recognition of the fact that the issues to be resolved in investigative medicine are not solely within the competence of the medical profession.

It is difficult to assess the effectiveness of the review committees. Barber and his associates, in a preliminary report on their intensive study of such committees, questioned the efficacy of the review process when it is carried out:

> Efficacy is, of course, a hard concept to define and measure in any field of human action. We have used two rough measures: what the committees have done with research protocols and how researchers feel about the efficacy of their committees.
>
> As to action, our respondents tell us that in 36% of the institutions, the committees have never required any revisions or made any rejections; another 38% tell us that some revisions were required, but that after revision the protocols were all approved; another 26% report one or more outright rejections; and, finally, 18% told us that there have been one or more instances where an investigator withdrew his proposal when he sensed that revision or rejection was likely. As to how researchers feel about the committees, some 76% of our individual respondents say they felt the committees were very effective. Clearly, on both measures, the review committees have a considerable degree of social control efficacy, yet it is also clear that there is room for improvement. Our data show that the committees are more likely to be effective by these measures when the institution has additional controls over research using human subjects; when the committee retains continuing review; and when the review processes include formal appeal procedures. These are all social control structures and processes which could be set up, where they do not now exist, to increase the efficacy of peer-group review.[27]

It stands to reason that the mere fact of having to submit a written research protocol to a group of one's peers will provide better protection of patients in catastrophic disease research, if only because it forces the investigator to pause and give thought to the impact of his research proposal not only on his subjects but on his colleagues as well. Moreover, the review conducted by knowledgeable peers may reveal deficiencies in design or unnecessary hazards, and turn up better safeguards or related research efforts overlooked by the investigator, which once communicated to the physician-investigator may also benefit his subjects and science.

At the same time, the review committee structure as promulgated by HEW has many inherent weaknesses. The guidelines given to the com-

---

[27] B. Barber, J. Lally, J. Marushka & D. Sullivan, *Experimenting with Humans: Problems and Processes of Social Control in the Bio-Medical Research Community* (unpub. manuscript, 1971).

mittees are sufficiently vague that their implementation, in the absence of further specification, will demand of the committees a considerable investment of time not to mention intellectual commitment, if substance is going to be put into HEW's general pronouncements. For example, the review is supposed to assure that "the risks to the individual are outweighed by the potential benefit to him or by the importance of the knowledge to be gained."[28] Many questions are hidden in this complex but all too brief prescription: *E.g.,* how are risks and benefits to be measured and, if such measures exist, how are they to be weighed against one another; what criteria, with what degree of certainty, would satisfy "potential benefit" and "importance of knowledge"; does the balancing of "knowledge to be gained" require an evaluation of research design and, if so, by whom and by what criteria; to what extent is greater risktaking made acceptable by what kind of consent? Review committees cannot be expected to find answers to these questions unless they devote more time to the enterprise than most committee members are likely to want to spend. Being confronted with these questions repeatedly and being able to give only unsatisfactory answers, committee members may become discouraged, cynical, and neglectful.

To remedy this weakness, the Secretary of Health, Education and Welfare should appoint a body charged with preparing documents that would give greater substance to the general principles.[29] This committee could also assist local review committees with respect to any troublesome decisions they have to make, review selected protocols each year, publish its opinions on protocols from both these sources so that they will be readily available to local review committees and for general scrutiny and study, and preserve these opinions as precedents for future deliberation and (eventually) newly articulated counterprecedents. As a national body it would in effect serve as one possible vehicle for communication among the local committees which at present work too much in isolation of one another, leading to a tremendous duplication of effort. If the national committee's membership is broadly representative, it may resolve a criticism levelled at the prevailing composition of institutional review committees, namely that they consist primarily, if not exclusively, of physicians.[30] Perhaps there is

---

[28] PROTECTION OF THE SUBJECT, note 22 *supra,* at 1.

[29] The staff of the Division of Research Grants at the National Institutes of Health has already begun this task with its statements of policy and commentary in THE INSTITUTIONAL GUIDE TO DHEW POLICY ON PROTECTION OF HUMAN SUBJECTS (1971).

[30] Barber reports that "only 22% altogether of the institutions have *any* kind of outsider (in this sense of nonmember of the institution) as a committee member," and the vast majority of these are other physicians, especially those who do clinical research in an area related to the institution's specialty. BARBER, note 3 *supra,* at 153. Thirteen percent of the committees are made up *solely of clinical researchers* from the same institution. *Id.* at 152.

an inherent wisdom in keeping the local committees which administer the research process staffed largely by medical professionals. Nevertheless, at the stages of formulating policy and reviewing decisions and consequences, there is a need for a much fuller representation of nonmedical personnel in order to bring other viewpoints to bear and to better protect all interested parties, including society at large.

It is beyond the scope of this book to examine in detail all aspects of the review committee concept. We have touched on some major issues and will make a few additional observations in the next section. The review committees represent the most formal mechanism devised so far for supervising the research process. To remain viable, their functions and their specific assignments in the overall human research process must be better conceptualized. Particularly for catastrophic diseases, for example, their decisions cannot be left in the hands of physicians alone since the issues to be resolved touch so vitally on the interests of a much broader constituency. The problems of defining death and of selecting patients for hemodialysis—discussed in Chapter Eight—are only two of the more prominent issues with profound social ramifications that have arisen from medicine's ever-increasing ability to treat catastrophic illness.

B. PUBLIC BODIES

1. Congressional Hearings

Congress has from time to time taken an active interest in medical problems and conducted extensive hearings, particularly in moments of crisis. A much celebrated instance was the inquiry by Senator Estes Kefauver's Subcommittee on Antitrust and Monopoly into FDA supervision of research. These hearings assumed great importance because of the occurrence of terrible infantile deformities in Western Europe caused by thalidomide which was then being tested extensively as a tranquilizer with American patients. Senator Kefauver's hearings led to the enactment of a strong drug control bill which provided for controls over the investigational use of drugs and a requirement of "patient consent," through an amendment offered by Senator Jacob Javits.[31]

Such hearings have the advantage of bringing a variety of divergent views and interests before the Congress and, through news media coverage, before the public. They also permit the public's elected representatives to determine whether remedial legislation is required to protect the interests of society. Thus, such hearings allow the participation of society in medical decisionmaking, although often over the objections of the professional

---

[31] See note 20 *supra* and accompanying text.

community. The weakness in these proceedings lies in the climate of crisis that generally surrounds them. The call for controls, engendered by a tragic case before the public, is vociferous, but the consequences of such controls for the overall administration of the research process are often insufficiently considered. The hearings clearly have a significant "informing" as well as a "policy-making" function by encouraging representatives of society to participate in the medical decisionmaking process.[32] We wonder, however, whether in between these two steps a third one need not be introduced, for example, through the appointment of a special committee, again broadly representative, which between hearings could in less hectic surroundings make recommendations to Congress as to needed legislation.[33]

2. Commissions—Congressional and Presidential

On occasion, congressional and presidential commissions are convened to explore existing and anticipated medical problems considered of great importance to society or to give additional momentum to health issues which require societal support. In recent years, Senator Walter F. Mondale, Chairman of the Subcommittee on Government Research of the Senate Committee on Government Operations, has repeatedly introduced a bill to establish a National Advisory Commission on Health Science and Society.[34] The bill specifies that the commission "shall be composed of fifteen members to be appointed by the President from among the fields of medicine, law, theology, biological science, physical science, social science, philosophy, humanities, health administration, government, and public affairs [and that it] shall undertake a comprehensive investigation and study of the ethical, social, and legal implications of advances in biomedical research and technology." Within two years the commission is charged "to submit a final report, containing detailed statements of the findings and conclusions . . . , together with its recommendations, including . . . recommendations for action by public and private bodies and individuals. . . ."[35]

---

[32] We note in passing that the published records of these hearings offer a wealth of fascinating and thought provoking material for teaching purposes, a resource which has been infrequently exploited.

[33] *See* note 53 *infra*.

[34] *See, e.g.,* Senate Joint Resolution 75, 92nd Cong., 1st Sess., 117 *Congressional Record* 7670-78 (1971). The resolution was adopted by the Senate on Dec. 2, 1971, *id.* at 43951-56, but Congress adjourned without House action on the resolution. It has been incorporated into H.R. 7724—National Research Act, Title II—Protection of Human Subjects of Biomedical and Behavioral Research—which was passed by the Congress and has become law. 120 *Congressional Record* H5725 ff (June 25, 1974) and S11776 ff (June 27, 1974).

[35] 117 *Congressional Record* S3710 (March 24, 1971).

In support of this resolution Senator Mondale noted that:

advances in biology and medicine make it increasingly clear that we are rapidly acquiring greater powers to modify and perhaps control the capacities and activities of men by direct intervention into and manipulation of their bodies and minds. Certain means are already in use or at hand—for example, organ transplantation, prenatal diagnosis of genetic defects, electrical stimulation of the brain. Others await the solution of relatively minor technical problems, while still others depend upon further basic research. All of these developments raise profound and difficult questions of theory and practice, for individuals and for society.

• • •

While holding forth the promise of continued improvements in medicine's abilities to cure disease and alleviate suffering, [recent] developments also pose profound questions and troublesome problems. There are questions about who shall benefit from and who shall pay for the use of new technologies. Shall a person be denied life simply because he does not have enough money for an organ transplant?

There will be questions about the use and abuse of power. When and under what circumstances can organs be removed for transplanting? Who should decide how long a person is to be kept alive by the use of a machine? . . .

There will be questions about our duties to future generations and about the limits on what we can and cannot do to the unborn. . . .

We shall face questions concerning the desirable limits of the voluntary manipulations of our own bodies and minds. Some have expressed concern over the possible dehumanizing consequences of increasing the laboratory control over human procreation. . . .

We shall face questions about the impact of biomedical technology on our social institutions. What will be the effect of genetic manipulation or laboratory-based reproduction on the human family? If laboratory fertilization can produce children for sterile couples, what will be the consequences for those orphaned or abandoned children who might otherwise have been adopted by these couples? What will be the effect on the generation gap of any further increases in longevity?

We shall face serious questions of law and legal institutions. What will the predicted new-fangled modes of reproduction do to the laws of paternity and inheritance? What would happen to the concept of legal responsibility if certain genetic diseases were shown to predispose to anti-social or criminal behavior? What would be done to those individuals with such traits?

• • •

Finally, we as legislators will face problems of public policy. We shall need to be informed of coming developments, of the promises they hold forth and the problems they present, and of public attitudes in these matters. We shall need to decide what avenues of research hold out the most promise for human progress. And we shall need to help devise the means for preventing undesirable consequences.

. . .

[W]e can ill afford to wait until the crush of events forces us to make hasty and often ill-considered decisions. . . . As Dr. Watson said in his testimony: "If we do not think about the matter now, the possibility of our having a free choice will one day suddenly be gone."[36]

Those comments graphically illustrate the range of problems that require consideration in the light of the rapid advances in biology and medicine. Whether such commissions are the best vehicles to provide answers and direction is another question. Much will depend on the competence of the staff and their consultants. Equally important is the willingness of the commission members to devote the time which such an enterprise entails. All too often, they accept these assignments in addition to their many other duties, and the final work produced suffers accordingly. If participation in the deliberations of the commission were to require the members to devote a major portion of their time to the project, being consequently relieved of other duties, better results might obtain.

Senator Mondale stressed the fact that we cannot "wait until the crush of events forces us to make hasty and often ill-considered decisions."[37] This observation underscores the need for anticipating advances, a subject to which we shall return in Part Three. The range of questions posed by Senator Mondale also makes it crystal clear that the issues to be considered go beyond the expertise of the medical profession. This is often not understood by physicians. During earlier hearings on the proposed resolution, Dr. Christiaan Barnard, one of the invited witnesses, viewed the commission primarily as an attempt to hamstring the medical profession. "If I am in competition with my colleagues of this country, which I am not, and were completely selfish," he testified, "then I would welcome such a commission, because it would put the doctors who embark on this type of treatment so far behind me and hamper the group of doctors so much that I will go so far ahead that they will never catch up with me."[38] Later on

---

36 117 *Congressional Record* 7670-71 (1971).

37 *Id.*

38 *Hearings on S. J. Res. 145 (National Commission on Health Science and Society) before the Subcommittee on Government Research of the Senate Committee on Government Operations,* 90th Cong.,2d Sess.(1968). [Hereinafter cited as *National Commission on Health Science and Society.*]

he conceded one value to such a commission, "to give money for research and problems like that," but he immediately went on to say,

> I think we must distinguish between what this commission is going to do. Is this commission going to decide on medical problems, and how the various transplant teams should handle a medical problem? If you ask me whether I think a commission should be necessary for that, I would disagree. But if you think that one should have a commission to decide whether money should be poured into research because we now have these new techniques, and this may need more money, and aspects like that, I would agree that there you need a commission; but not to help the doctor to make his decision.[39]

Dr. Barnard's responses to questions from various Senators whether he did not consider these problems "public issues," not only highlight medicine's concern about being controlled by outsiders but also reveal a fundamental confusion. Within limits Dr. Barnard may be quite correct that the administration of the research process should be left to the private ordering between physicians and their patients. But research and its consequences pose not only medical issues but societal ones as well and, as we have suggested before and will explore further in Part Three, at the stages of formulating policy and reviewing decisions and consequences, other representatives of society should assume a crucial role. Indeed, if at those stages of the decisionmaking process adequate policies can be established for the administration of research, which are acceptable to the professionals, society may rest easier in leaving them alone at the administrative stage in pursuing the activities traditionally assigned to them.

Presidential commissions, like legislative ones, can make an important contribution to informing legislators and the public of and making recommendations about the nation's health needs that require greater attention. Thus, the President's Commission on Heart Disease, Cancer, and Stroke asked, among other things, for the establishment of a "national network of regional centers each primarily oriented toward the solution of a specific disease problem, [for] a more general research attack on the fundamental problems of human biology, to which all the sciences basic to medicine can contribute, [and for] the establishment of Specialized Research Centers for intensive study of specific aspects of heart disease, cancer and stroke to supplement the research and training efforts of the regional centers previously described."[40] Though such commissions, looked at from a broader perspective, suffer from their special interest pleadings, they dramatically

---

[39] *Id.*

[40] PRESIDENT'S COMMISSION ON HEART DISEASE, CANCER, AND STROKE, A NATIONAL PROGRAM TO CONQUER HEART DISEASE, CANCER, AND STROKE 47-52 (1964).

bring to the attention of the government and the public the problems which must be solved, especially in terms of economic costs, in order to meet the health needs encompassed by their specialties.[41]

3. Public Funding Authorities

The financial resources required for the treatment of and research in catastrophic diseases are staggering. The magnitude of the problem is strikingly brought home by a glance at the available, though incomplete, data on the costs of hemodialysis and organ transplantation. The Committee on Chronic Kidney Disease, under the chairmanship of Dr. Carl W. Gottschalk, appointed by the Director of the Bureau of the Budget, estimated in 1967 that the total cost to the nation for all uremia patients for whom chronic dialysis or transplantation is medically indicated, would range from $800 million to $1 billion during the first six years of an all-out treatment program. This included the costs for the construction of facilities, training, and patient care as recommended by the Committee. By the year 1975, care for 22,000 patients was estimated to range from $180 to $237 million annually. "Annual yearly costs after 1975 are difficult to predict but are expected to continue to rise until a steady state is reached when the number of patients admitted to the program equals the number leaving through cure by transplantation plus those who die."[42] The Ad Hoc Task Force on Cardiac Replacement under the chairmanship of Dr. James V. Warren, appointed by the National Heart Institute, estimated that 32,168 persons might qualify each year as candidates for a heart transplant.[43] Dr. Theodore Cooper, Director of the National Heart Institute, estimated the costs for the care of a cardiac transplant patient to be $20,000, but experience has put the figure considerably higher.[44] Thus, the total bill for new hearts could come to over $900 million annually. We do not wish to make too much of these figures in themselves because as medical research advances and, for example, the immunological problems become solved or smaller and less complex dialyzers are developed, the costs may decrease substantially. However, with rising hospital costs and physicians' fees, as

---

[41] The great impact that special groups can have in "lobbying" to influence the composition and recommendations of commissions, as well as legislatures, is discussed at pp. 195-205 *infra*.

[42] COMMITTEE ON CHRONIC KIDNEY DISEASE, U.S. BUREAU OF THE BUDGET, REPORT 30 (1967).

[43] AD HOC TASK FORCE ON CARDIAC REPLACEMENT, NATIONAL HEART INSTITUTE, CARDIAC REPLACEMENT: MEDICAL, ETHICAL, PSYCHOLOGICAL AND ECONOMIC IMPLICATIONS 15 (1969).

[44] *What Price Transplanted Organs?* MEDICAL WORLD NEWS, June 28, 1968, at 28; *see also* p. 12 *supra*.

well as the increasing number of patients who are offered such therapies as medical science advances, the total funds required will always remain substantial.

All committees and task forces which have addressed themselves to the economic problems have concluded that the federal government will have to bear most of these costs and have recommended that funds be made available.[45] At the same time questions have been raised about priorities. Senator Mondale, for example, put it this way: "A public commitment of $1 billion could buy enough kidney dialysis centers to serve 25,000 persons in the next decade—or it could provide ambulatory care of a general nature for 1.2 million poor people."[46] Consequently, questions must be posed and answered about the allocation of resources: How and by whom should priorities for therapeutic care be formulated; should societal support for therapy be limited until per capita costs have come down to a reasonable level and if so, what is reasonable; should maximal support be given to research and if so with what priorities to which diseases, especially since there is every reason to believe that successful breakthroughs in medical knowledge will eventually affect the cost of therapy? In finding answers to these questions one first has to make assumptions about society's commitment to preserving human life. The course of action preferred may depend, for instance, on whether one agrees or disagrees with the position of Guido Calabresi:

> . . . Accident law indicates that our commitment to human life is not, in fact, so great as we say it is; that our commitment to life-destroying material progress and comfort is greater. But this fact merely accentuates our need to make a bow in the direction of our commitment to the sanctity of human

---

[45] In some instances, even major work in catastrophic disease treatment has, however, been supported entirely through non-federal sources. For example, Dr. Denton Cooley received no governmental funds for his research on heart transplantation and the artificial mechanical heart. According to Harry Minetree, this was not merely a matter of principle with Cooley; rather, he realized that his disagreements and competition with his senior colleague, Dr. Michael DeBakey, would preclude his sharing in Baylor-administered federal grants. H. MINETREE, COOLEY: THE CAREER OF A GREAT HEART SURGEON 39 (1973). Making a virtue of necessity, "in an effort to gain the support of individuals who were opposed to government give-and-control methods," Cooley spoke out against "the stifling bureaucratic ineptitude imposed on medical science by agencies of the U.S. Public Health Service." *Id.* Yet, while Cooley preferred private support, he was not opposed to government aid for his Texas Heart Institute. He worked with Dr. Domingo Liotta, who had been given federal funding at Baylor, to develop the latter's artificial cardiac devices to the clinical investigations stage; this resulted in some ticklish problems of "ownership" and necessitated negotiations with officials of the National Heart Institute, who were both impressed by and wary of Cooley's dramatic operations.

[46] *What Price Transplanted Organs?*, note 44 *supra*, at 29.

life (whenever we can do so at a reasonable total cost). It also accentuates our need to reject any societal decisions that too blatantly contradict this commitment. Like "free will," it may be less important that this commitment be total than that we believe it to be there.

Perhaps it is for these reasons that we save the man trapped in the coal mine. After all, the event is dramatic; the cost, though great, is unusual; and the effect in reaffirming our belief in the sanctity of human lives is enormous. The effect of such an act in maintaining the many societal values that depend on the dignity of the individual is worth the cost. Abolishing grade crossings might save more lives and at a substantially smaller cost per life saved, but the total cost to society would be far greater and the dramatic effect far less. I fear that if men got caught in coal mines with the perverse frequency with which cars run into trains at grade crossings, we would be loath to rescue them; it would, in the aggregate, cost too much. Lest this remark seem unduly cynical, we might consider our past unwillingness to keep all but a few victims of renal failure alive by use of artificial kidneys. Until now, artificial kidneys have cost too much, and people perversely have suffered kidney failure too frequently, so even though the victim was as clearly known to those who had to decide whether to save him as is the man in the mine, the answer quite frequently was no.[47]

4. Regulatory and Administrative Agencies

The two major federal agencies concerned with medical research are the Food and Drug Administration (FDA) and the United States Public Health Service, particularly the National Institutes of Health (NIH), both units of the Department of Health, Education and Welfare. The responsibilities of those agencies are quite different. The FDA, a regulatory agency, is charged with protecting consumers in the use of foods, drugs, and cosmetics, while the NIH supports through grants much of the nation's medical research and conducts some research at its own facilities.[48]

a. Food and Drug Administration. Prior to 1938 no controls existed over new drugs entering the market. It took a tragedy involving elixir-sulfonilamide, similar in extent to the later misfortune with thalidomide, to move Congress to insert in the law shortly before final passage the requirement of testing before marketing. Though under the 1938 law the FDA had the statutory authority to regulate the use of investigational drugs, it did not exercise this power. Not until 1962, following the enactment of the Drug Act amendments, did the FDA begin to regulate the ethical drug industry in earnest. The new law required the Secretary of HEW (and, by delegated

---

[47] Calabresi, *Reflections on Medical Experimentation in Humans*, 98 DAEDALUS 387, 388-89 (1969).

[48] For a detailed description and evaluation of these two agencies, *see* Curran, note 23 *supra*.

authority, the FDA) to promulgate regulations for the investigational use of new drugs and to obtain informed consent (see Chapter Six) from patient-subjects before such drugs could be dispensed. In this connection it is interesting to note that at that time not a single state had any statute which "covered the use of an experimental drug and required the physician to inform the patient of such use."[49]

It is not within the scope of this report to give a detailed description of the operation of the FDA and its relationship to the pharmaceutical industry. Suffice it to say that since 1962 it has promulgated detailed requirements for the testing of drugs through the various phases of preclinical testing and clinical trials.[50] Moreover, the original informed consent provisions have been elaborated over the years, and the interest of the FDA in consent attests to its concern over protecting the rights of patient-subjects. Finally, though the FDA essentially follows the PHS requirements with respect to review committees there is one important variation with respect to the composition of membership:

> The membership *must be* comprised of sufficient members of varying background, that is, lawyers, clergymen, or laymen as well as scientists, to assure complete and adequate review of the research project. The membership *must* possess not only broad competence to comprehend the nature of the project, but also other competencies necessary to judge the acceptability of the project or activity in terms of institutional regulations, relevant law, standards of professional practice, and community acceptance.[51]

b. Public Health Service—National Institutes of Health. As already indicated, the NIH is not a regulatory agency, and its function is mainly to award research grants and contracts to institutions and investigators as well as to conduct its own intramural research programs. Until 1966, when the Surgeon General promulgated his policy statement on institutional review committees, the policy of the NIH was to leave ultimate responsibility for the use of human subjects with the investigators themselves. It saw its primary function as evaluating the scientific merits of the project submitted for funding and, in the spirit of academic freedom, leaving everything else to the investigators' judgment. We have already discussed the PHS guide lines whose cornerstone is the requirement that each institution conducting federally funded research establish a peer review committee. The review committee system, as envisioned by the PHS, continues in the spirit of its basic philosophy of professional freedom. The committees are

---

[49] 108 *Congressional Record* 17395 (1962).

[50] *See generally* 21 C.F.R. (1972).

[51] 36 FED. REG. 5038 (1971), amending subparagraph (2), Form FD-1571, *see* 21 C.F.R. §130.3(a) (1972) (emphasis added).

given a great deal of discretion to chart their own course, and there is little regulation or review from above.[52] We have already commented on some of the implications of this policy.

   c. *A Comparison of the Two Agencies.* The FDA, whose primary focus is on the regulation of business concerns in interstate commerce (including their "research and development" components), originally took a stronger stand in its promulgations to protect the interests of the individual patient-subject and society than the PHS–NIH did, since the focus of the latter was on promoting research. Critics have argued that the FDA's concern is misplaced, an expression of unwarranted distrust in the integrity of investigators and only results in slowing down scientific progress. The PHS–NIH, on the other hand, is more clearly aligned with science and investigators and very much concerned not to hamper their activities unduly. The relevant officials at NIH have traditionally been drawn from the same group as the researchers who are obtaining the grants, and the practice of having protocols reviewed by "study sections" and national advisory councils further weds the NIH to the interests of the researchers. In putting it this simply we do not wish to suggest that either agency is not concerned with the other side of the coin; both are, of course, but their allegiances are different and this results in different emphases. Thus, each agency makes a valuable contribution in its own right to the research enterprise, but each has largely gone off in its own separate direction. What may be needed for overall decisionmaking in investigative medicine in general, and the catastrophic disease research process in particular, is another federal agency which, among other things, combines the spirit of the two existing agencies—facilitating the acquisition of knowledge and protecting the rights of individuals and society.[53] This would require the presence of representa-

----

[52] But recently HEW has proposed that "[e]ach DHEW agency shall appoint an Ethical Review Board to provide rigorous review of ethical issues in research involving human subjects by people whose interests are not solely those of the scientific community." 38 FED. REG. 31738, 31741 (1973). The Ethical Review Boards' relationship to the existing institutional review committees was not clearly spelled out in these proposed regulations.

[53] Amendments to H.R. 7724, introduced by Senator Edward Kennedy, came very close to establishing such a new agency. For a complete text of the bill and the subsequent Senate discussion, *see* 119 *Congressional Record* S16333-16353 (September 11, 1973). Section 1201 of the bill provided for the establishment within the Department of Health, Education and Welfare of a National Commission for the Protection of Human Subjects of Biomedical and Behavioral Research. The eleven members "appointed by the President from persons who are especially qualified to serve on the Commission by virtue of their training, experience, or background," shall represent the general public and such disciplines as law, ethics, theology, physical science, social science, and philosophy, as well as medicine and biology, but no more than five mem-

tives of these differing interests who could formulate policies which reconcile these varying viewpoints.

5. Courts

Investigators working in the area of catastrophic diseases and looking to the courts for guidance in resolving the problems which arise in investigative medicine will find little to assist them. There have been few pronouncements by the judiciary about medical research. Of course, numerous recent judicial opinions have dealt with informed consent (see Chapter Six), negligence, and assault arising in therapeutic situations and, should such causes of action arise in research settings, as they did in one recent case,[54] there is every reason to believe that courts will apply similar reasoning to research "malpractice" as they have in cases of medical negligence in con-

---

bers shall "have been engaged in biomedical or behavioral research involving human subjects." Section 1202 specified the following duties for the Commission:

(1) undertake a comprehensive investigation and study to identify the basic ethical principles and develop guidelines which should underlie the conduct of biomedical and behavioral research involving human subjects and develop and implement policies and regulations to assure that such research is carried out in accordance with the ethical principles identified by the Commission in order to assure the full protection of the rights of the subjects of such research;

(2) develop procedures for the certification of Institutional Review Boards;

(3) develop and recommend to the Congress the implementation of an appropriate range of sanctions (and the conditions for their use) for the failure of certified Institutional Review Boards to respond to Commission rules, regulations, and procedures;

(4) develop and recommend to the Congress a mechanism for the compensation of individuals and their families for injuries or death proximately caused by the participation of such individuals in a biomedical or behavioral research program; and

(5) develop and recommend to the Congress within one year after the date of enactment of this section an appropriate mechanism to broaden the scope of the Commission's jurisdiction in order to assure that all human subjects in biomedical and behavioral research programs, demonstrations and activities are protected.

The bill was passed, with amendments, by the Senate on September 11, 1973. *Id.* at 16349-16353. The Senate-House conferees subsequently reached a compromise agreement on the legislation which "calls for a temporary commission to function for two years. Thereafter it would be replaced by a national advisory council for the protection of subjects of biomedical and behavioral research. This would retain many of the functions of the commission." N. Y. Times, June 8, 1974, at 1, col. 4. As included in Title II of the National Research Act, Pub. Law No. 93-348 (1974), the Commission was given a more general mandate to investigate biomedical advances.

[54] Halushka v. University of Saskatchewan, 52 W.W.R. 608 (Sask. C.A. 1965).

ventional treatment.[55] Moreover, a number of cases, resulting from noncompliance with the FDA regulations of 1962 have been adjudicated, although these cases have not addressed themselves specifically to the problems raised at the frontiers of knowledge.

However, there exists a series of older cases which speak about medical experimentation. It should be noted though that the fact situations have little to do with true experimentation but rather with unorthodox medical practices for therapeutic purposes. The pursuit of research, in its contemporary sense, was not usually the motivation of these physicians. In the earliest English case, *Slater v. Baker and Stapleton, C. B.*[56] a noted surgeon employed a novel bone-breaking method to refracture an improperly healed leg. The court, holding for the plaintiff, said:

> For anything that appears to the Court, this was the first experiment made with this new instrument; and if it was it was a rash action, and he who acts rashly acts ignorantly. [I]n this particular case [he has] acted ignorantly and unskillfully, contrary to the known rule and usage of surgeons.[57]

The leading American case is *Carpenter v. Blake.*[58] Here plaintiff recovered from a surgeon for alleged malpractice in setting and healing a dislocated elbow and in failing to instruct the patient concerning aftercare. The court held:

> Much was said on the argument, as to the right of a surgeon to exercise his own judgment as to the mode of treatment he will adopt in the case of a wound, or of a disease which he is called upon to treat; that neither the rules prescribed by writers, nor those acted upon by other physicians or surgeons, can apply to every case, and hence latitude must be allowed for the application of remedies which the attending physician or surgeon has found to be beneficial. If this is not allowed, the argument is, that all progress in the practice of surgery or physic must cease, and the afflicted lose altogether the benefits of experience and of remedies that science furnishes for the alleviation of human suffering. It must be conceded that if a surgeon is bound, at the peril of being liable for malpractice, to follow the modes of treatment which writers and practitioners have prescribed, the patient may lose the benefits of recent improvements in the treatment of diseases, or discoveries in science, by which new remedies have been brought into use; but this danger is more apparent than real. Some standard, by which to determine the pro-

---

[55] Some of the reasoning would not necessarily be applicable, of course, since the underlying question (discussed hereafter) of the "innovative" and "not yet accepted" nature of the treatment differentiates research and therapeutic contexts.

[56] 95 Eng. Rep. 860 (1797).

[57] *Id.* at 862-63.

[58] 60 Barb. 488 (N.Y. Sup. Ct. 1871), *reversed on other grounds,* 50 N.Y. 696 (1872).

priety of treatment, must be adopted; otherwise experience will take the place of skill, and the reckless experimentalist the place of the educated, experienced practitioner. If the case is a new one, the patient must trust to the skill and experience of the surgeon he calls; so must he if the injury or the disease is attended with injury to other parts, or other diseases have developed themselves, for which there is no established mode of treatment. But when the case is one as to which a system of treatment has been followed for a long time, there should be no departure from it, unless the surgeon who does it is prepared to take the risk of establishing, by his success, the propriety and safety of his experiment.

The rule protects the community against reckless experiments, while it admits the adoption of new remedies and modes of treatment only when their benefits have been demonstrated, or when, from the necessity of the case, the surgeon or physician must be left to the exercise of his own skill and experience.[59]

In subsequent cases, though again there were no allegations made of experimentation, the courts commented on "experimental" practices as follows:

. . . There must be some criterion by which to test the proper mode of treatment in a given case; and, when a particular mode of treatment is upheld by a consensus of opinion among the members of the profession, it should be followed by the ordinary practitioner; and, if a physician sees fit to experiment with some other mode, he should do so at his peril. In other words, he must be able, in the case of deleterious results, to satisfy the jury that he had reason for the faith that was in him, and justify his experiment by some reasonable theory. . . .[60]

We have little doubt that, if the first case of vaccination had proved disastrous and injured the patient, the physician should have been held liable. Nor do we believe that a physician of standing and loyalty to his patients will subject them to mere experiment, the safety or virtue of which has not been established by experience of the profession, save possibly when the patient is in extremis, and fatal results substantially certain unless the experiment may succeed.[61]

We recognize the fact that, if the general practice of medicine and surgery is to progress, there must be a certain amount of experimentation carried on; but such experiments must be done with the knowledge and consent of the patient or those responsible for him, and must not vary too radically from the accepted method of procedure. One who claims to be a specialist in so far as diagnosing a case is concerned must also be held to the above rule.[62]

---

[59] 60 Barb. at 523-24.
[60] Jackson v. Burnham, 20 Colo. 532, 39 Pac. 577 (1895).
[61] Allen v. Voje, 114 Wis. 1, 12, 89 N.W. 924, 931 (1902).
[62] Fortner v. Koch, 272 Mich. 273, 261 N.W. 762 (1935).

We are of the opinion that, under the facts and circumstances disclosed by this record, including the fact that no immediate emergency existed, the defendant physician was obligated to make a disclosure to the parents of his infant patient that the procedure he proposed was novel and unorthodox and that there were risks incident to or possible in its use. . . .[63]

It should be noted that as time went on, the courts increasingly acknowledged the need for experimentation as well as the importance of disclosure if novel procedures are to be employed. The case law has thus moved from the position that the physician-investigator "experiments at his peril," to holding that he may expose patients to novel risks if they have consented. Yet this does not, of course, sufficiently demarcate the bounds of permissible medical experimentation. Cases which raise questions about the extent of the authority of investigators· to pursue research with human subjects, and under what conditions, have not yet come before courts except for the recent Detroit psychosurgery litigation.[64] When they do in greater numbers, Louis L. Jaffe's prediction may turn out to be correct:

> Judges are sensitive to the ethos of the time. Our society places a high premium on scientific experimentation and the pursuit of knowledge. To a greater extent than was formerly true, judges will be conscious of the conflict of interests and will seek to give due weight to each of them in any case involving experimentation carried on pursuant to current standards of propriety. The courts, for example, have been willing to take account of the conditions of modern surgery in permitting a further operation without consent where unexpected and serious pathology turns up in the course of an operation performed under anesthesia. We should proceed on the hypothesis, therefore, that in framing our ethical principles the common law will be hospitable to procedures that recognize the social value of human experimentation without sacrificing the interests of patients and subjects.[65]

Accordingly, the courts may hold back from placing obligations on physician-investigators that their colleagues would require, since judges "ordinarily allow a considerable latitude for the exercise of conscience and skill."[66] As Jaffe observes:

> A committee may demand safeguards that the law does not require. It may, for example, require experiments to be performed by a group or demand that the therapeutic and experimental functions be kept separate and be per-

---

[63] Fiorentino v. Wegner, 26 App. Div.2d 693, 272 N.Y.S.2d (Sup. Ct. 1966), *reversed as to defendant hospital,* 19 N.Y.2d 407, 227 N.E.2d 296 (1967).

[64] Kaimowitz v. Department of Mental Health for the State of Michigan, Civil Action No. 73-19434-W (Circ. Ct. for the County of Wayne, State of Michigan, 1973). For further discussion of this case, *see* note 70 *infra.*

[65] Jaffe, *Law as a System of Control,* 98 DAEDALUS 406, 416 (1969).

[66] *Id.* at 414-15.

formed by different personnel. A court, on the other hand, would probably not impose such conditions even though it believed them to be wise. A committee might veto a project on the ground that it did not hold sufficient promise of fruitful results. It is unlikely that a court would feel qualified to make such a judgment, and if the experimental subject had been fairly treated, it would not condemn the experiment. Thus, there is a significant area of discretion within which conscience and technical judgment are to be exercised.[67]

Courts, which play a major role in the allocation of burdens in many other areas of risk-creation,[68] are thus not major participants in the area of risktaking in human experimentation. They have grappled with the issue of liability for improperly tested drugs,[69] but generally have not engaged in any deep analysis of the societal costs and benefits of various allocations of risk. As human experimentation in general, and catastrophic disease research in particular, comes to be governed by more extensive administrative mechanisms, the major function of the judiciary will probably be limited to ruling on the reasonableness of the administrative or committee determinations, as they relate to the rights of both investigator and subject.[70]

---

[67] *Id.* at 415.

[68] *See generally* G. CALABRESI, THE COSTS OF ACCIDENTS (1970); W. BLUM & H. KALVEN, PUBLIC LAW PERSPECTIVES ON A PRIVATE LAW PROBLEM (1965).

[69] *See* pp. 148-50 *infra*, where we focus on the private litigants as the moving parties in attempting to right an abuse arising from poor or fraudulent experimentation.

[70] The recent psychosurgery case in Detroit involved a prisoner (John Doe) under a life sentence who had "consented" to experimental psychosurgery. The case was brought before the court by Gabe Kaimowitz, a legal aid attorney, who represented himself and the Medical Committee for Human Rights. Subsequently the court appointed Professor Robert Burt of the Michigan Law School as counsel for John Doe. Before the psychosurgery issue was decided, the issue of the constitutionality of Doe's detention was raised, and on March 23, 1973, the Court rendered an opinion that his detention was unconstitutional and ordered his release. Since it appeared possible that the research project would go forward with other patients at some point, the Court felt that the case was appropriate for a declaratory judgment. The two issues framed for decision in this judgment were as follows:

1. After failure of established therapies, may an adult or legally appointed guardian, if the adult is involuntarily detained, at a facility within the jurisdiction of the State Department of Mental Health give legally adequate consent to an innovative or experimental surgical procedure on the brain, if there is demonstrable physical abnormality of the brain, and the procedure is designed to ameliorate behavior, which is either personally tormenting to the patient, or so profoundly disruptive that the patient cannot safely live, or live with others?

2. If the answer to the above is yes, then is it legal in this State to undertake an innovative or experimental surgical procedure on the brain of an adult who is involuntarily detained at a facility within the jurisdiction of the State Department of

C. QUASI-PUBLIC GROUPS

In addition to the express authority wielded by the many official and professional bodies, a less formal, but in some instances equally influential, role in catastrophic disease decisionmaking is assumed by a number of private individuals and organizations which take on a public aspect through their activities. These include newspapers, private participants in the legal process, organizations which "lobby," and nongovernmental sources of funding.

1. The Press

The interest shown by journalists in heart transplantation is familiar to all, but it is interesting to note that chronic hemodialysis and kidney transplants also continue to make front-page news. The coverage provided by the press increases; this reflects the public's interest in such dramas as physicians agonizing over the patient whose dialysis treatments have to be terminated for lack of funds[71] or kidneys being flown to waiting patients

---

Mental Health, if there is demonstrable physical abnormality of the brain, and the procedure is designed to ameliorate behavior, which is either personally tormenting to the patient, or so profoundly disruptive that the patient cannot safely live, or live with others?

After extensive hearings the court held that:

... the answer to question number one posed for decision is no.

In reaching this conclusion, we emphasize two things:

First, the conclusion is based upon the state of the knowledge as of the time of the writing of this Opinion. When the state of medical knowledge develops to the extent that the type of psychosurgical intervention proposed here becomes an accepted neurosurgical procedure and is no longer experimental, it is possible, with appropriate review mechanisms, that involuntarily detained mental patients could consent to such an operation.

Second, we specifically hold that an involuntarily detained mental patient today can give adequate consent to accepted neurosurgical procedures.

In view of the fact we have answered the first question in the negative, it is not necessary to proceed to a consideration of the second question, although we cannot refrain from noting that had the answer to the first question been yes, serious constitutional problems would have arisen with reference to the second question.

Kaimowitz v. Department of Mental Health for the State of Michigan, Civil Action No. 73-19434-W (Circ. Ct. for the County of Wayne, State of Michigan, 1973). In this instance the court did not rule on the reasonableness of the administrative or committee determinations, though there was extensive testimony on these issues. Instead it based its decision only on the question of the capacity of the inmate-research subject to give legally adequate consent for experimental neurosurgery.

[71] *See, e.g.,* Altman, *Artificial Kidney Use Poses Awesome Questions,* N.Y. Times, Oct. 24, 1971, at 1, col. 6.

in distant cities.[72] While the tempo of media coverage has decreased markedly from the barrage of news stories, to say nothing of radio and television reporting, which marked the early days of cardiac replacement, there can be no question that the communications media perform an important function in the process of decisionmaking about catastrophic diseases.

Indeed, the way in which the media played out their role when it came to heart transplants caused not a little distress, especially among physicians. Complaints were raised that rather than presenting the case of heart grafts in the medical literature and meetings, they were aired among the "circus trappings and glitter"[73] accorded to exciting and fashionable items of news.

> When [the first human transplant] was described as "the miracle in Cape-town" and followed by a triumphal worldwide tour by the head of the surgical team, Christiaan Barnard, M.D., thereby becoming a folk hero, it is not surprising that the more conservative physicians drew back in consternation. As though this were not enough, there ensued what appeared to be an international race to be a member of the me-too brigade. There has never been anything like it in medical annals, nor has it been an edifying spectacle for some of us.[74]

Although the press can hardly be held solely responsible for the conduct of transplant surgeons, the amount of publicity given to the cardiac operations certainly fed the flames of ambition and fame which burned in the breasts of numerous surgeons and hospital directors.

While some physicians were aesthetically offended by the publicity, it served many useful functions. The attention paid to the challenge of unsolved medical problems may have attracted some young people to research medicine; the purses of many people were probably opened to medical centers engaged in transplantation,[75] thereby providing funds which would also support other research efforts. Basic "public policy" issues of medicine, like the definition of death, were also brought to the forefront of lay interest. Although the issue had arisen in medical circles previously, the advent of heart transplantation, with its rush of press coverage, marks the

---

[72] *See, e.g.,* Thomas, *One Victim's Kidneys Aid Pair: Transplants Performed Here, Boston,* N.H. Register, Feb. 13, 1971, at 1, col. 3.

[73] Page, *The Ethics of Heart Transplantation: A Personal View,* 207 J.A.M.A. 109 (1969).

[74] *Id.*

[75] For example, the "celebrity" of both Drs. Michael DeBakey and Denton Cooley is a major factor in their ability to finance their multimillion dollar cardiovascular research and treatment centers in Houston. *See* T. THOMPSON, HEARTS: OF SURGEONS AND TRANSPLANTS, MIRACLES AND DISASTERS ALONG THE CARDIAC FRONTIER (1971).

point at which the public was first educated about the new criteria which provide the basis for declaring death in a patient whose brain had been irreversibly damaged while his heart and lungs continued to function. Finally, the mass media were probably indirectly responsible for saving many lives, since the attention given to the need for more organs probably lay behind the willingness of relatives to give a deceased person's organs, and it definitely stimulated the offer of kidneys by living, unrelated donors in a number of instances.[76]

Nevertheless, the enthusiastic coverage given to cardiac transplantation was not without its liabilities. Inevitably some of the difficult scientific facts or close medical issues were oversimplified in the popular press, with the result that the public had too rosy a view of the prospects of transplantation at first, which turned into bitterness and distrust (and a decrease in the number of donors) as the difficulties came home to roost. Part of this phenomenon was plainly of the press's making: The transplanters were made out to be larger-than-life characters capable of defying natural laws and holding death at bay. Another part may have had its origin in the physicians' understandable desire to present their operations as therapy;[77] the press for the most part accepted this characterization, while in fact physicians would have done better to stress the highly experimental aspect of transplantation.

A more fundamental problem with the media's role centers on the detailed "personal interest" stories which each operation seemed to generate: the private lives of the donor and his family, the recipient and his, and the whole life story of the transplant surgeon were usually set out for public view. This served as a painful reminder to some physicians of the major changes which have come about in the medical profession's attitude toward confidentiality and privacy. "Only a few decades ago probably the majority of those concerned would have been censured but today there is only minor grumbling."[78] It may be that it was this kind of story which was most successful in stirring up support, both fiscal and physical, among the general public, and the need for money and willingness to participate in an experiment may overcome the usual rules of confidentiality, as some suggested.[79] It is less likely that many physicians would have any reason to applaud another unfortunate consequence of the detailed and extensive coverage given to transplantation procedures: the creation of the image of the phy-

---

[76] *See* Sadler, Davison, Carroll & Kountz, *The Living, Genetically Unrelated, Kidney Donor*, 3 SEMINARS IN PSYCHIATRY 86 (1971).

[77] Fox, *Heart Transplants: Treatment or Experiment?*, 159 SCIENCE 374 (1968).

[78] Page, note 73 *supra*, at 111.

[79] *See, e.g.,* Hessel, *Heart Transplants and Public Information*, 278 NEW ENG. J. MED. 797 (1968).

sician as a man not to entrust one's life to, since he may be after one's organs.[80]

In sum, the news media in the process of carrying out their normal functions gave an unprecedented amount of coverage to dialysis and transplantation, especially cardiac. In doing so, they played the important role of public educator, but because the boundaries of proper conduct were not well-defined, it also seems to have harmed individuals and perhaps to have distorted decisionmaking about catastrophic diseases.

Ironically, there is no real indication from the type of coverage given that there was much intention on the part of journalists to wield this sort of influence in the process. This is not always so, of course. For example, the media on occasion expose abuses in medicine and research very effectively. In January 1969, Harold E. Martin, editor of the *Montgomery Advertiser-Journal,* ran a series of highly critical articles about the drug testing programs being conducted by Southern Food and Drug Research, Inc., in Alabama prisons. These reports were subsequently given national prominence through Walter Rugaber's coverage in the *New York Times* of the prison testing and plasmapheresis programs in which he stressed the federal government's failure to exercise its responsibility for supervising the quality of products tested and produced, and the conditions under which the work took place.[81] Shortly thereafter, the FDA Commissioner announced that all drug testing in institutional settings would be subject to peer group review.[82] Similarly, a number of science and medicine reporters, particularly Morton Mintz of the *Washington Post,* persisted in raising questions about the safety of the oral contraceptives at a time when the pharmaceutical companies were inundating the medical profession (and thereby the consuming public) with assurances that "the pill" was the most carefully tested drug ever marketed.[83] Mintz was also responsible for after-the-fact coverage of the abuses which had been turned up by the Food and Drug Administration in the testing of MER/29, an anti-cholesterol drug marketed by the William S. Merrell Co. in the early 1960s, which caused serious side-effects in many of its users including "usually operable cata-

---

[80] *See, e.g.,* Kass, *A Caveat on Transplants,* Washington Post, Jan. 14, 1968, at B-1, col. 1—transplant surgeon may be seen as "vulture hiding at the foot of the bed."

[81] *See, e.g.,* Rugaber, *Prison Drug and Plasma Projects Leave Fatal Trail,* N.Y. Times, July 29, 1969, at 1, col. 5.

[82] *See* F.D.A., Notice of Proposed Rulemaking, 34 FED. REG. 13552 (1969); Rugaber, *F.D.A. Will Require Drug Test Review,* N.Y. Times, Aug. 13, 1969, at 1, col. 5.

[83] *See, e.g.,* Mintz, *Are Birth Control Pills Safe? Some Doctors Doubt that the Drug Has Been Tested Well Enough for Possible Side Effects,* Washington Post, Dec. 19, 1965, at E-1, col. 1; *see generally* J. KATZ, WITH THE ASSISTANCE OF A. CAPRON & E. GLASS, EXPERIMENTATION WITH HUMAN BEINGS 736-92 (1972).

racts in both eyes, loss or thinning of hair, and severe skin reactions."[84]

The activities of these reporters demonstrate the function the media can serve in bringing to public attention the faults as well as the successes of research medicine. On the whole, however, the media's effect is an indirect one: It can expose conduct, which is then judged according to the standards held by the reader, but it is probably less effective in establishing its own standards beyond deploring conduct which is clearly unethical or has been determined to be improper by a recognized authority as the MER/29 testing was held by the FDA and the courts.

2. Private Parties

The MER/29 episode also gives a glimpse of the role which private parties assume in instigating official action. Although the Food and Drug Administration officers in charge of the MER/29 application had been critical of the drug's animal tests, they approved the drug for sale after a year of negotiation with the company during which time the latter submitted additional experimental data to substantiate its position. After the drug had been on the market for a couple of years, with occasional reports of adverse side-effects occurring among its users, the FDA learned from a former employee of the company that some of the animal data had been fabricated. The information supplied by this person was crucial in prompting a much needed investigation of the drug and in leading to its suspension.[85]

In addition to initiating such a process, private individuals were also involved in the MER/29 affair as litigants seeking damage payments from the manufacturer for the injuries they had suffered. Several hundred claims were filed in courts across the country, and a number led to substantial awards.[86] Although the Food, Drug and Cosmetic Act does not in itself provide for private remedies for its violation, such actions may be brought for the tort of negligence, a means by which private litigants have traditionally "policed" conduct dangerous to the public. In support of their claim of negligence, plaintiffs may show that the defendant's conduct violated applicable statutes or regulations; if, as in the MER/29 cases, the relevant law was intended to protect the plaintiffs (as indeed the drug

---

[84] M. MINTZ, THE THERAPEUTIC NIGHTMARE 257 (1965).

[85] *See generally Hearings on Competitive Problems in the Drug Industry before the Subcomm. on Monopoly of the Sen. Comm. on Small Business,* 91st Cong., 1st Sess. (1969).

[86] *See* Roginsky v. Richardson-Merrell, Inc., 378 F.2d. 832, 834 n.3 (2d Cir. 1967), which also reports three other cases decided as of that date with cumulative compensatory and punitive awards of $2,147,500 for the four cases, reduced by the judges to $1,047,500.

testing provisions were intended to safeguard drug users), then proof of a deviation from the standard established by the statute would be proof of negligence.[87] Where, as in the MER/29 cases, the proof also demonstrates intentional fraud on the part of the defendant, punitive as well as compensatory damages are appropriate.

Although it seems improbable (but, of course, not impossible) that a member of a transplant or dialysis treatment "team" would "blow the whistle" on the team's activities, as the Merrell employee did, in part because of the nature of the activities and in part because of the lack of a clear regulatory structure, private litigation is certainly a possibility. Much concern has been expressed of late about the adverse effects of malpractice litigation.[88] As it relates to our topic, the complaint most frequently made is that the substantial sums which are paid in these cases have a depressing effect on the level of activity and innovation in medicine, and that they lead to much useless and perhaps harmful precautionary conduct (such as ordering many extra unnecessary tests on all patients) on the part of all doctors; moreover, a portion of the rise in the cost of medical care is ascribed to the increase in malpractice insurance premiums. While such cries of alarm are doubtless somewhat excessive, serious questions can be raised whether individual litigants can serve as effective and efficient agents of review in the catastrophic disease process. The difficulties faced in her malpractice action against Denton Cooley by the widow of Haskell Karp, the recipient of the only artificial heart implanted in a human being to date, suggest that beyond problems of proof and of the burden of persuasion, special difficulties will be encountered by litigants who attempt to challenge decisions and actions taken by the select physician-investigators on the edge of catastrophic disease research.[89] Unlike the drug manufacturer who deals with many unknown consumers on a strict buyer-seller basis, the transplant surgeon is probably more concerned with his reputation among his fellow physicians and the few patients he actually sees and treats than he

---

[87] *See, e.g.,* Toole v. Richardson-Merrell, Inc., 251 Cal. App.2d 689, 702-04, 60 Cal. Rptr. 398, 408-09 (1967).

[88] *See, e.g.,* Halberstam, *The Doctor's New Dilemma: "Will I Be Sued?"* N.Y. Times, Feb. 14, 1971, §6 (Magazine), at 8; *Federal Panel Urges Reform to Diminish Malpractice Suits, id.,* April 18, 1972, at 20, col. 4; *Medical Report: Malpractice Crisis,* 38 INS. COUNSEL J. 521 (1971).

[89] See Karp v. Cooley, 349 F.Supp. 827, 829 (S.D. Tex. 1972), *aff'd,* 493 F.2d 408 (5th Cir. 1974). *See also* Capron, *Informed Consent in Catastrophic Disease Research and Treatment,* 123 U. PA. L. REV. 340, 431-35 (1974); R. FOX & J. SWAZEY, THE COURAGE TO FAIL 210-11 (1974)—concluding that although the lawsuit was "the strongest action taken in the case of the artificial heart" its inadequacies make it doubtful that the subjects of therapeutic innovation "are adequately protected by the present legal process."

is with whether his insurance company has to pay an award in a particular case.[90]

Private parties operating on a "class" basis can probably play an even more useful role in the process. For instance, when the FDA issued its preliminary statement on peer group review, the Council on Health Organizations, represented by a "public interest" law firm, submitted comments which were influential in having the rule as finally promulgated take into account certain factors ignored by the FDA.[91]

3. Lobbies

In addition to providing funds for research and treatment (discussed hereafter), private groups have also played an important part in the catastrophic disease process through the influence they have exerted on legislative and administrative decisionmaking. The great energy and dedication that the participants in such "lobbying" efforts bring to their task is often the result of firsthand experience with the disease in themselves or members of their families. Drs. Samuel Bessman and Judith Swazey describe the "paradigm of a crusade"[92] in the movement in the mid-1960s to enact state laws requiring the screening of newborns for an inborn error of metabolism:

> By taking a very active role in an important field of medicine, a small group of determined and highly motivated parents of mentally retarded children, together with a few equally dedicated physicians, needed less than three years to persuade forty-one states to pass laws requiring the testing of newborn children for phenylketonuria (PKU), a rare and imperfectly understood cause of mental retardation.[93]

The forceful nature of this type of special interest lobbying was well illustrated recently with the passage of H.R. 1, the 1972 Social Security

---

[90] Drug houses are also, of course, concerned with their reputation. But there is less likelihood of serious injury to that reputation through the adverse results of lawsuits since the drug company's "reputation" is probably largely a result of advertising in lay and professional media rather than of the "referral" type common for physicians.

[91] *See* FDA, *Institutional Committee Review of Clinical Investigation of New Drugs in Human Beings*, 36 FED. REG. 5037 (1971).

[92] Bessman & Swazey, *Phenylketonuria: A Study of Biomedical Legislation*, in HUMAN ASPECTS OF BIOMEDICAL INNOVATIONS 49, 50 (E. Mendelsohn, J. Swazey & I. Travis eds. 1971).

[93] *Id.* at 49. In addition to their concern about PKU children, the interest of the physicians may have been based on the potential support for their clinical research or on a desire for medical prominence from their work on the disease and its detection.

Act amendments.[94] The concerted efforts of groups, such as the Kidney Foundation, and of leading clinicians—which included the demonstration to congressmen of a patient on hemodialysis who needed financial support to continue his life-sustaining treatment—were successful in getting the bill amended to provide for Medicare payments for hemodialysis and kidney transplantation for persons with chronic kidney failure.[95]

4. Private Funding Sources

The funds for transplantation, and especially for research on immunology which is needed for transplantation to advance, come largely from clinical research grants awarded by the National Institutes of Health, although it is difficult to know exactly what part indirect financing by university medical schools still plays. Private sources of funds, in addition to the patient's own resources and health insurance coverage,[96] probably played a particularly important role in the early years of long-term dialysis. The relative importance of such philanthropy for chronic hemodialysis as applied to a much larger patient population is probably decreasing, although there are presently no exact figures on this. Nevertheless, the importance of private decisionmakers for the catastrophic disease process should not be underestimated; the willingness of wealthy individuals or foundations[97] to underwrite a particular line of research or innovative therapy[98] should not be ignored. So long as the tax laws encourage such private decisionmaking, it may be relevant to inquire whether this is the most effective and wisest way to allocate funds (*i.e.,* money not collected in taxes is equivalent to funds allocated legislatively). It is not clear whether any discernible pattern

---

[94] Act of October 30, 1972, Pub. L. No. 92-603, 86 Stat. 1329.

[95] The lobbying focused initially on the Rehabilitation Act of 1972 (since support for dialysis had come in the past through the vocational rehabilitation offices in some states). The pressure generated there resulted in amendments to the Social Security bill, H.R. 1. *See Hearings on H.R. 8395 Before the Subcomm. on the Handicapped of the Senate Comm. on Labor and Public Welfare,* 92d Cong., 2d Sess., pt. 1, at 310-50 (1972).

[96] The Gottshalk Report in 1967 concluded that "voluntary health insurance, on its face, looks much more promising" as a source of private funds, but noted that only about 35 percent of the population is covered by plans which would provide any adequacy of coverage for chronic treatment. COMMITTEE ON CHRONIC KIDNEY DISEASE, U.S. BUREAU OF THE BUDGET, REPORT 87-89 (1967).

[97] Especially notable in this regard are the special purpose foundations established as a result of a public concern with a particular disease entity, such as the Kidney Foundation, Hemophilia Foundation, National Tay-Sachs and Allied Diseases Association, etc.

[98] *See note 75 supra.*

would emerge from an examination of private giving in the area of catastrophic disease treatment and research.

In this part we have moved from an analysis of the authority of the physician-investigator as decisionmaker in the catastrophic disease process to the authority of the patient-subject and finally to the authority of professional and public institutions. All these participants have important roles to play, and the debate whether decisions in the catastrophic disease process should be private or public can no longer be answered as "either/or," since they clearly encompass both private and public decisionmaking. When Christiaan Barnard and his patient Louis Washkansky agreed to a heart transplantation they probably had every right to make such a private agreement—but this decision, like many others in catastrophic diseases, has affected the professions and society in a great many ways, and in dealing with the reverberations which followed and are yet to follow, professional and public institutions have an important role to play.

To define these roles will require much thought, but for thought to be relevant, data are needed. Thus Chief Judge David L. Bazelon was correct when, following participation in a closed door session in which it was decided who should be selected for hemodialysis at a medical center that he was visiting, he concluded that "mechanisms will be needed for recording all these decisions."[99] He admonished the group of decisionmakers, "let everybody know what went into [the decision]. . . . Over time the public [and one hopes all the participants are] going to react but they are not going to know with that door closed."[100] The issues raised by that challenge provide the springboard for our consideration of the three stages of decisionmaking in the following chapters.

[99] *National Commission on Health Science and Society*, note 38 *supra*, at 279.
[100] *Id.* at 280.

PART THREE

Stages of Decisionmaking—
Proposals and Recommendations

In Parts One and Two of this book we endeavored to identify the major problems confronting decisionmakers in the catastrophic disease process and to explore the capacities of the major participants to resolve these problems. Building on this examination, we will now propose a number of general and specific recommendations for the ordering of the catastrophic disease process. Though we shall continue to make reference to issues that have arisen in hemodialysis and organ transplantation, most of our recommendations are framed independently enough of these specific issues to make them relevant to other existing or newly arising issues created by medical progress.

As we have already suggested, the problems which require resolution by physician-investigators, patient-subjects, the professions, and the state are sufficiently disparate throughout the catastrophic disease decisionmaking process that the analysis of the roles which these participants should play will be facilitated by introducing distinctions among several stages in this process. We have therefore divided the process of research on and treatment of catastrophic diseases into three decisional stages—the formulation of policy, the administration of research and therapy, and the review of decisions and their consequences. We believe that such a scheme will prove useful, and it provides the framework on which the final three chapters are built.

153

A review of the literature reveals the absence of any distinctions between policy and administration decisions. For example, when commentators complain about the unwelcome intrusion of "outsiders" in the domain of the professionals,[1] it is not at all clear whether they refer to the day-by-day administrative research and therapy decisions which have to be made or to the more general policy decisions, such as the allocation of resources for all medical care or the determination of the extent and limits of patient-subject participation in hazardous experimentation. We believe that once such distinctions are introduced, physician-investigators can accept more readily, and even welcome, the participation of "outsiders" in formulation as well as review decisions. While some may remain concerned about the possibility of becoming too hampered in their pursuits by *any* regulation by outsiders, they too should recognize that one of their major objections has been based on the fear of undue direct intrusions into the clinical or laboratory decisions which they believe they alone must be allowed to make. If rules and procedures that provide adequate protections and well-articulated procedures can be promulgated for the formulation and review of the catastrophic disease process, all concerned may feel more comfortable leaving the actual administration of research and therapy in the hands of the immediate participants—physician-

---

[1] Representative of the attitude of many physician-investigators is the following exchange between Dr. Christiaan Barnard and members of the Subcommittee on Government Research of the Senate Committee on Government Operations holding hearings in March 1968 on a proposal to establish a commission to study the problems raised by biomedical advances.

Dr. Barnard: [L]et me give you something to compare that with.

Who pays for the cost of war? The public. Who decides where the general should attack and how he should attack? . . .

. . . The general is qualified to make that decision. And, therefore, he is qualified to spend the public's money the best way he thinks it is fit to spend it.

You cannot have control over these things. You must leave it in the people's hands who are capable of doing it.

Senator Ribicoff: So not only the operation, but the person who would be the donee, in your opinion, should be left entirely to the medical team?

Dr. Barnard: Yes, sir.

. . . Commissions have been set up to decide on various medical advances in the past. These commissions . . . have hampered the progress of medicine in nearly every case where such commissions intervene; because they were not qualified to deal with the various aspects.

Hearings on S.J. Res. 145 (National Commission on Health Science and Society) before the Subcomm. on Government Research of the Senate Comm. on Government Operations, 90th Cong., 2d Sess., at 82 (1968).

investigators and patient-subjects—and thus reverse an ever-increasing trend to supervise ongoing medical interventions. For example, the "continuing review of *ongoing* projects and activities"[2] now required by HEW could then be limited to particular situations, including regular spot checking, specified at the formulation stage, and be evaluated again at the review stage once the project has been completed. Of course, it is important that the review mechanisms established not only permit careful and sensitive evaluation of the decisions and their consequences but also, in the light of such evaluation, lead to revisions in existing policies. Accordingly, in what follows we shall have more to say about the first and third stages and less about the second stage of the catastrophic disease process.

[2] U.S. DEP'T OF HEALTH, EDUCATION & WELFARE, INSTITUTIONAL GUIDE TO HEW POLICY ON PROTECTION OF HUMAN SUBJECTS [HEW Publication No. (NIH) 72-102] 8-9 (1971).

CHAPTER EIGHT

The Formulation of Policy

Any proposals for structuring the catastrophic disease process, especially recommendations that address themselves to the overall policies which should shape this process, immediately arouse concerns about their impact on physician-investigators' freedom of action which is considered so essential for the pursuit of knowledge. These concerns cannot be brushed aside, and all promulgations for the ordering of the research and therapy process must be examined in terms of their effects on the advancement of science, an important societal value as was noted in Chapter Three. Nevertheless, the problems posed by the catastrophic disease process can be resolved neither by physician-investigators alone nor by them in conjunction with their patient-subjects unless these participants are granted a degree of freedom and immunity not enjoyed in comparable areas by other groups in our society. Once the issue is raised, it is unlikely that professional or public institutions will be disposed explicitly to delegate such authority to investigators and/or subjects; nor would such a position have merit. The burdens imposed on individual investigators in deciding on their own, for example, what risks to take in order to seek benefits for science or the community would be so awesome to most that they themselves would ask for guidance from the profession or the state. And even if this were not to happen, a variety of informal mechanisms would quickly be created by their colleagues to preclude practices which they, for good or bad reasons, found intolerable. For example, the constraints imposed by codes of ethics and traditional professional practices are indications of the fact that physician-

157

investigators, as well as the professions and state, do not believe that research and therapy can be carried on *carte blanche*. Though obvious, this background is needed to place in perspective the views of those commentators who lament the imposition of any restrictions which invade the freedom of investigators. Since such freedom does not and cannot exist, the real question which requires answering is: What controls will least infringe or neglect the values of all participants engaged in the catastrophic disease research and treatment process? We start from the assumption of the inevitability of controls, which leads to the further assumption that the catastrophic disease process is better served *as a rule* if greater clarity exists about the nature, implications, and consequences of such controls.[1] Thus, we seek to bring to the surface the problems which require resolution so that policies can be formulated and reformulated with greater conscious recognition of the values to be preferred and those to be neglected. Throughout we ask: Who among the various participants should have what kind of authority to make what decisions in a way that will lighten rather than increase existing burdens?

There is another reason for our interest in formulating better policies for the catastrophic disease process. In recent years, due to the dramatic disclosures of harm inflicted on patient-subjects as well as the spectacular and awesome advances made or about to be made by medical research, much legislation has been either promulgated or proposed for the control of human investigations.[2] Since most likely this trend will continue, it will prove useful to have available for study not only our proposals but others as well for the ordering of this process. Such documents may inform decisionmakers of the many interlocking problems which require consideration and lead to legislation which takes these issues into account rather than

---

[1] In some situations, conscious or unconscious obfuscation of the nature, degree, etc., of such controls may be desirable, particularly when no resolution of the issues involved seems likely to satisfy all (or even most) of the participants. It is our belief, however, that as to most of the troublesome issues raised by catastrophic diseases the questions are already out on the table and cannot be successfully ignored.

[2] For example, the revelations in the press concerning the Tuskegee Syphilis Study prompted a number of congressional proposals, including one by Senator Jacob Javits to enact the current HEW guidelines into law, S. 3935, 92d Cong., 2d Sess. (1972), and one by Senator Hubert Humphrey to establish a National Human Experimentation Standards Board to provide independent review of all medical research on man. S. 3951, 92d Cong., 2d Sess. (1972). Similarly, Assemblyman Leonard P. Stavisky introduced a bill in New York following the Southam-Mandel cancer experiment at the Jewish Chronic Disease Hospital in Brooklyn "to Amend the Education Law in Relation to Scientific Research on Human Subjects, to Provide for the Advancement of such Research through the Protection of its Subjects, and to Establish a State Board on Human Research." Ass. Bill No. 1837 (1971).

being solely influenced by one particular tragic event. More often than not decisions reached in a crisis create more problems than they resolve.[3]

Finally, we should make a few orienting comments about our underlying assumptions with respect to theories of decisionmaking, which naturally have a major impact on our proposals for the "formulation" stage (and which, of course, also influence our treatment of the other two stages). Braybrooke and Lindblom caution against use of "rational-comprehensive planning," which tends to operate as follows:

> Let ultimate values be expressed in general principles satisfactory to everybody who is ready to attend to the arguments identifying them—or, if there is no hope of that, satisfactory at least to those who are now undertaking a specific job of evaluation. Let these principles, which may embody notions of happiness, welfare, justice, or intuitive notions of goodness, be stated so exactly that they may be arranged intelligibly in an order of priority that indicates precisely which principles govern the application of others and when. Then derive within the limits of such a system intermediate principles that are suitable for application in particular cases, and that—allowing for rare cases of equality in net benefits—will indicate unambiguously which of alternative policies is to be chosen, according to the values they would promote.[4]

Although we believe it is useful to identify the relevant values and goals involved in catastrophic disease decisionmaking[5] and to explore allegiance of the participants to these values and their competence and authority to act, we engage in this process for purposes of *analysis* not for *constructing* a "rational comprehensive" system. Instead, more in line with Lindblom's approach,[6] we have built our proposals on the basis of incremental, self-correcting changes. Thus we do not consider our proposals a final edifice but rather a scaffold from which major building can take place.

---

[3] I submit that these are problems which medicine cannot solve within the intellectual boundaries of its own discipline. I submit that from lawyers and physicians laboring at what has been called the interface of medicine and law, with such ancillary experts as forensic medicine is accustomed to assemble, are most likely to come pragmatic solutions to these problems. . . . [W]ithout organized pressure from the discipline of forensic science for a judicial, a contemplative, an investigative, or even a committee approach to these problems, the law of medical practice will again be plagued by ad hoc precedents and emergency legislation hastily contrived in response to public pressure and emotional reaction to particular medical calamity.

Matte, *Law, Morals, and Medicine: A Method of Approach to Current Problems*, 13 J. For. Sci. 318, 331-32 (1968).

[4] D. Braybrooke & C. Lindblom, A Strategy of Decision 9 (1963).

[5] *See* Chapter Three *supra.*

[6] *See generally* C.E. Lindblom, *New Decision-Making Procedures Governing Research on and Treatment of Catastrophic Diseases* (1970) [Appendix C].

A. ANTICIPATING MEDICAL ADVANCES

In his presidential address to the American Political Science Association, Harold Lasswell admonished his colleagues for not appreciating long before atomic weapons were introduced

> the political consequences of sudden and stupendous increases of fighting effectiveness [and for not clarifying] in advance the main policy alternatives open to decisionmakers in this country or elsewhere. We did not create a literature or a body of oral analysis that seriously anticipated these issues. As political scientists we should have anticipated fully both the bomb and the significant problems of policy that came with it.[7]

Similarly, a Lasswellian contemplating our topic could chide the medical community for not anticipating organ transplantation and the development of means for purifying blood long before their first clinical trials and for not seriously considering "the significant problems of policy" which would then require resolution. Had physicians addressed themselves to this task, they would have created a literature, which might have explored such issues as the extent to which scarce resources should be supplied for costly but life-saving interventions both for experimental and therapeutic purposes, the criteria and procedures which should govern the selection of recipients and donors, or who should decide when resources must be made available, and at what cost, to those in need of them. Such deliberations would have been extremely useful to the so-called "Life or Death Committee" in Seattle which had no documents to consult on how to select a few candidates for hemodialysis from the many applicants and instead asked itself at one of its first meetings "where do we begin—the universe? the solar system? the earth?"[8]

A brief glance into the future readily reveals new problems about to be created by the rapid advances in medical science and technology which require careful and thorough analysis. In the field of organ transplantation, once the mysteries of rejection are understood and successfully mastered, many questions will have to be posed and answered. For example, who should receive organs as long as resources remain scarce, under what circumstances should organs be made available to all in need of them, by what means should much needed organs be acquired, etc.? What holds true for catastrophic diseases is even more relevant to the problems soon to be created by the anticipated breakthroughs in the fields of genetics and

---

[7] Lasswell, *The Political Science of Science*, 50 AM. POL. SCI. REV. 961 (1956).

[8] Alexander, *Who Decides Who Lives, Who Dies*, LIFE, Nov. 9, 1962, at 103 [hereinafter cited as Alexander].

psychosurgery.[9] Past experiences make it only too evident that we have been, and remain, ill-prepared (and therefore ignorant) in dealing with such medical issues once they arise. We believe that mechanisms need to be constructed to promote anticipating medical advances, undertaking prior analysis of the anticipated problems, and preparing background materials to be consulted once decisions have to be made. Thus, we seek to emphasize here the scholarly and not the decisional dimension of the task.

The task of anticipating and analyzing the problems created by medical science is, of course, not the sole province of the medical profession. Political scientists, economists, and lawyers, to name a few, can make valuable contributions to such efforts and indeed their services must be enlisted, for the medical aspect of these issues is only one facet of the total picture. Thus the question immediately arises, within what settings can these activities be carried out optimally? One might turn to such groups as the National Academy of Sciences and suggest that they appoint committees to study these issues and prepare position statements. Indeed, a three-year study into four areas (sex determinism, *in vitro* fertilization, behavior modification, and aging) was recently completed by the NAS–NRC's Committee on the Life Sciences and Social Policy, chaired by Milton Katz of Harvard Law School and staffed by biochemist-physician Leon Kass.[10] Comparable studies are being undertaken by ongoing task forces of the Institute of Society, Ethics and the Life Sciences in Hastings-on-Hudson, N.Y. Similarly, Congress has mandated a national commission, based on the suggestion of Senator Walter F. Mondale, to undertake "a comprehensive investigation and study of the ethical, social and legal implications of advances in biomedical research and technology."[11] The recommendation that the members of this commission include persons from "the fields of medicine, law, theology, biological science, physical science, social science, philosophy, humanities, health administration, government, and public affairs,"[12] suggests the range of interdisciplinary contributions envisioned by the Congress. While such bodies have their usefulness, their often limited life span and the part-time efforts of their members reduce their value. The present national commission, for example, must attempt to complete its "special

---

[9] *See, e.g.,* ETHICAL ISSUES IN HUMAN GENETICS (B. Hilton, et al. eds. 1973); THE NEW GENETICS AND THE FUTURE OF MAN (M. Hamilton ed. 1972); A. ROSENFELD, THE SECOND GENESIS (1969); Salpukas, *Caution is Urged in Psychosurgery,* N.Y. Times, Apr. 6, 1973, at 24, col. 4.

[10] The Committee's report, entitled "Assessing Biomedical Technologies: An Inquiry into the Nature of the Process," was held up for a number of years; *see* Holden, *Ethics: Biomedical Advances Confront Public, Politicians as well as Professionals with New Issues,* 175 SCIENCE 40 (1972) but was released in mid-1975.

[11] National Research Act, Pub. Law No. 93-348, § 203 (1974).

[12] *Id.* at S3710.

study" of the implications of biomedical advances under Section 203 of the Act within the two-year period in which it is also conducting its "comprehensive study" of the principles and practices of human experimentation in this country, pursuant to Section 202 of the Act. The major thrust of our recommendation goes in a different direction and, if implemented, could even enhance the value of such commissions, for they would then have available better background material to aid their deliberations.

The impetus for the study of the anticipated problems posed by medical advances should come from medicine and have its locus in its centers of learning—medical schools.[13] We appreciate that the implementation of such a recommendation requires a shift in emphasis, or at least an additional dimension, for medical education which has increasingly become clinically oriented (on both the research and service sides) and less attentive to the systematic exploration of issues which—like the anticipation of medical advances—delve into the ways biomedical activities impinge on individuals and society at large. To accomplish such an objective, faculty will need to be recruited who have a scholarly interest in pursuing these problems. Since they will be hard to find, their number will probably be few initially. But there is every reason to believe that through their teaching and writing they will stimulate medical students and younger colleagues to develop similar interests and thus provide a growing scholarly output.

Though we envision the impetus for such efforts to originate within the medical community, we expect that academic physicians will seek collaborative relationships with colleagues from other disciplines, some of whom will be given permanent appointments to medical school faculties and others of whom will remain members of the departments within their disciplines, yet devoting a considerable amount of their time to this work. From such beginnings in a few medical centers a significant flow of important basic contributions may emerge which in turn will stimulate other medical schools to institute similar programs.[14] The resulting work should

---

[13] A number of such programs have recently been begun, including the Interfaculty Program in Medical Ethics at the Harvard Medical School and the Joseph and Rose Kennedy Institute of Bioethics, which was established by a $1.3 million grant to Georgetown University from the Joseph P. Kennedy, Jr., Foundation to provide "on the job" training for graduate students.

The Kennedy Institute, according to director Andre Hellegers, will be an unusual experiment in reuniting long-fragmented disciplines. Under one roof will be all the clinical, scientific, psychological, and sociological aspects of reproduction, genetics, and obstetrics.

Holden, note 10 *supra*, at 41.

[14] There are still only a handful of universities across the country that offer courses with an interdisciplinary approach to ethics. The only full-fledged program is a 4-year course offered at Columbia University's College of Physicians and Surgeons.

prove invaluable to all decisionmakers who are called upon to formulate policy relatively quickly once the issues come before them.

B. THE RELUCTANCE OF EXISTING INSTITUTIONS TO FORMULATE POLICY

In principle, there is no reason why existing institutions, whether governmental (such as the National Institutes of Health), interdisciplinary (the National Academy of Sciences), or professional (the American Medical Association) could not formulate policies more vigorously and consistently than they have done in the past, even though they are not the only groups who should have such authority. Indeed, they have from time to time assumed this function albeit with apparent hesitation and reluctance.

The most conspicuous efforts in the past have involved codes of ethics to guide physicians and researchers. Although considered by some commentators to be sufficient guideposts, such codes are of limited value for the complex decisions physician-investigators have to make, as we noted in Part Two. Even if they were written in less visionary language, they would need to be surrounded with commentary as well as to be supported by mechanisms allowing for their constant interpretation and reinterpretation. Moreover, mechanisms are also needed for constantly formulating new policies for the many new questions that are raised as soon as such guidelines are promulgated. As yet, procedures have not been devised for these tasks. For example, in 1966 the American Medical Association promulgated its *Ethical Guidelines for Clinical Investigation*,[15] patterned after the World Medical Association's *Declaration of Helsinki*[16] which had been adopted by that body two years earlier. Ironically, it is the significant discrepancy between these two documents that highlights the need for mechanisms which would clarify their meaning and permit their reconciliation.

Unlike the Helsinki Declaration, the AMA guidelines propose that

---

But ethics seminars, where available, are increasingly popular with medical students.

It has been more through the activities and symposia sponsored by such interdisciplinary groups as the Hastings institute than through the efforts of organized medicine that public attention has been focused on questions raised by new biomedical technology. .'. .

Id. More interdisciplinary work is being undertaken at law than at medical schools. *See, e.g.,* J. KATZ, WITH THE ASSISTANCE OF A. CAPRON AND E. GLASS, EXPERIMENTATION WITH HUMAN BEINGS (1972), one recent tangible result of the law-medicine collaboration at the Yale Law School.

[15] AMERICAN MEDICAL ASSOCIATION, OPINIONS AND REPORTS OF THE JUDICIAL COUNCIL 9 (1969) [hereinafter cited as *AMA Guidelines*].

[16] 271 NEW ENG. J. MED. 473 (1964) [hereinafter cited as *Helsinki*].

"[m]inors or mentally incompetent subjects may be used as subjects only if [t]he nature of the investigation is such that mentally competent adults would not be suitable subjects."[17] On the other hand, the *Declaration of Helsinki* states, and the AMA guidelines do not, that "[a]t any time during the course of clinical research the subject or his guardian should be free to withdraw permission for research to be continued."[18] No explanation is provided for the differences nor is any mechanism available to guide physician-investigators in adopting or rejecting part or all of either document, based on its disagreement with the other or for any additional reasons. Beyond their discrepancies, both documents suffer from vagueness of language which generally afflicts all such prescriptions. Take the following from the AMA statement: "Ordinarily consent should be in writing except where the physician deems it necessary to rely upon consent in other than written form because of the physical or emotional state of the patient."[19] This prompts such unanswered questions as: If the emotional state of the patient requires "consent in other than written form," is the only difference between the two the signature of the patient to such a document? If so, why should the emotional state preclude that? Or does it mean that the consent differs in other ways as well, and if so how? Moreover, what are the criteria for the nature of the physical or emotional conditions which allow for dispensing with written consent?

An initial attempt to provide a mechanism for elaborating on the generalized advice contained in codes of ethics has been made by the Surgeon General of the United States Public Health Service through a requirement of "peer group review" committees in institutions conducting PHS-funded research; this method was subsequently taken up, with modification, by the National Institutes of Health and the Food and Drug Administration.[20] As described in Chapter Seven, each institution is required to establish procedures for prior approval of research protocols involving human subjects. The basic development is a hopeful one, in that physician-investigators are provided with some organized means of testing their ideas, on both scientific and ethical grounds, prior to commencing their intervention. As has been noted, however, there are a number of weaknesses: First, the system only extends to research; second, there are indications that in a large majority

---

17 *AMA Guidelines,* note 15 *supra,* at 11.

18 *Helsinki,* note 16 *supra,* at 473.

19 *AMA Guidelines,* note 15 *supra,* at 11.

20 W. H. Stewart (Surgeon General), *Memorandum to the Heads of Institutions Conducting Research with Public Health Grants* (1966); PUBLIC HEALTH SERVICE, U.S. DEP'T OF HEALTH, EDUCATION & WELFARE, PROTECTION OF THE INDIVIDUAL AS A RESEARCH SUBJECT (1969); Food and Drug Administration, *Institutional Committee Review of Clinical Investigations of New Drugs in Human Beings,* 36 FED. REG. 5037 (1971).

of the institutions the guidelines have been less than vigorously applied;[21] third, strong commitment to the committee mechanism is necessary to counterbalance all the natural incentives to avoid it;[22] fourth, the guidelines by which the institutional review committees work are sufficiently vague that if the committees are left to their own devices, as they have been, the members would have to devote an inordinate amount of time and intellectual commitment to the task of putting substance into the general promulgations made by HEW and contained in ethical codes if they were to take their assignment seriously and be successful at it. This can hardly be expected and in fact has not occurred.

An example in the catastrophic disease area of a policy formulation which goes beyond an ethical code addressed to individual physicians is provided by the National Academy of Sciences' statement on cardiac transplantation in man.[23] This document sets forth very well criteria that should be met by institutions before their staff attempts to carry out cardiac transplants. But with respect to the selection of donors and recipients the statement only noted that this "extremely sensitive and complicated subject is now under intensive study by a number of well-qualified groups in this country and abroad" and admonished each institution that "it behooves [it] to assure itself that it has protected the interests of all parties involved to the fullest possible extent."[24]

What emerges from these examples is a picture of policies which need procedures to breathe life into them and to overcome the vagueness of their prescriptions. We appreciate the expressed concern that more definitive policies will prematurely freeze positions, but we suspect another reason for this state of affairs—namely, that existing bodies have given insufficient consideration to the possibility of formulating policies which are meaningful and yet allow for flexibility, because to do so would be to invite greater societal scrutiny of their conduct which has until now been largely beyond the purview of nonprofessionals.[25]

---

[21] *See* B. BARBER, J. LALLY, J. MAKARUSHKA & D. SULLIVAN, RESEARCH ON HUMAN SUBJECTS 163 (1973). The review committee was more likely to be "very well received," however, when it reviewed *all* (not just NIH-sponsored) research and when unanimous agreement among committee members was needed for a project to be approved. *Id.* at 165-66.

[22] Melmon, Grossman & Morris, *Emerging Assets and Liabilities of a Committee on Human Welfare and Experimentation*, 282 NEW ENG. J. MED. 427 (1970).

[23] Board of Medicine, NAS, *Statement on Cardiac Transplantation*, 18 NEWS REPORT OF THE NATIONAL ACADEMY OF SCIENCES, March 1968, at 1 [hereinafter cited as *NAS Statement*].

[24] *Id.* at 3.

[25] *Cf.* K. DAVIS, DISCRETIONARY JUSTICE: A PRELIMINARY INQUIRY (1969); Shapiro, *The Choice of Rulemaking or Adjudication in the Development of Administrative Policy*, 78 HARV. L. REV. 721 (1965).

C. FORMULATING POLICY—WHO AND WHAT?

A major task confronting decisionmakers in the catastrophic disease process is the formulation of better policies. It is beyond the scope of this book either to specify all the policies which need to be formulated or to work out in detail all the issues that need be considered for each problem area. Nevertheless, by selecting a few of these issues for more detailed discussion, we would like to indicate the direction of our thinking and of the analytic work which needs to be done. Three general questions should be kept in mind: What policies should be formulated, how should these policies be formulated, and who should formulate them?

A major objective of this book is to identify those decisions that most fully promote and protect the interests, values, and ends of the catastrophic disease participants. Nevertheless, concern with the ultimate outcome should not diminish the attention given to the means of decisionmaking for a number of reasons. First, the content of any decision is largely dependent on the people and institutions that make it and the procedures they follow. Since all the issues which deserve resolution cannot be anticipated, achieving "good" decisions requires designing a system which employs the means and participants most likely to advance the interests one believes are correct. Second, the choice of decisionmakers and methods is itself a value choice which can have a greater impact, for better or worse, on the interests of medicine, subject, and society than that of any particular decision. Finally, the focus on "who" and "how" highlights the need to examine decisionmaking from the vantage points of those who are given authority and of those who give the authority.

What follows is largely formed and informed by what seems to us a central fact of catastrophic disease treatment: scarcity. Of course, on closer examination scarcity exists in all areas of medicine. But the dramatic aspects of such scarcity are especially pronounced when it can lead to disabling illness and death, and this drama throws a spotlight on the importance of the pervasive question: Who will make the decisions and by what means? We begin our exploration with an examination of the distinctions which can be drawn along the wide range of medical interventions (from basic research to unquestioned therapy). Even that discussion is influenced, though not determined, by the problems raised by scarce resources.

1. Drawing Distinctions between Points in the Process

a. Basic v. Applied Research. The distinction often drawn in scientific circles between basic and applied research is of little significance for our inquiries. The amount of "basic" as compared to "applied" research is much smaller in medicine than in other scientific fields. In large part this simply reflects the fact that all of medicine is primarily an applied science focused on the tasks of curing disease and alleviating the suffering it causes.

Moreover, the possible distinction between fundamental and applied research is of little use in this context for a number of reasons. First, the same issues of risks v. benefits to the human subjects occur no matter what the research is labelled. Second, if a theoretical difference does exist, it is very difficult to make out in practice. The movement along the spectrum from very theoretical to very applied biomedical research appears to be more rapid than in other areas of science. Some of this results from the nature of the science being pursued, and some seems to be a consequence of the fortuitous fact that most medical research (except pharmacology) is conducted in university settings in close proximity to other research in the life sciences. As a committee of the National Academy of Sciences recently observed:

> The hospital-based medical school is constantly concerned with the human problems that present themselves daily. But the clinical faculty lives cheek by jowl with the medical sciences faculty, and they, in turn, are a bridge to the chemistry, physics, and biology departments of the campus. There need be no organizational barrier to progress from initial observation, to research, to development, and then to skills and knowledge of the others. In this sense, medical research may be unique in that fundamental research in virtually all other disciplines must leave the campus for its development, application, and field testing.[26]

The NAS committee shows that the interaction which takes place flows in both directions. Laboratory findings are rapidly applied in clinical settings and observations made in the clinic shed light on biological theories and suggest avenues for further inquiry. The area of immunology, which is so centrally related to organ transplantation, as was discussed in Chapter Four, illustrates this phenomenon well. Clinical experience with skin grafting demonstrated the process of tissue rejection and particularly the "second set" phenomenon; these processes were then explored at length in animals, especially the inbred strains of mice developed at the Jackson Memorial Laboratory in the 1920s. The resulting theoretical explanations of the natural phenomena involved were subsequently employed in kidney transplantation, at first with identical donors, using immunosuppressive drugs; this, in turn, has shed light on the whole immunological process and may provide valuable data for cancer therapy.

The difficulties one would thus face in deciding whether a particular

---

[26] BIOLOGY AND THE FUTURE OF MAN 654 (P. Handler ed. 1970).

piece of research is "basic" or "applied" at any moment serves to underline our position that *any* explorations involving human beings should be subject to the policies discussed in this chapter and the administration and review mechanisms described in the succeeding chapters.

b. Bases for Distinguishing Research and Therapy. We also find the traditional distinctions between the experimental and therapeutic stages of biomedicine of limited value. Research has usually been distinguished from therapy on the basis of its unknown risks and on whether pursuit of knowledge (or, more concretely, the accumulation of data) is a major reason for the medical intervention. The recognition that *all* medicine entails unexpected risk has led to such formulations as "the treatment of every patient is an experiment."[27] This, in turn, often shifted the emphasis from risks to a common sense distinction between therapy and biomedical research, based on the finding that a particular procedure has been accepted and is being employed regularly by clinicians in the treatment of their patients.

The "acceptance" criterion raises many problems, *e.g.,* how general must it have become, what weight should be given to what kind of opposition, and the like? At this point, however, instead of seeking answers to these questions, we wish to turn to another issue. Acceptance has often been equated in the literature with availability and thus the label "experimental" has been attached to those procedures which are not yet widely available, although the lack of availability may reflect not only hesitation or ignorance on the part of most physicians about the value of the procedure but also the inability of the health care system to provide the procedure to all who are "suitable" for it. For instance, one member of the so-called "Life and Death Committee" in Seattle (a committee which was established to select hemodialysis recipients because of the scarcity of resources) explained that he was able to reconcile himself to choosing one person over another for dialysis because he could regard the procedure as research, not treatment.

> [W]e are not making a moral choice here—we are picking guinea pigs for experimental purposes. This happens to be true; it also happens to be the way I rationalize my presence on this committee.[28]

This mode of line drawing has the advantage of permitting decisionmakers to avoid facing the fact of deviation from the myth that good health care is "a universal human right."[29] Yet at some point, when a new procedure has moved from experiment to therapy in the primary sense of those

---

[27] *See, e.g.,* Jonas, *Philosophical Reflections on Experimenting with Human Subjects,* 98 DAEDALUS 219, 241 (1969).

[28] Alexander, note 8 *supra,* at 117.

[29] BIOLOGY AND THE FUTURE OF MAN 627 (P. Handler ed. 1970).

words (*i.e.,* greater certainty), strain on continued use of the term "experimental" in the second sense (*i.e.,* scarcity) becomes too great.

A more functional reason for employing the second meaning of the terms research and treatment (*i.e.,* scarce v. available) is that under it research efforts are viewed as being appropriate on a smaller scale than is customary for treatment, and the decision to undertake a research program is seen as a more restricted commitment than one to begin support of therapy. This attitude has merit because in the initial stages of a new medical procedure, scientific and ethical principles require that it be applied to only a limited number of carefully supervised and controlled cases.

Yet such line drawing is hard to maintain in any particular instance. An expenditure of funds for medical research is similar to a capital expenditure; most of its value (and hence its justification) is derived once the capital good, or the new means of treatment, is put to use. Hence, there is tremendous pressure to move from the research to the treatment modality once the possibility of usefulness is suggested. In addition to the desire not to "waste" the investment made in research,[30] an even stronger impetus toward therapeutic application arises from physicians' traditional desire to help their patients in any way they can. This impetus is reenforced not only by curiosity but also by a real sense of frustration over the limitations of existing therapeutic approaches. This is not to say physicians always act upon this desire; on the contrary, every day patients are probably denied hundreds or thousands of potentially beneficial interventions because the personnel or equipment necessary to perform them have been allotted to other patients who are in graver danger or have a more "interesting" case medically or simply have more money or "pull." For the most part these are low visibility decisions involving, for example, patients who are turned away from a hospital because they cannot show financial ability in advance, or patients who are never even referred to a specialist for the same reason; the treatment at issue is often not a new or particularly complicated one. Sometimes—as with organ transplantation or dialysis—the decision to employ or not to employ a new and valuable modality is more visible to the physician, his peers, and the community at large. In such cases it would be extremely difficult to stick to a ruling that a proven biomedical innovation should simply be ignored.

c. The Significance of the Research v. Therapy Distinction. In dwelling on these distinctions it should be clear that more is at stake than merely a couple of labels—"experimental" and "therapeutic." What has commonly been posited is that a great many *consequences* flow from these designa-

---

[30] The knowledge gained by research may be valued by some in its own right, and as such would not, of course, be "wasted" even if it were never used in therapy.

tions: (1) once an intervention has been classified as "therapeutic," it is assumed that the benefits-risks calculation has been resolved decisively in favor of "benefits" so that an individual physician can feel free to employ the procedure with his patients on the basis of his own judgment and without peer review; and (2) greater freedom is delegated to the physician within the traditional physician/patient model of decisionmaking, under which physicians exercise a "therapeutic privilege" to withhold information from patients that would have to be disclosed to subjects in research.

Both of these bases—"risk-benefit" and "consent"—for distinguishing research and therapy have been all too uncritically accepted. As to the former, the degree of risk-benefit cannot consistently be taken as a benchmark for labeling an intervention experimental or therapeutic. First, in situations in which a procedure is without risk or poses only negligible risks it is labelled "experimental" whenever it is carried out primarily to accumulate knowledge, and so forth; thus, some interventions which are called "experimental" have a "better" risk-benefit ratio than some which are "therapeutic." One difference in risks does probably exist, however, in that the risks in research are likely to be less well defined than those in therapy (if we take as one basis of a valid description of research that it involves the exploration of new techniques). But with proper laboratory and animal testing, such "unknown" risks can (and should) nevertheless be kept within a narrow range. And, as is well known, unexpected consequences to patients of many so-called "established" treatment modalities are considerable and therefore therapeutic risks are not always predictable.[31]

The second problem with using "risk-benefit" to differentiate research and therapy is that the view that a procedure labelled "therapeutic" has few risks may lead to its being applied inappropriately precisely because it is no longer subjected to the careful scrutiny which is applied to experimentation.

> Fields of surgery that become separated from a biosciences mission have shown a pernicious tendency to revert to a service-oriented craft—inflexible and misapplied. After 50 years of criticism, routine tonsillectomy in children bewilders the onlooker.[32]

----

[31] A recent example is provided by the discovery, twenty years after the fact, that diethylstilbestrol when used to prevent miscarriages may cause cancer in female offspring when they reach maturity. *See, e.g.,* Langmuir, *New Environmental Factor in Congenital Disease,* 284 NEW ENG. J. MED. 912 (1971); Folkman, *Transplacental Carcinogenesis by Stilbestrol,* 285 NEW ENG. J. MED. 404 (1971).

[32] Moore, *Scientists and Surgeons,* 176 SCIENCE 1100, 1102 n.2 (1972).

Where careful scrutiny is absent or is overwhelmed by the drive to proceed no matter what, experimental procedures may also be carried out in which the risks are not worth taking when compared with the benefits. For example, Dr. Dwight Harken

"Consent" likewise provides an insufficient basis on which to differentiate experimentation and therapy. The bases of this argument were presented at some length in the discussion of the informed consent model of decision-making in Chapter Six. In brief, it is our belief that the therapeutic setting requires as much attention to the full requisites of informed consent as does the experimental. Indeed, in therapeutic contexts the danger is greater that the patient will be unable (for internal and external reasons) to exercise his role as decisionmaker unless the physician is genuinely committed to involving and informing him.[33] Consequently, it would be fallacious to define "therapeutic" as those interventions in which physicians are free to make decisions for their patients because they supposedly know what is in their "best interests."

d. The Transition from Research to Therapy. The central difficulty, however, is not that the significance of the research-therapy distinction has been misunderstood but that it has been accepted almost unquestioningly by physicians under criteria that have never been spelled out. The criteria could not be spelled out because such distinctions serve different functions and the prior question was never raised: For what purposes is the distinction being made? A prime example of the resulting confusion is found in the history of heart transplantation.

From the beginning of their experience with the clinical application of cardiac transplantation techniques in man, surgeons labeled the procedure "therapeutic." Dr. Christiaan Barnard stated that he did not like to call the operation on Louis Washkansky, the first recipient, "an experiment—it was treatment on a sick patient."[34] After three more operations had been performed, he told a national group of transplant specialists in Chicago that "we must now consider heart transplantation as a therapeutic procedure. It is not an experiment that we perform on someone who is otherwise dead— but a form of treatment we offer seriously ill patients."[35] Even after it

---

mentioned at our consultants' meeting that in examining the hearts which had been removed from cardiac transplant recipients in centers around the world, he found that a large number could have been restored through valvular surgery, which carried a risk of about 10 percent, far below that associated with transplantation.

[33] *See* pp. 98-99 and 102-03 *supra.*

[34] TIME, Dec. 29, 1967, at 32.

[35] *Medical News,* 203 J.A.M.A. 39 (Jan. 15, 1968). According to Dr. Denton Cooley, the leading cardiac transplanters assembled at the international Cape Town Conference in July 1968 similarly reached the judgment that the procedure was "an effective therapeutic measure to prolong and improve . . . life [for the patient with end-stage heart disease]." *Minutes of the Cape Town Meeting,* MEDICAL WORLD NEWS, Aug. 9, 1963, at 23. Some scientists took marked exception to this view of the status of cardiac transplantation. *See, e.g.,* A. Fox, *Heart Transplants: Treatment or Experiment,* 159 SCIENCE 374 (1968).

became apparent that few of the transplants were functioning for more than a couple of weeks, the surgeons continued to refer to the operation as therapy.[36] If the function of the distinction between research and therapy is success of the intervention, then clearly it was not therapy; if it is viewed as an attempt to maintain life in an otherwise hopeless situation, it can be labelled therapy.

The problems created by such a lack of clarity of purpose are manifest. Most importantly, many patients—both recipients and donors (and their next of kin)—were apparently seriously misled by unqualified statements on the transplanters' part. Consent was given on the basis that a life was going to be saved—when in fact the real good (if any) which could be expected was an increase in knowledge.[37] As Paul Ramsey has observed:

> When some physicians say that a new radical therapy promises to extend the life of a patient "indefinitely," they mean "unpredictably." Such a physician would be minimally satisfied (while hoping for more) by any length of days that is somewhat more (or maybe longer) than present prognosis or by any available alternative treatment. A member of the public hears him promise more, and this conspires "to push the patient onward" into investigative therapeutic surgery, perhaps without exercising full freedom of human decision that this is a good thing for him to do.[38]

---

[36] N.Y. Times, Sept. 29, 1968, at 10, col. 2 (quoting Dr. Denton A. Cooley). In an article appearing in May 1969 of which he was coauthor, Cooley wrote that cardiac transplantation "is still an investigative procedure with minimal clinical application." Nora, Cooley, et al., *Rejection of the Transplanted Human Heart: Indexes of Recognition and Problems of Prevention*, 280 NEW ENG. J. MED. 1079, 1085 (1969). As Paul Ramsey has observed, there is no way to "know what to make" of Cooley's apparent reversal of views. P. RAMSEY, THE PATIENT AS PERSON 232, n. 20 (1970) [hereinafter cited as RAMSEY].

[37] *See, e.g.,* RAMSEY, note 36 *supra,* at 225:

> The medical profession needs to listen attentively to the words people use, in their ordinary meanings, when they speak about what they have been doing in giving and receiving hearts. Mrs. Virginia May White was overheard by her family to say, while watching a TV news report concerning heart transplants, "How marvelous to give someone a chance to live." Upon her accidental death a few days later, her husband and children quickly agreed that her heart could be transplanted at the Stanford Medical Center into the chest of Mike Kasperak, a 54-year-old retired steel worker, who died 15 days later. Kasperak's wife told reporters that she urged her husband to "go ahead, don't waste any time; I want you alive and with me." Helen Krouch, of Patterson, New Jersey, told her parents while in perfect health, "If I could save someone's life, I would do it. If I knew I were going to die, I'd like to die that way." Upon her death or while dying, she was, as a consequence of this statement, moved so that her heart could be implanted in Louis Block at Maimonides Medical Center in Brooklyn, N.Y. Thereby she may have contributed to the advancement of medical science and the benefit of future patients, but she did not accomplish what she said she was willing to do for Louis Block.

[38] *Id.* at 235.

The greatest problem with the present mode of judging the transition from research to therapy, as illustrated by the heart transplantation example, is not this dislocation of the consent model but the fact that there are no generally agreed upon criteria by which the transplant surgeons' statements can be measured or criticized. Thus, no one else really participates in the determination that a procedure has moved from one category to the other.

We propose that the issue of when an intervention moves from research to therapy should first raise the question: For what purposes need such a distinction be made? Once purpose is articulated it may be easier to establish criteria. For example, if the purpose is to determine which medical interventions should be given prior review by an institutional advisory committee, then distinctions based on risk and consent should largely determine whether committee scrutiny is necessary. Hence, for this purpose we believe the question of the transition to therapy should be reframed in terms of the spectrum from complex high risk procedures for which informed consent will be difficult to obtain to those which are "low risk/easy consent." Under this formulation, interventions (whether labelled "experimental" or "therapeutic") at the former end of the scale would be subject to prior committee review. Such a procedure would have a number of functions. First, it would permit appraisal of the relative risks and benefits of a procedure as to any group of patients (subjects) and evaluation of the capacity of investigators to provide meaningful information to patient-subjects in order to obtain their consent for participation. On the basis of its informed knowledge about the procedure, the institutional advisory committee[39] could also make recommendations on whether and when specific procedures need no longer be regularly reviewed, because the combination of the risk and consent factors are now within an acceptable range.

Second, the policy formulated by the committee could take account of the expertise necessary to conduct a high risk procedure. This seems to be what the Board on Medicine of the National Academy of Sciences had in mind when it issued its guidelines on cardiac transplantation in February 1968. Since, as has been noted, the bases and significance of the labels "experiment" and "therapy" are not clear, the NAS statement first had to argue that while it was appropriate (given prior knowledge) to undertake cardiac transplantation in man, "the procedure cannot as yet be regarded as an accepted form of therapy, even an heroic one."[40] The Academy group then went on to argue that since "there are considerably more institutions whose staffs include men with the surgical expertise appropriate for the

---

[39] *See* Chapter Nine *infra* for a discussion of the proposed functions of the institutional advisory committee.

[40] *NAS Statement*, note 23 *supra*, at 2.

first step of the investigation—the actual transplantation—than have available the full capability to conduct the total study in terms of all relevant scientific observations,"[41] the institutions carrying out the procedure should be limited to those which could meet certain criteria.[42] We believe that such policy guidelines are very much needed, since the lack of definitive therapy for many diseases means that new modalities will be proposed which require a properly qualified and authorized body to indicate the conditions under which the new procedures should be tested and the point at which they can be taken to have superseded prior methods as "standard therapy."

Clearly all novel procedures will have to be evaluated as to where they fall along the "high risk/difficult consent" or "low risk/easy consent" spectrum. This will present no problem for new procedures, but it will require a review of a great many procedures now being employed with human beings in order to determine whether they fall in one group or another. We would like to make clear, if it is not already, that by "difficult consent" we do not mean difficulties encountered with individual patients in obtaining consent which is another issue that must be given separate treatment. We only mean problems of consent arising from either (1) a lack of knowledge about consequences inherent in many novel procedures, (2) the heavy psychological burdens placed on some patients by the nature of their ailment, or (3) a need not to disclose some or all of the background to the patient-subjects because the value of the study would be undermined by such disclosure.

Finally, our suggested method for formulating policy would permit representatives of the general community to participate in the decision about the conditions under which a new procedure would be limited to a trial basis in a few institutions, because society is not yet willing or able to expend the funds necessary to make the procedure generally available to all who may require it.

Thus, in a sense we have not discarded the distinctions between research

---

[41] *Id.*

[42] In brief, the NAS criteria were:

1. That the "team" have had "extensive laboratory experience" so as to possess not only surgical but also biological expertise.

2. That all data on recipients (including lifetime follow-up) be readily available to other investigators through an organized communications network.

3. That the institution protect "the interests of all parties involved to the fullest possible extent," since the procedure is intended to produce new knowledge and is not yet accepted therapy, and the choice of donors and recipients should be reviewed by an independent panel of physicians.

The concept of a board "to determine the surgical and research capabilities of the surgical team and institution" was criticized by some. *See, e.g.,* Brewer, *Cardiac Transplantation: An Appraisal,* 205 J.A.M.A. 691, 692 (1968).

and therapy but substituted for a particular purpose a set of factors along a spectrum which better reflect the need for such distinctions in the evaluation of those aspects of research protocols concerned with safeguarding the rights and welfare of human subjects. In the next section we turn to allocation of resources, and here too we maintain the distinctions between research and therapy. But functionally we now define research as an innovative technique that is being applied to a limited number of cases, and treatment as the application of this technique to larger segments of the patient population.

2. Allocation of Resources for Research

A distinction between research and therapy based on the number of patient-subjects involved, as already discussed, has two consequences for the formulation of policies on the allocation of resources for research. First, to the greatest extent possible, an effort should be made at the time that research is contemplated to evaluate the cost of implementing the therapeutic advances which are the aim of the research. Such predictions will often be difficult to make and their accuracy will frequently be problematic, since the full scope of a research project and all the applications of its products are often hard to anticipate. Yet the effort is a vital one if we are not simply to repeat the errors of the past; in some instances the "social cost" of developing a new treatment and then failing to make it widely available may be much greater than simply permitting the disease in question to go untreated or to be treated by the less successful means already at hand. Given the immediacy of the suffering experienced by persons afflicted by the kinds of illnesses discussed in this book, such an assertion is hard to make and may even seem inhumane. Yet it may be better to die of thirst in a barren desert than within sight of an oasis at which others are drinking—better, in the sense of being less painful and less destructive of value adherence, both for the individuals involved and for the society which countenances the spectacle. Perhaps this is too extreme a posture for it could impede research which may eventually turn out to be less costly than initially contemplated. At least, however, this approach facilitates a clear-headed attitude toward the costs of new procedures and will encourage decisionmakers to restrict a new procedure to a limited, "experimental" scale until there is public support for the cost of implementing the procedure on a broad clinical scale.

Second, in order to know when to proceed with research, policy also needs to be formulated on the types of societal "side-effects" which are either unacceptable or which at the least require advance discussion by persons outside the biomedical research establishment. For example, if a totally implantable artificial heart were to be developed, what would happen to our present concepts of life and death and how would the decision be reached when to recharge or replace (or *not* to recharge or replace) such a unit? Should a patient's unwillingness (for religious or other reasons) to consent to an autopsy be a valid reason for refusing to give him an artificial heart? Such questions deserve advance discussion, and the policies which will govern the application of this type of innovation should be articulated, at least in an initial formulation, before the first case is presented as a medical *fait accompli.*

   a. *Judging Research on the Basis of Future Benefits.* Little need be said here about the policies which require formulation to guide the setting of priorities for the allocation of funds and personnel for research. The adequacy of the methods and standards employed by the Public Health Service have been addressed elsewhere.[43] We note in passing that since Congress appropriates the majority of funds for medical research, at least these elected representatives of the public can be involved in this aspect of decisionmaking. Suffice it to say that it is difficult to base allocation on predicted "usefulness," since a so-called "useless" pursuit may illuminate a problem in another research area. If the research phase is limited to a small number of patient-subjects, costs may not be very great and thus it may prove to be wise rarely, if ever, to preclude the exploration of a new area of applied research entirely but instead to restrict the funding to a few investigators if the project is considered of low priority.

   The difficulties in attempting to calculate the amount to be spent on research are illustrated by the work of the President's Commission on Heart Disease, Cancer, and Stroke. The commissioners first calculated the direct expenditures made for patients with these three conditions by way of hospital and nursing home care, professional fees, drugs, and so forth. This amounted to some $4.28 billion as of 1962. But, as they noted, "direct costs are only the beginning."[44] By far the largest component of their $42.8 billion estimated total was the "burden to the economy, owing to loss of output"[45] of all those who would have been alive during 1962 had they not died during the previous 60 years of these three conditions. Such a calculation seems questionable at best, however. First, it assumes the complete elimination of all effects (including disabilities short of death) of these diseases. Second, when one is talking about diseases which account

---

   [43] *See, e.g.,* R. Zeckhauser, Some Thoughts on the Allocation of Resources in Bio-Medical Research (1967) (Occasional Paper No. 4, Office of Ass't. Secty. for Planning and Evaluation, HEW).

   [44] President's Commission on Heart Disease, Cancer, and Stroke, A National Program to Conquer Heart Disease, Cancer, and Stroke 5 (1964).

   [45] *Id.*

for 70 percent of all deaths, it is questionable to presume that all persons saved from death by these diseases would live out a full work-life, and if they did not that any loss of their expected years of productivity should be counted as the "cost" of another disease instead. Third, there are obvious difficulties in estimating the value of lost labor in an economy which has a surplus, rather than a shortage, of manpower.

A graver problem with such an approach is that it values lives only in terms of their productive output for society, without taking account of the intangible value which is usually given to life itself and to the relief of suffering. Moreover, a policy which decided which *research* to pursue on the basis of predicted economic and productive gains to society would spell trouble once the innovation moved beyond research to *therapy:* There are strong indications (which will be discussed hereafter) that society is uncomfortable in having decisions about the allocation of lifesaving treatment based on the relative productivity or economic output of the persons needing care. In sum, then, policies for deciding about the "scientific payoff" of competing research proposals may raise problems if they rely, even implicitly, on valuations of how much economic benefit society will reap from the successful development of the technique being studied. On the other hand, policies formulated simply in terms of lives saved or suffering reduced may appear too vague to stand up against competing demands (medical and nonmedical) for the scarce dollar, especially in an age which places such great faith in "cost/benefit analysis" and other tools of rational, economic planning.

b. Choosing Subjects for Research. Thus far we have spoken of research in terms of the "usefulness" of its results rather than the "propriety" of its process. Too often it seems to be forgotten that policy also needs to be formulated on the selection of subjects for research. In practice, research subjects are usually chosen by the same mechanism as patients are selected for scarce treatments, since the present system does not draw a firm line between the stages in the process of developing a new modality. For example, the committee in Seattle which chose people with renal failure for the first chronic dialysis program is usually viewed as a device for "patient" selection (and is discussed as such in subsection 3(c) later in this chapter). But, as has already been noted, it viewed itself as a mechanism of selection for an experiment as well.[46]

The basic failure in this area has stemmed from our collective unwillingness to discuss openly the obligation of members of society to participate in experiments. It is rarely stated forthrightly that patients (especially in "hopeless" cases) should participate in research when asked to do so,

---

[46] *See* text accompanying note 28 *supra.*

although this is the message which is conveyed, directly or indirectly, to individual patients. A patient may prefer an existing treatment with a known risk over an experimental technique of unknown risk, or vice versa, although for the good of *all* patients (especially future ones) new techniques should be tested if there are reasonable indications that they will provide a better benefit/risk ratio than present treatments. Rather than leaving it up to individual physician-investigators to select groups of patients for participation "for the good of mankind," we believe a rational policy should be developed to control subject selection. Questions must be asked and answered as to whether subjects should be drawn from the category of "patients" or from a broader group; whether all who consent to treatment at designated centers should be randomized for assignment to conventional or experimental modalities; and whether it is proper to offer subjects compensation, perhaps in the form of not charging them for the experimental therapy and paying for any resulting injuries. Such policies must be formulated by a broadly constituted body.

3. Allocation of Resources for Therapy

The extent of support for research on catastrophic diseases raises some problems, but even greater difficulties have to be faced at the stages of allocating funds for treatment. Indeed, to recapitulate, some of the most important questions about research support are posed by the eventual development of new and expensive treatment modalities which the health care system does not have the financial ability (or desire) to deliver to all who need them. In this section, we address directly questions of choice about treatment: what to treat and whom to treat?

a. Choosing Diseases to Treat. A fundamental question immediately arises: *Should* policies about which diseases to treat[47] be formulated at all? As a society, we believe in rationality and orderliness. Yet we also possess the capacity to deny reality and to cling to myths whenever the price dictated by rationality is too high. The conscious articulation of a policy by which we collectively decide which types of suffering to treat and which not to treat may be a very costly undertaking emotionally and politically. If this endeavor holds no real probability of success or would be too disruptive, we might wish to abandon it. Then the decisions made will remain

---

[47] It should be noted that policies on which *diseases* to treat may be formulated in such a fashion that they in fact become disguised decisions about which *people* to treat, since many diseases occur with much greater frequency among certain, definable population groups. While this factor may have important ramifications, we do not address it here; the problems raised by acknowledged and unacknowledged choices between patients are discussed in subsection c *infra*.

ambiguous and their bases and the relationships among them will remain unclear to decisionmakers and public alike.

The absence of a clearly formulated policy does not necessarily mean that "good" decisions cannot be reached. We have no societal policy on the relative levels of consumption of most products, and yet orderly decisions are made on them through the market. In his consultant's report, Guido Calabresi remarks:

> We feel relatively comfortable with this decisionmaking device (a) because we believe that the demand for each type of shoe [for example] and the cost (in other activities foregone) and hence the supply of shoes can be expressed adequately in money terms; (b) because in this area we believe that societal costs and benefits from each type of shoe can on the whole be made a part of the market structure facing individual buyers and producers (*i.e.*, there are few externalities, either monetary or moral); (c) because little present-future choice is involved; (d) because whatever effects unequal income distribution has on choices can probably be more effectively handled directly through income redistribution than by collective decisions as to the number of resources to be dedicated to leather shoes v. sneakers.[48]

If the choice of which diseases to treat were a decision that met Calabresi's criteria, then decisionmaking could be left to the market. Medical decisions have traditionally been handled in this fashion, with the portion of national income devoted to health care and the portion of health care allocated for the treatment of each disease reflecting the interaction of patient's demands, physicians' wishes, and the opportunity costs of the goods and services employed. This method has obvious advantages, primarily by avoiding the expense and other burdens of a collective decisionmaking mechanism and relying on individuals as the best rankers of their own preferences.

There are, however, problems in leaving allocation of medical resources to the "invisible hand" of the market, and these are exacerbated in dealing with catastrophic diseases. First, it is difficult to place a dollar value on life and health, since neither can "be expressed adequately in money terms." Hence, the "supply" of patients who are willing to die at a given "price" (or, rather, would choose not to be saved at a cost above that point) is hard to evaluate.

Second, "externalities" influence the decisions (*i.e.*, costs which must be borne by someone, often society at large, but which do not enter the calculations of the primary decisionmakers in the market). Moreover, in deciding about which diseases to treat, many of the externalities are difficult to state in monetary terms. For example, the community's professed devotion to the preservation of human life "at any price" has a value, although it

---

[48] Calabresi, consultant's memorandum, at 2 (1970) [Appendix A].

would be difficult to quantify that value or specify the amount by which it is eroded through any particular choice of which diseases to treat and which not to treat. On the other hand, some externalities may cause too many resources, rather than too few, to be devoted to the treatment of a catastrophic disease. Richard Zeckhauser points out that the "markets for medical services are plagued by all sorts of imperfections."[49] Since most health services, particularly in the area of major illness, are provided through nonprofit institutions, concern for the prestige associated with a "diverse" and "innovative" treatment capability may have a greater impact on decisions than economic considerations do, since "the medical services and prices offered by hospitals may not reflect even approximate real resource costs. Hospital charges should hardly be used as a guide to policy decisions."[50]

Third, as Calabresi notes, the choice of saving X lives now rather than $X + Y$ lives in the future complicates decisionmaking. Outside of such rudimentary areas as saving money for the benefit of our potential descendants or our own "rainy day," we are not particularly adept at weighing future versus present costs and benefits:

> To the extent that the benefits of our allocation result from the saving of future rather than present lives (i.e., research), we can expect difficulties apart from the problem of preserving more general values. . . . The decision for research expenditures with respect to casastrophic diseases . . . forces us to decide how many lives today we are willing to forego (by funding research and thus failing to use for present life saving all the resources which we will dedicate to catastrophic diseases) in order to save more people in future generations.[51]

A further difficulty with total reliance on the market is that the harsh effects of income inequality make us particularly uncomfortable when they differentiate access to a service as essential as health care. In such circumstances, we may not be satisfied to wait until the problem is "handled directly through income redistribution," especially since even with equal income distribution not all people would have to devote a large share of their finances to health care but a few will need sums for lifesaving therapy which exceed the financial capabilities of any but the very wealthy.

A final reason, not mentioned by Calabresi, why the market system is likely not to be very satisfactory is that the goods and services in question, particularly the new and scarce ones, are regarded to a certain extent as

---

[49] Zeckhauser, *Catastrophic Illness* (consultant's memorandum), at 15 (1972) [Appendix L].

[50] *Id.* at 33.

[51] Calabresi, note 48 *supra*, at 4-5.

public goods, especially since they were developed with direct or indirect public support.[52] Furthermore, physicians see themselves as the guardians of the public as well as healers of individual patients; due to their expertise and to legal protections, they can enforce a "monopoly" over certain procedures. For example, when chronic hemodialysis was begun in Seattle, the physicians involved clearly regarded this new-found capability as a community asset, to be given to those who would derive "the most benefit" and not to be allocated by individual physicians on the basis of attempting to save only "their own" patients. Moreover, while members of the medical profession are well rewarded in the marketplace, they seem to regard the idea that the market could allocate all health care funds as distasteful if, for example, it were to involve a marketplace in organs, with suppliers offering paired and unpaired organs at a price.[53] Consequently, the profession chooses to keep a tight rein on the way the "game" is played to prevent such practices from developing, although they would follow from a logical extension of the market model.

If in place of the market we turn to collective decisionmaking to determine at least some of the allocation decisions on the treatment of disease, what sorts of policies can be formulated to guide these decisions? C. E. Lindblom sounds a cautionary note:

> For the design of improved decision-making processes to govern research and therapy for catastrophic diseases, there are no available formulae, no established guidelines, no standard blueprints, no decision-making procedures in comparable problem areas that can simply be copied. We know a good deal about organizations, collective problem solving, decision-making proc-

---

[52] Collective funding of research represents an attempt to overcome the market's inability, noted earlier, to take into account individuals' desire that new treatments be developed for which they are unwilling to pay since they may (or may not) actually need these treatments themselves in the future.

[53] When the question of allowing donors to sell *paired* organs arose at our consultant's meeting, the physicians dismissed the idea as unthinkable. The conflict was highlighted in a recent article:

> If it is permissible to remove organs from living persons with their consent, may such persons sell their organs? Today blood is often sold by blood "donors." Commentators are not agreed as to whether the sale of an organ that could produce a permanent deficiency in the donor should be permitted. In a recent symposium, G. A. Leach, science correspondent of the *New Statesman*, suggested "that selling one's organs is ethically acceptable (though perhaps not socially desirable)." However, Dr. Jean Hamburger of Paris, one of the leading transplant surgeons, thought that the "basic rule must be to avoid any kind of pressure (including financial) on the prospective donor," and therefore sales should not be permitted.

Sanders and Dukeminier, *Medical Advance and Legal Lag: Hemodialysis and Kidney Transplantation*, 15 U.C.L.A. Rev. 357, 390 (1968).

esses, public administration, public policy making and politics; but all our information taken together is far from giving us specific design and guidelines for complex decision making. What is required, therefore, is the art of practical judgment, at best only supported but never displaced by our social scientific knowledge.[54]

With this advice in mind, we believe that general conclusions can be reached on two points. First, that representatives of the public must be involved in the formulation of policy on allocation. Such a suggestion is often proposed these days, but usually without any attempt to articulate the basis on which decisions are to be made other than those which physicians and other scientists are already competent to handle. An elementary reason for including nonphysicians is that they hold the purse strings. For example, Senator Abraham Ribicoff met Christiaan Barnard's insistence for a "hands-off" policy with the argument that heart transplantation "has become a public issue because the public is paying the cost—society as a whole is paying the general costs. . . ."[55] A more significant reason is that since the judgment of which types of diseases most threaten societal well-being rests more on value choices than scientific knowledge, it is appropriate for it to be made by the public rather than by physicians alone.[56] Indeed, this sort of allocation decision is handled, at least in broad outline, by Congress already, with further refinements provided by the officials of the Department of Health, Education and Welfare.

A second general conclusion is that the treatment of a catastrophic disease is more likely to be supported as its marginal cost decreases compared with its marginal return, a calculation which generally includes the benefit derived from a visible affirmation of society's commitment to saving life. In other words, the more identifiable both the patients and the means of treatment are, the greater the percentage allocation of funds to that disease. "As we approach a situation where all or virtually *all* the lives in an acceptable category come close to being saved, given the resources we are willing to make available, the value of the remaining lives will increase dramatically so that a jump to 'total' life saving (in the category) is likely to

---

[54] Lindblom, *New Decision-Making Procedures Governing Research on and Treatment of Catastrophic Diseases* (consultant's memorandum), at 1-2 (1970) [Appendix C].

[55] *Hearings on S. J. Res. 145 (National Commission on Health Science and Society) before the Subcomm. on Government Research of the Senate Comm. on Government Operations,* 90th Cong., 2d Sess., at 8-82 (1968) [hereinafter cited as *National Commission on Health Science and Society*].

[56] The need for a collective choice is a further reflection of the problem of "externalities" mentioned earlier. For example, an increase in the level of treatment may not only benefit those treated but also other members of society, since it is more pleasant to live in a society without certain kinds of distressing illnesses.

occur."[57] The extension of Medicare payments to pay for hemodialysis or renal transplantation under §2991 of the 1972 Social Security Act Amendments bears out this analysis.[58]

b. Catastrophic v. Other Diseases. The foregoing suggests that certain particular characteristics of catastrophic diseases will tend to distort the process of collective formulation of policy about allocation of resources for treatment. The immediacy and avoidability of death as a consequence of nontreatment, particularly when the lives of known individuals are at stake, puts these decisions on a different level than many other medical ones. Consequently, it is not surprising that one of the major questions raised by the treatment of catastrophic diseases is whether or not too many resources are being devoted to this area. As one commentator queried during the early enthusiasm over transplantation:

> The development of borrowed and artificial vital organs presents a new instance of an old problem; how to distribute scarce resources justly. Medical care is a scarce resource; quality care, especially so. Is large-scale transplantation the best use of these limited resources?[59]

The cost of treating catastrophic illness is by definition so great that many people could receive ordinary medical attention for the same amount that is needed to care for one with a catastrophic disease. The federal government, the major single source of medical funds, does not usually cover a citizen's medical bills, unless he is indigent[60] *or* is receiving innovative therapy supported by a research grant. Thus, the question is clearly posed whether the health needs of the ordinary patient or of the person burdened by a catastrophic illness should be met. "A public commitment of $1 billion could buy enough kidney dialysis centers to serve 25,000 persons in the next decade—or it could provide ambulatory care of a general nature for 1.2 million poor people."[61]

---

[57] Calabresi, consultant's memorandum, at 5-6 (1970) [Appendix A]. Zeckhauser describes this as a function of the preservation of life at all costs myth being an "on-off variable," which operates on an all-or-nothing (rather than graduated) basis. Zeckhauser, *Catastrophic Illness* at 23-24 (1972) [Appendix L].

[58] Pub. L. No. 92-603, §2991 (October 30, 1972).

[59] Kass, *Caveat on Transplants*, Washington Post, Jan. 14, 1968, at B-1, col. 5.

[60] An indigent person's medical expenses may be met by the government in a number of ways—through various forms of public assistance ("welfare"), Medicaid, Vocational Rehabilitation payments, or by treatment at Veterans' Administration hospitals, at public or private hospitals supported under the Hill-Burton Act which mandates "a reasonable volume of services to persons unable to pay therefore," 42 U.S.C. §291 (c) (3) (1970), or at community health centers established by the Office of Economic Opportunity, 42 U.S.C. §2811 (1970). *Cf.* Euresti v. Stenner, 458 F.2d 1115 (10th Cir. 1972).

[61] Sen. Walter F. Mondale quoted in *What Price Transplanted Organs?*, MEDICAL WORLD NEWS, June 28, 1968, at 29.

In outline, the issue can be stated as a choice between giving full treatment (which will often be lifesaving) to the few who suffer from terminal and devastating illnesses or providing routine medical care to a far greater number of persons, some of whom may not even really need medical attention and almost none of whom would be conspicuous enough by the nature of his or her condition at that time to come into the public eye were treatment not given. Of course, general medical care and catastrophic disease treatment are not unrelated: Greater attention to the preventive aspect of regular medical care might reduce the incidence of some types of catastrophic illness substantially. Such considerations should not be disregarded, but they cannot alone determine the outcome of choices concerning *current* sufferers. The policy choice thus turns on the question: Which is worse, severe suffering and death for a few or minor suffering with perhaps some disability for many? The answer presently being given is: Both are bad, and the "solution" appears to be to increase the amount of money spent on health care, with the goal of providing care, of both routine and extraordinary types, to all, regardless of ability to pay.[62]

Until such time as full health protection, including "major medical" coverage, is provided to all, questions of choice will remain. In deciding which diseases to treat, economic evaluations are possible, but they will probably not provide very exact guides.[63] Thus, the choice to fund certain treatments and neglect others will probably continue to remain largely a matter of chance and politics, which lends further support to our basic argument that the allocation should be handled by public bodies rather than by "experts" alone.

c. Selection of Treatment Recipients. As long as support of catastrophic disease treatment remains inadequate or depends on nonfinancial factors (such as the availability of organs for transplantation), choices will have to be made among possible recipients of treatment. Unlike the resolution of the "macroeconomic" questions discussed in the preceding subsections, a policy of "muddling through" seems less likely to be satisfactory in making the "micro" choices involved in, for example, allocating time in a dialysis treatment center's schedule to *A* rather than to *B, C,* or *D.* What we need are statements of policy on who should be selected and on the means by which they should be chosen. In what follows we examine the strengths and weaknesses of a number of possible avenues of patient selection and conclude with suggestions on the way in which policy should be formulated.

---

[62] This is the stated purpose of all the health care proposals currently being considered in Congress.

[63] *See* the discussion at pp. 241-45 *supra.*

i. THE MARKET. Perhaps it would be simplest to make the treatment resources available to those who wish to purchase them. Kidney dialysis is presently being handled in this fashion on a limited scale by a number of "health care" corporations. The most active of these, National Medical Care, Inc., is in the process of doubling its present capacity of 4,500 dialysis treatments a week in 29 "satellite" centers across the country.[64] Although most of the patients cared for in such facilities are not paying for their treatment entirely out of their own funds (*i.e.,* they receive some support from health insurance, federal funds, and state vocational rehabilitation), the system is still a "market" one, with the price charged being set roughly by the interplay of the cost of providing the services and the demand for them.

Rather than having individuals bid for the limited number of treatment slots available, an alternative market system would extend the right to each person for a portion of the treatment, the size of the portion calculated so that the number of options would use up, but not exceed, treatment capacity. Those who needed the treatment and had the funds would then buy from others the portions necessary to get treated. Although the price would lead some of the poorer patients to sell their options rather than purchasing the whole treatment, this market system, however unacceptable, is slightly better than the first, "since the effect of income distribution is somewhat mitigated where people are allowed to sell rights to life instead of having to buy them."[65] Calabresi goes on to note that nevertheless,

> as the choice more obviously involves lives, even the right-to-sell market becomes unacceptable. We can, for instance, usefully contrast whether we allow (1) people to sell their blood (minimal risk to life), (2) sell a kidney (somewhat greater risk to life), (3) be one of three people who for a price take one chance in three of having to give their heart for a transplant (⅓

---

[64] This discussion is based largely on information obtained in a 1972 interview with Dr. George L. Bailey of the kidney dialysis unit at the Peter Bent Brigham Hospital in Boston. The artificial kidney center run by National Medical Care, Inc., in Brookline, Mass., is operated as an affiliate of the hospital under a contract which provides for the supervision of the center's operations by that hospital. The affiliate relationship was required by Massachusetts law (subsequently amended); similar regulations on out-of-hospital dialysis exist in California. The conflict-of-interest charges raised concerning the participation of hospital staff members in a profit-making health care company (when physicians responsible for the hospital's own dialysis program are officers and substantial shareholders in the company providing dialysis) are not germane to our analysis. Since the adoption of the 1972 Social Security Act amendments the number of private, profitmaking dialysis centers has grown rapidly; National Medical Care, Inc., estimates that approximately 95 percent of all patients have their dialysis paid in whole or in part by Medicare.

[65] Calabresi, consultant's memorandum, at 13 (1970) [Appendix A].

chance of selling a life) and (4) a straight deal under which a man sells his heart for a transplant.[66]

In the present hypothetical case, of course, the confrontation with life-selling is less direct than in Calabresi's examples, since what is being sold is an option on a portion of a potentially lifesaving treatment. On balance, however, this distinction, and indeed the distinction between the "selling" and "buying" markets, probably makes little difference in our evaluation of the primary characteristic of the market: While it permits individuals to give expression to their desire to expend their resources on preserving their own lives versus other expenditures, the spectacle of desperate patients bidding against each other for limited treatment facilities would be destructive of the myth of our collective attachment to the incomparable value of human life.

The market could also be modified from one in which catastrophic disease treatment is purchased to one trading in "contingent claims,"[67] that is, the purchase of insurance so that treatment resources will be available if one needs them. Since people would not be in actual need at the time of purchase, the problems of desperation bidding and of placing a dollar value on life would be avoided. The future nature of the payoff creates some difficulties, however. For one, there is the practical difficulty of knowing the quantity of treatment resources needed at any future time.[68] Second, a contingent claims market is biased in favor of the cautious person, the per-

---

[66] *Id.*

[67] *See* Zeckhauser, *Catastrophic Illness*, at 5 (1972) [Appendix L]. Calabresi refers to the same arrangement as a "market in risks." Calabresi, consultant's memorandum, at 17 (1970) [Appendix A]:

In effect a market in risks permits (and requires) the individual to view his own life in statistical terms. It thus has consequences similar to those observable in all calculations concerning "statistical lives": it avoids the distortions caused by the extreme concern (perhaps brought on by fear, guilt, etc.) manifest for the identifiable threatened life but it decreases the ability to view potential injuries as affecting human lives at all. The latter aspect may be somewhat mitigated in the case of an individual thinking about future risks to *himself* rather than the collectivity contemplating potential injury to unidentified people in his midst (e.g., victims of accidents at grade crossings).

[68] The problem of "adverse selection" (*i.e.*, sickly people buy more health insurance than healthy people), which always complicates prediction on insurance, is somewhat mitigated, because people are unlikely to know of their own increased (or decreased) likelihood of needing treatment of this type. Similarly, "adverse incentives" (*i.e.*, a person with insurance is more likely to develop the insured-against condition) will also probably not interfere here as much as with insurance for less serious health problems. *See* Zeckhauser, *Catastrophic Illness* at 6-8 (1972) [Appendix L].

son willing to forego present enjoyment for future safety.[69] Consequently, a third problem arises: At the time of the "payoff," treatment resources may be devoted to saving A, who is only moderately attached to living but enough so that he will accept treatment since he has already paid for it through insurance, rather than saving B, who wants desperately to live but who failed to insure against catastrophic illness. If the "contingent claims" market is strictly enforced so that there is no way for B to obtain treatment, there would probably be few public reverberations from his desire to do so, since there would be no present forum in which he could make a spectacle of himself frantically bidding (against C and D and other noninsureds) the price of treatment higher and higher.[70] But an open system of sales, or a black market, could arise in which some "winners" in the insurance scheme (*i.e.,* those who purchased a contingent claim on catastrophic disease treatment and then developed such a disease) would sell their rights to the highest bidder. That practice could be equally, or more, destructive than ordinary "desperation bidding." To avoid this phenomenon, the payoff could be in monetary terms (like the "major medical" coverage some people now have), rather than directly as a share of treatment resources. Unfortunately, such a system would not guarantee adequate facilities and would therefore leave open the danger of desperation bidding, by both the insured and (depending on their means) the uninsured.

As disconcerting as the spectacle would be, it might still be tolerable if we felt that it were the method most likely to reach the "right" allocation of treatment resources. But it does not represent a true expression of a desire to live, since a rich person would have to devote only a small percentage of his wealth to offer a price for the treatment which would exceed the amount which could be offered by a poor person who was willing to give all that he possessed to purchase the treatment. The economist's theory of the market in part postulates that through the expression of individual choice a distribution of goods and services can be arrived at which is optimal for society. Thus the market in catastrophic disease treatment would be less bothersome if we were confident that a man's wealth accu-

---

[69] If people's willingness to take risks vary (as one might suppose) by their wealth category, further difficulties are presented in constructing a "wealth neutral" market when the goods traded are "contingent."

[70] For this to be true, the policy against giving treatment to noninsured persons would have to be strictly, even ruthlessly, enforced. Any deviation would open the prospect that a patient could—if he were sufficiently importunate—get the treatment without insurance. One obvious potential hole in the dike is research: Some uninsured patients would be offered experimental treatment; indeed this is not too different from the current situation where patients in research programs are often treated "free" and regardless of their ability (or inability) to pay for conventional therapy.

rately reflected his worth to society, so the fact that a large percentage of rich people received the scarce lifesaving treatment could be said to result from their being more valuable. Yet such a premise would be dismissed out of hand by most people today, both as a factual matter and as a deviation from our collective ethic of equality of all persons.

To eliminate the distortion of wealth variation a number of alternatives could be tried. The modification closest to the simple market model would be the creation of a wealth distribution neutral market, as described by Calabresi in the following terms:

> The price at which scarce lifesaving resources were allocated would vary with the wealth of the recipient. . . . Wealth neutrality could only be achieved by setting rules for each wealth category so that the same proportion of potential users would buy the scarce resource in each wealth category. The prices would be set so that only the total resources allocated would be bought.[71]

In addition to some theoretical difficulties,[72] this method of treatment distribution faces many practical objections. First, there is the general problem of cheating or falsification of wealth status, and particularly the likelihood of black markets. More important, it would be exceedingly difficult to construct such a system, and the more precisely it was calculated the more offensive the regulation would seem. There is something very unattractive about a governmental agency expending great energy and intellectual resources to be constantly adjusting the price of the treatment for each wealth category (and perhaps redefining categories as well) so as to be able to announce that "we have found just the price where enough of you, whether rich or poor, will choose to die rather than avail yourselves of this treatment."

In sum, modifications in the market—by changing what is bargained for or people's ability to bargain—do not seem likely to solve the problems inherent in the market system. In particular, we doubt that people's own willingness to pay for and undergo a lifesaving treatment corresponds very exactly to the value of their lives to society, and, even if it did, the market does a poor job of allowing them to express their valuation. Therefore, further modifications in, or abandonment of, the market system are necessary.

---

[71] Calabresi, consultant's memorandum, at 14 (1970) [Appendix A].

[72] Prime among these is that such a system "only works to the extent that high life valuation is itself evenly spread across wealth distribution categories. . . . There is no special reason to assume such an even spread, as cultural factors and attitudes toward life are not independent of wealth." *Id.* at 15.

ii. COLLECTIVE DECISIONS. Rather than leaving the allocation of treatment resources to individual decisions in the marketplace, we could assign this task to a group appointed by the community which would pick treatment recipients according to their importance to society. There are two ways to go about this: either to formulate standards openly and then employ them to select among the applicants for treatment or to combine these two steps and have a single body make the selections according to whatever criteria it finds appropriate for judging the case before it. The defining characteristic of the second method is that no set of standards is ever publicly articulated by the selecting group; indeed, that is the advantage of such a system in its proponents' eyes.[73]

The system of explicit formulation is the one most common among federal regulatory bodies. Regulatory agencies formulate sets of standards, derived from general policy statements contained in enabling legislation, by which the regulated individuals or groups will be judged in the performance of their activities. The criteria are publicly promulgated, either in the course of adjudication or as a result of rulemaking proceedings, and are finally applied individually or in comparative hearings when a scarce resource must be allocated to one among a number of applicants. Failure to decide according to the promulgated standards exposes an agency's decision to reversal upon judicial review.

"Social value" can play an explicit role in administrative standards, both in the case of companies (*e.g.,* in deciding which broadcaster should be licensed for a channel because he will best serve the "public interest, convenience or necessity," etc.) and of individuals (*e.g.,* exemptions from military service for men employed in defense industries or otherwise "in the national interest," etc.). On a similar basis, standards might be established to select for lifesaving treatment those persons whose continued lives would provide the greatest "return" to society for each dollar invested in their treatment. Depending on the precision with which standards could be promulgated,[74] more or less discretion might be left to the administering body to apply them according to its "expertise" and free of judicial review.

The ominous social reverberations which would inevitably resound from

---

[73] Since no policy is formulated, such an approach is not strictly within the scope of this chapter, but ought to be discussed in the chapter on administration which follows. We discuss it here, however, for reasons of convenience and because it is so closely tied in practice with the other method of collective decisionmaking.

[74] It seems probable that fairly exact standards could be drafted; it is a more difficult question whether the application of such standards would result in the selection of a group of treatment recipients which precisely optimized the "social return" of the amount invested in treatment. In other words, we can be exact and clear, but we may not be right.

such a scheme hardly require expatiation. The drafting of soldiers provides an illuminating comparison. In times of national emergency, when everyone or nearly everyone (especially males) is called upon to make sacrifices and take some risks, the drafting of some people into active service, with its accompanying higher probability (but not, of course, certainty) of death or injury, gives rise to some uneasiness but is generally accepted. When the effort in which the draftees are called upon to fight is, like the conflict in Southeast Asia, unpopular, the system of selection may come in for a great deal of criticism; otherwise, abuses of the system, rather than the system itself, are more likely to become the subject of disapproval. On the other hand, where the need for a method of selection is not based on national survival but on the accident of disease and where an adverse selection means certain death, a societally based ranking of persons would be difficult to accept. If the ranking were believed, it would be hard to confine it to the sphere of catastrophic diseases. More likely, the ranking would be doubted and criticized for being too arbitrary and lacking in ability to differentiate between people on any number of important points—in other words, it would be hard to reach collective agreement on what is a truly "valuable" life. Furthermore, any explicit ranking would either undermine, or be undermined by, our society's proclaimed devotion to the concept of human equality, adherence to which is very important for the just and efficient operation of many of our social institutions.

To overcome these difficulties a second alternative has been suggested, namely, reliance on a body which will select recipients without publicly declaring why it favors *A* over *B*. Probably the most notable example of this type of decisionmaking is the jury (particularly in a criminal case);[75]

---

[75] The analogy is most sharply drawn in the case of a jury sitting to determine punishment in a capital case. In McGautha v. California, the Supreme Court was faced with the contention that "to leave [a] jury completely at large to impose or withhold the death penalty as it sees fit is fundamentally lawless and therefore violates the basic command of the Fourteenth Amendment that no State shall deprive a person of his life without due process of law." 402 U.S. 183, 196 (1971). The Court affirmed the lower courts' rejection of this proposition on the ground that "committing to the untrammeled discretion of the jury the power to pronounce life or death" does not offend the Constitution, especially in light of "the present limitations of human knowledge" in drafting standards. *Id.* at 207. Neither Mr. Justice Harlan for the Court, nor Mr. Justice Brennan for the minority, discussed the strains placed on society by open articulation of the characteristics which deserve death versus life imprisonment. One may presume, from the standards proposed by the American Law Institute in Model Penal Code §201.6 (Proposed Official Draft, 1962), that in the case of capital sentencing these standards would relate primarily to a person's *conduct*, especially that which surrounded his crime (*i.e.*, elements of aggravation and mitigation, etc.); in the case of catastrophic disease patients, the bases for judgment are more likely to be characteristics of a *status* rather than *conduct* type.

judges in sentencing convicts and, to a lesser extent, local draft boards and hospital clinical investigation committees also provide useful analogues of this model.

> To the extent they are representative they may reflect societal rankings of value of lives. To the extent that they make individual decisions they can consider individual . . . desire to live (if they so choose) more readily than can be done under responsibly promulgated general standards. To the extent they are local, individualized and a-responsible (*i.e.*, they do not need to give the reasons for their decisions and answer for them), they avoid many of the demoralization costs. . . .[76]

These advantages seem to have recommended this model to the physicians at the Swedish Hospital in Seattle when they sought to establish a method for selecting patients for their pioneering chronic hemodialysis program in 1961. The device they developed was to give the power of choice to

> seven humble laymen. They are all high-minded, good-hearted citizens, much like the patients themselves, who were selected as a microcosm of society-at-large. They were appointed to their uncomfortable post by Seattle's King County Medical Society, and for more than a year now they have remained there voluntarily, anonymously and without pay.[77]

Without any formal guidelines and relying solely on their own opinions and consciences, they were assigned the task of selecting patients among those whom the physicians said were medically and psychiatrically suitable candidates for the limited number of dialysis beds available in the artificial kidney center. The Seattle committee drew up a list of factors it would weigh in making its selections, but since it was an "a-responsible" body, it did not have to publicize its criteria nor explain their interrelationship nor even provide assurance that they were adhered to in each case. In her *Life* article Shana Alexander did reveal some of the committee's thinking, particularly the broad exclusions it had adopted.

> For example, the doctors recommended that the committee begin by passing a rule to reject automatically all candidates over 45 years of age. Older patients with chronic kidney disease are too apt to develop other serious complications, the medical men explained. Also, the doctors thought that the committee should arbitrarily reject children. The nature of the treatment itself might cruelly torment and terrorize a child, and there were other purely medical uncertainties, such as whether a child forced to live under the dietary restrictions would be capable of growth. In any case, the doctors believed it would be a mistake to accept children and thereby be forced to reject heads of families with children of their own.
>   . . . Finally they agreed to consider only those applicants who were resi-

---

[76] Calabresi, consultant's memorandum, at 10-11 (1970) [Appendix A].
[77] Alexander, note 8 *supra*, at 106.

dents of the state of Washington at the time the feasibility trial got under way. They justified this stand on the grounds that, since the basic research to develop the U-shaped tube had been done at the University of Washington Medical school and its new University Hospital—both state-supported institutions—the people whose taxes had paid for the research should be the first beneficiaries. . . .[78]

Plainly these rules vary a great deal in their underlying rationale: To exclude all patients over 45 because "older patients" tend to have other diseases which complicate treatment seems quite a different rationale than excluding children because they would be taking up space which could be used for "heads of families with children of their own." In all likelihood none of the rules would meet the standards applicable to officially promulgated regulations. Yet, of course, they did not have to; they were arbitrary judgments made in an area in which rationally articulated decisions seemed to the committee either impossible of attainment or destructive in their impact. Even the *Life* coverage, which exposed the workings of the Seattle "Life or Death Committee" to greater scrutiny than is typical for an a-responsible body, served mainly to focus attention on the fact that such a group had to make the decisions it did, rather than to criticize the basis on which the group's decisions had been reached.

Although one does not want to admit it, however, even "high-minded, good-hearted citizens" make mistakes and may even be

> unrepresentative, corruptible, or simply arbitrary. Unless one knows why a decision is made to prefer *A* over *B*, or unless one has substantial faith in the decider's ability to know and apply societal values, one is bound to suspect that the preference did not reflect a sensible or even honest scale of values.[79]

A fine line separates the exercise of reasonable, albeit a-responsible, discretion from irresponsible and arbitrary judgment. On the other hand, if a pattern emerges from the choices made, so that a committee's criteria can be discerned by piecing together the characteristics of the people it selects, then such difficulties as having a system with an explicit societal ranking reappear, with the added problem that the ranking has not been subject to review and correction by agencies responsible to the community and sensitive to its wishes.

    iii. THE LOTTERY. When the burdens of using a selection system which depends on conscious choice, made either by those selected or by society or a combination of the two, seem too great, decisionmakers have some-

---

[78] *Id*. at 106-07.

[79] Calabresi, consultant's memorandum, at 11 (1970) [Appendix A]. Both the sense and moral acceptability of the values underlying the Seattle committee's decisions are doubted by Sanders & Dukeminier, note 53 *supra*, at 377-78.

times turned to chance as a basis for making choices. Our most recent military "draft" used a lottery as its primary means of selection.[80] As Calabresi has succinctly observed:

> The principal advantages of the lottery are that it is extremely cheap administratively, and that it fails to rank people's lives. Its principal disadvantage stems from its second advantage. The lottery treats the man who wants to live desperately, even with an artificial kidney, exactly in the same way as the man who other things being equal might prefer to live but for whom the burden of an artificial kidney (or of life in general) is such that he would almost as soon die.[81]

On this analysis, the "fairness" of the lottery may be seen to be deceptive—it is more blind than fair, for an evenhanded approach is desirable only insofar as it deals with like classes of individuals. A lottery probably represents the method of selection which causes the fewest pangs of conscience and which is the least destructive of fundamental values, but it is certainly not likely to produce the optimal set of treatment recipients, whether judged by individual or societal standards, unless it is used to select among a group of applicants who are relatively equal on relevant criteria.

iv. FORMULATING A METHOD OF SELECTION. As we indicated at the outset of section C of this chapter, this book cannot go in detail into all the *issues* which make up each problem area—rather, we are interested in suggesting the *means* of decisionmaking that seem best suited to producing good policy formulations while taking account of the value considerations set forth in Chapter Three. On the specific subject at hand—policies to guide the selection of treatment recipients—it would be a mistake for the National Institutes of Health, which are staffed mostly by physicians and scientists, to promulgate explicit standards on the social as well as medical characteristics required of recipients to become eligible for the scarce resources devoted to treating catastrophic diseases.

On the other hand, some means of collective decisionmaking is necessary, both because of its inherent advantages and because of the weaknesses of leaving policy to individual decisionmaking in this area. The market simply cannot handle the externalities involved, even if the problems of desperation bidding and income inequality were solved. Collective decisionmaking can better take into account the benefits derived by individuals from public health actions, which will affect not only the total amount which ought

---

[80] The military selection system also employed societal criteria (no one under 18 to serve), the market (voluntary enlistment), and personal choice (those whose numbers are selected in the lottery may postpone their obligation to serve until after completion of undergraduate education).

[81] Calabresi, consultant's memorandum, at 20 (1970) [Appendix A].

optimally to be spent on catastrophic disease treatment but also the distribution of the resulting resources among the potential recipients.

Accordingly, we suggest that treatment recipients can best be selected by a national system employing a mixture of collective standards and the lottery.[82] In brief, such a system would rely on medical criteria to narrow the initial field of persons suffering from a catastrophic illness down to a pool of those who can reasonably be said to be likely to benefit from treatment.[83] From this pool, regular drawings[84] would be held whenever additional treatment spaces became available. It would probably be necessary for the system, although national in scope, to be subdivided by region and locality; depending on the nature and expense of the treatment and on whether it has to be taken continually at a medical center or can be administered in patients' homes (perhaps after a training period at a center), the relevant pool for each drawing may be national, regional, or local.[85]

Although such a system would avoid the previously enumerated dangers which arise when a collective body goes beyond medical criteria to evaluate "social worth" as a basis for selecting people for lifesaving care, we recognize that it still threatens to undermine the myth of societal commitment to life as a "pearl beyond price" because the process itself shows that we as a society are only willing to commit limited resources to certain types

---

[82] Although we do not suggest using the market as a screening mechanism, this would not prevent fees from being charged for the treatment nor treatment centers from being run by private concerns on a profitmaking basis. The only requirement would be that the amount a patient is required to pay should be set so that he would not be foreclosed from being treated for financial reasons. The amount actually charged could be graduated according to income; the difference between that amount and the cost of services could be made up by public or private medical funds, including payments by persons in high wealth categories which exceed the cost of their treatment.

[83] Patient-applicants would be presumed to be qualified *for* inclusion in the treatment pool in cases of doubt. They would not have the power to challenge the qualifications of others who were included; although they are "competing" for the scarce treatment spaces available, the system is not an adversarial one and there are no *comparative* standards.

[84] The term "drawing" is used metaphorically. Rather than an actual drawing, a computer-operated random number selection or other such process could be employed. A patient chosen by this method could decline treatment but could not assign his right, a rule necessary to avoid the black market problems discussed previously.

[85] A detailed proposal for the selection of hemodialysis patients along these lines was prepared by one of our consultants, Al Katz [Appendix G]. *See* 22 BUFF. L. REV. 373 (1973). The selection method described here is appropriate for any scarce, high-technology medical treatment; to a large extent, the problem of scarcity has been overcome for hemodialysis. The administrative aspects of such a plan are discussed in the following chapter.

of medical care or to treat only a portion of those who suffer. Yet most people are already aware of our collective deviation from our professed beliefs. If the proposed system serves to reduce some of the obfuscation which has surrounded this point, we find its advantages as a method of selection more than outweigh the resulting loss in societal peace of mind and self-image. Indeed, it is not clear that making people more aware that increased medical resources are needed is not a strength, rather than a weakness, of the proposed system. If this tends to increase the pressure, noted by Calabresi and confirmed by the passage of "H.R. 1" in 1972,[86] to commit further resources as the proportion of those saved increases in order to achieve "total" treatment for a particular disease, this may not be a bad result. Should the fear be that such a phenomenon amounts to a diversion of unwarranted resources to a particular "high-visibility" disease, that factor should be considered at an earlier time: namely, as we have previously suggested, when the decision is made to cease regarding a treatment modality as an experiment for a few patient-subjects and to employ it instead on a wider basis as regular therapy.[87]

Since various bodies (mostly local) already perform the screening function on a formal or informal basis, the major changes wrought by our suggestion would be (1) that the basic medical criteria would be subject to prior publication so they could be known and criticized by all concerned and so that their application would be more easily reviewable; (2) that socioeconomic considerations would not enter into selection of patients, except to the extent (probably inevitable, even if small) that they contaminate the medical criteria in some disguised form; and (3) that the "choice" of the individuals involved would be somewhat reduced. It is this last point which probably poses the greatest obstacle for the proposal. If we believed that the present system actually gave every patient the opportunity to make choices among a number of options and thereby to decide the amount and distribution of catastrophic disease treatment, we would be reluctant to suggest departing from it. As set forth earlier, however, the market system's numerous problems prevent individual patients from exercising

---

[86] *See* text accompanying notes 57-58 *supra.*

[87] In order to avoid stagnation, research into new methods of disease treatment will also need to be conducted. Whenever practicable, subjects for such research (such as variations in the treatment modality, etc.) should be selected by the same method as that regularly used for patient selection; like patients, subjects' participation is always dependent on their informed consent and right to withdraw. One matter on which flexibility is vitally necessary concerns the medical criteria used in the initial screening. With increases in knowledge, it should be possible to offer treatment to persons previously thought to be "unsuitable" for medical reasons. Subjects for such research should also be selected through the "drawing" mechanism from those applicants who were excluded from the regular drawings on medical grounds.

this sort of control. The relevant decisions are actually made by physicians and hospitals in what they judge to be patients' best interests. Our proposal, then, simply recognizes the fact that the decisions are in fact going to be made by someone other than solely the individual involved, and it offers a rational, and we hope fair, system for making decisions collectively.

4. Selection of Donors

One resource for the modern treatment of the catastrophic illnesses discussed here is unique: organs for transplantation. Since this resource is so unusual, we have chosen to treat it separately from the discussion of those resources (including artificial organs) whose supply is largely dependent on economic factors. We begin with a discussion of formulating policy on how to obtain organs (which is brief in light of the similarity of the issues to the questions discussed concerning the distribution of resources); this is followed by sections in which donations from living and dead persons are discussed.

a. Policies on Obtaining Organs. As is true for other resources, the central fact about transplantable organs is their scarcity. Consequently, well thought-out policies are required to increase the supply. The least expensive and most readily available sources consists of cadaver organs, primarily from accident victims.[88]

Prior to 1968, organ donation in this country was complicated by anachronistic legal provisions designed to prohibit graverobbing and by the absence of clear rules specifying the interests which could exist in a dead body and who could exercise them. The promulgation of the Uniform Anatomical Gift Act (UAGA) in the summer of 1968, and its subsequent adoption by all states and the District of Columbia, went a long way to cut through the fog which had enshrouded the subject. Under the Act, a person has the right during his lifetime to permit or forbid the use of his organs for purposes of treatment, research, and teaching after his death; if he fails to act, the organs can be donated by his next-of-kin (according to an order of priority established by the Act) after the person has died. The donee can be an individual patient or a physician or hospital, with the latter being free to use the organs as needed locally or elsewhere.[89]

---

[88] *See, e.g.,* Dukeminier, *Supplying Organs for Transplantation,* 68 MICH. L. REV. 811, 814-15 (1970)—citing statistics that 10,000 kidney transplants could be performed per year in this country if immunological problems are solved, and that there are approximately 10,600 suitable cadaver kidneys available each year.

[89] Thus, the organ-typing and patient-matching program operated for kidneys by Dr. Paul Terasaki's group at U.C.L.A. provides for hospitals to share the kidneys available to them on a nationwide basis, for which they receive "credits" that put them higher on the list for a cadaver organ the next time a "compatible" one is available. *See* Terasaki, Wilkinson & McClelland, *National Transplant Communica-*

In effect, the UAGA creates a "market" system with a zero price for organs (although the donee, by custom or contract, sometimes pays the cost of the donor's final hospitalization as well as the expense of removing the organ). The system relies on individual choice, with a leading role being taken by physicians who in most circumstances are the initiators of the donation. While no reliable figures are yet available to establish the impact the UAGA has had on the level of donation, it is generally agreed that not enough organs are being donated to meet present need, and some commentators doubt that the current method will ever produce sufficient donations.[90]

In its place a number of alternatives are possible. The first would simply add a payment procedure to UAGA-type organ transfers. Although the Act speaks of "donations," its terms do not prohibit sales as well. It is uncertain, however, that individuals would express much interest in an offer to sell a right to one's organs after death (with present payments), since the purchaser would have little assurance that the seller would die at a time and place or in a manner conducive to useful organ donation.[91] It would be possible, however, to make payment to a terminally ill patient, or, after his death, to his estate. Sales of this type might, however, pose serious psychological threats for dying patients and impose unwanted pressures on the next-of-kin.

The sale of "spare" organs by living donors for immediate delivery raises fewer logistical and psychological problems. Jesse Dukeminier, Jr., found "no statute in an American state expressly prohibiting the sale of a spare organ"[92] but nevertheless suggested that making a payment to a live donor raises the prospect of civil and criminal liability for the physician removing the organ. While we do not share his concern on these points, we doubt that payment is wise for policy reasons. As Richard M. Titmuss has argued with considerable force, a major fault with the American system of collecting blood is that the existence of paid donors discourages volunteers.[93] While all the data necessary to support his argument are not available, the

---

tions Network, 218 J.A.M.A. 1674 (1971). This type of arrangement is discussed in greater detail in Chapter Nine.

[90] *See, e.g.*, Sanders & Dukeminier, note 53 *supra*, at 394 *ff.*; Note, *Compulsory Removal of Cadaver Organs*, 69 COLUM. L. REV. 693 (1969) [hereinafter cited as *Compulsory Removal*].

[91] If the purchaser is the state (or other national organization) the problem of location is reduced somewhat. Were *A* to buy the right to *B*'s organs at the time of the latter's demise, *A* would not want *B* to die in a distant city where his organs would do *A* no good. Were the government to purchase the organs, it might be less concerned, since they could probably be put to use in any of a number of locations.

[92] Dukeminier, note 88 *supra*, at 850.

[93] R. TITMUSS, THE GIFT RELATIONSHIP: FROM HUMAN BLOOD TO SOCIAL POLICY (1971).

danger that payment for organs (kidneys in particular) would decrease "altruism" among donors and their next-of-kin is one reason for not permitting payment for organs.[94] Furthermore, since the poor would probably sell organs disproportionately, this system would probably be subject to a charge of "exploitation."

An alternative which is likely to increase the supply would be to presume that organs may be removed from any corpse unless a prior objection has been raised. In the proposal made by Dukeminier and Sanders,[95] objection could be raised "either by the decedent during his life or by his next-of-kin after the decedent's death."[96] Giving a role to the relatives is intended to permit them to protect their religious beliefs and is also a recognition that most transplanters would hesitate to go ahead if relatives were to claim that the deceased objected to the removal of his organs—even if they could produce no "proof" of this fact within the short time in which organs remain "viable" after a person's death. Yet as others have noted, by requiring the transplanters to make sure that the relatives do not object, the Dukeminier-Sanders plan places as much of a burden (in terms of effort to secure consent and danger of delay) on the system as the existing procedure.[97] The debate thus turns on whether society would find a system of choosing to give ("opting-in") or choosing not to give ("opting-out") more acceptable.

If the right to object were to be left solely with the person whose organs are to be removed, the process of obtaining organs could be greatly simplified and the number of available organs would doubtless increase greatly. The presumption in favor of routine salvaging would have to be widely publicized and "opting-out" made as simple as sending a preaddressed postcard to a central computer registry which could be consulted by a surgeon prior to organ removal.[98] Before the enactment of the UAGA, questions

---

[94] If the government purchases the organs, would it do so in every case (at a high cost in resources thus diverted from lifesaving therapy)? If not, on what basis would it decide when to pay and when not? (If on the basis of wealth of the corpse, why not employ more direct means of income redistribution?) If individuals were to buy the organs, it would amount to the creation of a market system on the distribution side, with all the problems discussed earlier in subsection 3(c)[i].

[95] *See* Sanders & Dukeminier, note 53 *supra*, at 410-13; Dukeminier, note 88 *supra*, at 837-42; Dukeminier & Sanders, *Organ Transplantation: A Proposal for Routine Salvaging of Cadaver Organs*, 279 NEW ENG. J. MED. 413 (1968).

[96] Dukeminier, note 88 *supra*, at 837.

[97] Sadler, Sadler, Stason & Stickel: *Transplantation: A Case for Consent*, 280 NEW ENG. J. MED. 862 (1969).

[98] A central renal registry was part of a plan, along the lines outlined here, proposed by the Advisory Group on Transplantation Problems appointed by the Health Ministers in Great Britain and chaired by Sir Hector MacLennan, M.D. *See Advice*

might have arisen whether such an arrangement would give sufficient attention to the next-of-kin's rights over the corpse. The UAGA made clear, however, that these rights, if they ever existed, are subject to alteration or abolition by the legislature; the decedent's determination to give his organs for transplantation or other use is binding, despite any objection on the part of his relatives. It seems equally valid to reduce relatives' control so as to permit removal of the organs unless a deceased had objected. A more difficult question is raised if the relatives claim an objection on religious grounds. On the one hand, the deceased was in a position to forbid use of *his* body if he shared his relatives' view. On the other hand, the relatives may claim that their religion does not make requirements about the burial of one's *own* body but about those of one's kin. This argument may prove too much, however. On this logic, could not the relatives equally well claim a "right" to control *any* body, whether the deceased be a relative or a member of their church or not?[99]

A more far-reaching restriction on the right to object could abolish this right altogether, making donation compulsory,[100] as autopsies already are under certain conditions.[101]

> Moreover, if organs are treated as property of the decedent, the decedent may have no power to order destruction of his organs by burial or cremation so long as the organs have value. It has been held in a number of cases that a direction to destroy one's own property at death is against public policy and is therefore void.[102]

While these and other analogies suggest that the public interest in saving lives through transplantation is great enough to justify making organ removal automatic (when medically useful), the policy issues (such as impact of this method on the emotions and personal feelings of the survivors) need to be openly debated before legislatures take such a step. Furthermore, since the donor is also deprived of the right to object, the religious considerations mentioned previously would loom much larger. If it is possible for the government to "accommodate its purpose [*i.e.*, saving lives] by

---

on the Question of Amending the Human Tissue Act 1961 (Cmnd. 4106) National Health Service (1969). Their recommendations were embodied in a Renal Transplant Bill, which was not adopted.

[99] If the deceased had been a member of their church, he could have chosen to "opt-out" of donation himself.

[100] *See Compulsory Removal*, note 90 *supra*.

[101] *See, e.g.,* Young v. College of Physicians & Surgeons, 81 Md. 358, 32 A. 177 (1895); Sturgeon v. Crosby Mortuary, Inc., 140 Neb. 82, 299 N.W. 378 (1941).

[102] Dukeminier, note 88 *supra*, 834.

means which do not impose such a burden,"[103] then compulsory removal of cadaver organs would run afoul of the First Amendment.

The only way to establish the need for a compulsory system, in other words, is to try less restrictive systems and see if they will produce an adequate supply. We believe that, for the moment, present policy, as embodied in the Uniform Anatomical Gift Act, ought to be given a fair trial first. Studies should, however, be conducted to determine whether the Act is adequately facilitating donations and whether any of its features should be revised. The real need for a change in policy on the obtaining of organs will arise when and if transplantation technology overcomes the problem of rejection and establishes itself as a highly successful form of therapy. If, under these circumstances, it appears that a change in procedure is warranted, prime consideration should be given to the "opting-out" system proposed by the MacLennan committee in Great Britain.[104] While it might be objected that in the case of a patient who had *not* opted-out, the attending physician would feel unwarranted pressure to forego necessary treatment so as to speed death, it seems likely that the very much greater supply of organs that could be expected under such a system would on the whole *reduce* the pressure in each individual case.

b. Donation by Living Individuals. Thus far the policies under discussion have been ones which require a societal judgment, and we have spoken in terms of legislative action. As we turn now to issues that have been dealt with largely through the private ordering of physicians, hospitals, patients, donors, and their families, the question arises whether a need exists for more broadly representative groups to engage in formulating policy more openly and explicitly. The following discussion will treat separately the donation of paired and unpaired organs, with primary attention devoted to the formulation of policies concerning the former.

i. PAIRED ORGANS. As described in Chapter Four, living donors have been an important source of kidneys for transplantation since the earliest days of the procedure. Patients' relatives were the donors in more than 30 percent of all kidney grafts to date and they continue to provide an important source of organs. Unrelated living donors, by contrast, gave 14.5 percent of the kidneys in the 14 years prior to 1967 for which records are available, but have not been used as donors at all since 1969.[105] Since the

---

103 Braunfield v. Brown, 366 U.S. 599, 607 (1961).

104 *See* note 98 *supra.*

105 *See* Advisory Committee to the Renal Transplant Registry, *Ninth Report of the Human Renal Transplant Registry,* 220 J.A.M.A. 253 (1972). In addition to the 122 organs included in this figure for 1953-1966, and 144 to date, there have been to date 31 donations by spouses, who are also "unrelated" in the genetic sense. On the other hand, Dr. Carl Fellner concludes on the basis of the early reports (which contained a finer breakdown of donor categories) that more than half of the kidneys

failure to employ this source does not stem from any ready availability of organs from other sources (as has already been noted), it must be a result of transplant surgeons' choice—and, in fact, this situation provides a valuable illustration of policymaking by physicians.

The reasons physicians have difficulties in using unrelated donors are not hard to fathom. Outside of research settings, physicians are not used to dealing with persons who will derive no therapeutic benefit from an intervention. Although some transplanters made use of live, unrelated donors in the early days of renal grafting, perhaps because less was known about how to keep cadaver organs viable and because the experimental nature of the procedure meant that all (recipients as well as donors) were taking risks, gradually there emerged a "distrust and suspicion toward the motivation of such [unrelated live] donors and a definite repugnance concerning their use."[106] Dr. Harrison Sadler and his colleagues discovered from a careful study of 18 unrelated donors that the primary motive for their donation was not "the satisfaction of drives or the discharge of infantile impulses, but the very personal area of self-identity, a self-ideal quite unconscious to them at the time."[107] In spite of their published findings, the Sadler group "continued to hear the remark, 'they [unrelated donors] must be crazy to do such a thing, no matter what you say—they are perverted'."[108]

This kind of thinking on the part of transplanters has rarely been expressed in formal rules or statements.[109] Although no live related renal donors have been used for three years in the United States, the policy of physicians as publicly stated does not bar such employment and the International Transplantation Society even acknowledges "that the wish to donate an organ need not be a sign of mental instability."[110] The deviation of

---

from unrelated donors were "free kidneys" obtained from persons who had to undergo a nephrectomy for reasons unrelated to transplantation. Fellner, *Altruism Revisited: The Genetically Unrelated Living Kidney Donor* (consultant's memorandum), at 4 (1972) [Appendix E].

[106] Sadler, Davison, Carroll, & Kountz, *The Living Genetically Unrelated Kidney Donor*, 3 SEMINARS IN PSYCH. 86 (1971). *See also* pp. 93-94 *supra*.

[107] Sadler, *Summary Notes on a Clinical Decision-Making Model* (consultant's memorandum), at 1 (1972) [Appendix H].

[108] *Id.*

[109] The French position, as expressed before the National Academy of Medicine in October 1970 by Dr. J. Dormont, is that "the donor must . . . be chosen exclusively from among the close relatives of the recipient." Dormont, *Les Problèmes Moraux de la Transplantation d'Organs*, 154 BULL. ACAD. NAT. MED. (PARIS) 623 (1970).

[110] Hamburger, et al., *A Declaration of the International Society of Transplantation*, 12 TRANSPLANT. 77 (1971). *Cf. Bar Council Report on Organ Transplants*, 3 BRIT. MED. J. 716 (1971)—approving organ removal from a mentally competent donor over 16 years of age who has given his written consent after he had been fully advised of the risks.

practice (or one could say, tacit medical policy) from official policy is, at the moment, not too distressing because the success rate of kidney grafts from unrelated donors is still below that of any other category (including cadavers), since present tissue typing methods apparently do not permit the identification of certain important antigenic factors which are absent (although undetected) in related donors such as siblings. But, as Dr. Fellner notes,

> it is only a question of time before tissue matching with the help of HL-A antigen typing, and other typing systems yet to be found, will have progressed to the point where, for organ transplantation purposes, the equivalent of a monozygotic twin could easily be pinpointed in the population at large.[111]

Before such time arises, it will be necessary for policy to be formulated on this subject making clear whether genetically unrelated donors should be accepted. This is a question which cannot be resolved by physicians alone. It concerns such issues as: (1) Does society have any interests in preventing a person from making a gift (or, as discussed previously, a sale) of an organ if that creates risk to his own life? (2) What level of risk is acceptable? (3) What level of "success" of the transplant is necessary, if any, to justify the donor's risk? (4) How does the availability of organs from other sources, such as cadavers or living *related* donors, affect the decision? (5) What is the relevance of different success rates between living unrelated donors and other sources? And (6) what is the relevance of surgeons' beliefs with respect to the use of organs from unrelated donors?

While these questions must be addressed by a public policymaking body, such as a special advisory group to the National Institutes of Health or to legislatures, it is our opinion that evidence already exists to indicate that there are reasons of policy, if not of medicine, to prefer unrelated rather than related donors. Unlike Sadler's findings about unrelated donors (who were accepted only if they persisted on their own initiative in their offer, over a number of months and without encouragement from the transplant center), there are many indications that related donors were not true volunteers, participating of their own free will. One study showed that such donors did not reach their decisions in the thoughtful, rational manner which had been assumed by the theorists on consent.[112] Moreover, despite physicians' attempts to protect the donor from undue pressures, it is apparent that veiled or even open pressure from family members as well as

---

[111] Fellner, *Altruism Revisited,* at 1 (1972) [Appendix E].

[112] Fellner & Marshall, *Kidney Donors: The Myth of Informed Consent,* 126 AM. J. PSYCHIATRY 1245 (1970); *see also* Fellner & Marshall, *Twelve Kidney Donors,* 206 J.A.M.A. 2703 (1968); notes 27-36 & accompanying text *supra.*

unconscious feelings of obligation and other psychological factors weigh heavily on family donors.[113]

> In most instances, no real decision-making problem existed for the donor. Most commonly, he stated that he must give to save the life of the potential recipient or he could not face himself. In a sense, he is "called." It is not always a call about which he is enthusiastic, but it is one which he believes he is unable to refuse.[114]

From such observations by others and from a review of his own interviews with donors (who typically declared "I had to do it"), Dr. Fellner argues that "most donors do not act out of pity or altruism but out of a feeling that they have to do this for their own sake."[115]

If this analysis is correct, then physicians appear to have adopted an informal policy which excludes people as donors whom the physicians believe act from "improper" motives and must be "crazy," when in fact those people's donations are a far more "voluntary" expression of their own choice and a more "genuine" reflection of a well integrated person than are the donations made by family donors. There is thus a need for others, who themselves are not so emotionally involved as the transplanters clearly are, to participate in the formulation of policy in this area.

Some additional light on decisionmaking with respect to live donors is thrown by contrasting medical policy on unrelated donors with that on the use of related donors who are incapable of giving valid consent. In most circumstances, no thought would be given to using such donors; however, where a child in renal failure has an identical twin, physicians favor use of the twin as an organ donor since the prognosis is so favorable.[116] Since minors[117] cannot themselves consent to operations, and since it is believed that parents or guardians cannot give permission when the procedure is not

---

[113] *See, e.g.,* Simmons, Hickey, Kjellstrand, & Simmons, *Family Tension in the Search for a Kidney Donor,* 215 J.A.M.A. 909 (1971); Crammond, *Renal Homotransplantation: Some Observations on Recipients and Donors,* 133 BRIT. J. PSYCH. 1223 (1967).

[114] Eisendrath, Gultman & Murray, *Psychological Considerations in the Selection of Kidney Transplant Donors,* 129 SURG. GYNEC. & OBSTET. 243 (1969).

[115] Fellner, *Altruism Revisited,* at 8 (1972) [Appendix E]. He also believes that these donors experience a feeling of power from their act and gain in self-esteem.

[116] Since 1967, one- and two-year survival rate for monozygotic twin transplants has been 100 percent. *Ninth Registry Report,* note 105 *supra,* at 256. Dialysis is not favored as a method of treating children with kidney disease because of the adverse effects of the treatment and dietary regime on growth and possibly on the child's psyche.

[117] Customarily defined as persons under 21, although most states have now made 18 the age of majority.

intended to benefit the child,[118] refuge has been taken in court actions. In these cases, the judiciary has uniformly approved the physicians' and parents' request for permission to transplant a kidney from the well to the ailing twin. In the first cases,[119] the children were teenagers, who one may assume were old enough at least partially to comprehend the contemplated operation; thus, their consent and agreement to having their kidneys removed properly played a role in the courts' reasoning. More recent cases have involved much younger children.[120] Here, the weight of the decisions has been cast onto the argument that the child-donor *does* receive a benefit by avoiding the psychic harm which would arise from the loss of the twin. This seems to be an attempt on the part of the judiciary to avoid having to confront the policy question of using nonconsenting individuals as donors. Some commentators, such as David Daube, have been sharply critical of the present practice.[121] There is a pressing need to engage in an open policy debate on this subject, which will touch many of the same questions of comparative benefits and risks set forth previously in the discussion of unrelated donors and which will also raise the whole issue of the use of children in medical research. This debate should eventually lead to proposals by professional and legislative bodies alike as to the policies which are to guide these research activities.

ii. UNPAIRED ORGANS. The donation of an unpaired organ is tantamount to taking one's life. For this reason, we know of no situation in which such a donation has been permitted. Paul Blachly has suggested, however, that persons engaged in "suicide-prevention" discuss with those intent on sui-

---

118 Although, as was discussed in Chapter Six, the kidney cases in minors are usually taken to exemplify the problem of obtaining valid permission for a nonbeneficial intervention, they involve an additional element: namely, that the parents face a conflict-of-interest in desiring to help the ailing child through a donation by the well child. This conflict may becloud the parents' judgment more than would be true in other nonbeneficial (research) interventions.

119 The earliest cases are three unreported Massachusetts decisions growing out of operations performed at the Peter Bent Brigham Hospital. The cases are discussed in Curran, *A Problem of Consent: Kidney Transplantation in Minors,* 34 N.Y.U.L. REV. 891 (1959).

120 Hart v. Brown, 289 A.2d 386 (Conn. Super. Ct. 1972)—approval of transplant in seven-year-old twin girls. In Strunk v. Strunk, 445 S.W. 2d 145 (Ky. 1969), the donor was a 27-year-old inmate of a state mental institution; he was found to have a "mental age of approximately six years."

121 "Children should on no account be donors, and there should be no cheating by maintaining . . . that the child would suffer a trauma if he were not allowed to give his twin a kidney or whatever it might be." Daube, *Transplantation: Acceptability of Procedures and the Required Legal Sanctions,* in ETHICS IN MEDICAL PROGRESS: WITH SPECIAL REFERENCE TO TRANSPLANTATION 188, 198 (G.E.W. Wolstenholme & M. O'Connor eds. 1966) [hereinafter cited as MEDICAL PROGRESS].

cide that they donate a paired organ instead.[122] Blachly argues that since potential suicides usually involve depression and feelings of unworthiness, the opportunity to help others in a dignified fashion may be very therapeutic. Similarly, the attention given a donor has been viewed as very valuable in overcoming the inner forces leading a person to contemplate taking his own life. When it comes to the "inevitable case" that still insists upon suicide, the question arises whether we should overcome our present mores

> to permit such a person to end his own life in a dignified way which would permit utilization of his organs. . . . One would think that the stigma that the friends and relatives attach to a suicide would be much lessened if they knew several persons would live as a result.[123]

The issue of "positive euthanasia" which is raised in an oblique fashion by this suggestion was confronted directly a number of years ago by one of our consultants, Dr. Belding H. Scribner, in his presidential address to the American Society of Artificial Internal Organs:

> [I]f I knew that I had a fatal disease I would seriously consider volunteering to donate one of my kidneys while I was still well. As far as death is concerned, I would like to be able to put into my will a paragraph urging that when my physician felt that the end was near, I be put to sleep and any useful organs taken prior to death. . . . I think that ethical and legal guidelines should be devised to permit me and others to volunteer in these ways.[124]

At the present time a number of groups and individuals are drafting statutes on euthanasia and urging their enactment.[125] Although we doubt that such measures would meet with widespread approval today, and we have not seen any which avoid the conflict-of-interest problem without an impossibly cumbersome judicial mechanism, we think it is appropriate for persons working in the catastrophic disease area to show the effect which euthanasia could have on the treatment of disease.

c. The Definition of Death. Since an increasing majority of kidney transplants, as well as all transplants of unpaired organs, are done with organs from cadaver donors, the question, "When is a person dead?" is of great

---

[122] Blachly, *Can Organ Transplantation Provide an Altruistic-Expiatory Alternative to Suicide?*, 1 LIFE-THREATENING BEHAVIOR 6 (1971).

[123] *Id.* at 9. We would reject this specific proposal because it can easily lead to exploitation of the therapeutic relationship.

[124] Scribner, *Ethical Problems of Using Artificial Organs to Sustain Human Life*, 10 TRANS. AM. SOC. ART. ORGANS 209, 211 (1964).

[125] The primary concern of the euthanasia proponents is not, of course, organ transplants but the pain and expense involved in the prolonged care of terminal, debilitated and often unconscious patients.

importance to policymaking in catastrophic diseases. The greatest source of concern with this subject probably occurs outside the transplant context in decisions about when to turn off a respirator which is maintaining "life" in a terminal, unconscious patient.[126] But public and professional concern about the determination of death did not become a major issue until the new methods of maintaining life artificially were applied to patients who were to be prospective organ donors. Public sensitivity about this procedure is well illustrated by an exchange between Dr. Christiaan Barnard and Senator Carl T. Curtis during the 1968 congressional hearings on Senator Walter Mondale's proposed commission on health science issues.

Senator Curtis: [T]he young lady whose heart was transplanted into Mr. Washkansky's body received artificial respiration.
Dr. Barnard: Yes, sir.

• • •

Senator Curtis: Who made the decision to discontinue the use of the machine?
Dr. Barnard: The neurosurgeons and neurologist. Those are a group of four doctors—
Senator Curtis: Now, that coincided with the time you were ready to begin the surgery?
Dr. Barnard: Yes, sir; that is correct.
Senator Curtis: It did not necessarily coincide with the time they made the decision that she was going to die?
Dr. Barnard: This was a few hours later.
Senator Curtis: So the machine was continued and stopped, not in relation to the time that the knowledge was available that she would not live, but it was continued to a time and stopped at a time to fit in with the schedule of the heart transplant to another person?
Dr. Barnard: This is correct.
Senator Curtis: And her surgeons made that decision?
Dr. Barnard: The doctors who were caring for her, as she was a patient who had severe brain damage, and therefore was cared for by the neurologist and the neurosurgeons.
Senator Curtis: Did they represent the recipient of the heart?
Dr. Barnard: No; they were only representing the donor. Their names are not on this team that you see published as the transplant team.[127]

---

[126] The plight of such patients and their families could be—and often is—dealt with under the heading "catastrophic illness." Although the financial aspects of the care given such dying patients are similar to the problems created by the innovative treatments provided for renal and cardiac failure, we have chosen to concentrate on the latter category of diseases and treatments, as was explained at the outset.

[127] *National Commission on Health Science and Society*, note 55 *supra*, at 74.

In a polite fashion, Curtis was asking Barnard whether transplant surgeons were not deciding that a patient was dead whenever it suited their convenience.

Yet if Curtis thought that medicine or law could provide him with a definite standard by which the conduct of Barnard and other transplanters could be measured, he was mistaken. The traditional medical criteria for declaring death—the absence of cardiac and respiratory functions—were at that very time being challenged, especially in the light of transplant procedures, but no definitive statement has as yet emerged.[128] Since that time, however, physicians have generally agreed that certain criteria relating to an absence of nervous system functioning also provide a reliable basis on which to base a declaration of death. These criteria were given their most authoritative promulgation by an *ad hoc* committee of the Harvard Medical School, often referred to by the name of its chairman, Dr. Henry K. Beecher.[129]

The Beecher Committee described in considerable detail three criteria of "irreversible coma": (1) unreceptivity and unresponsivity to externally applied stimuli and inner need; (2) absence of spontaneous muscular movements or spontaneous respiration; and (3) no elicitable reflexes. In addition, a flat (isoelectric) electroencephalogram was considered to be "of great confirmatory value" for such a clinical diagnosis.[130] Though generally referred to as criteria for "cerebral death" or "brain death," these criteria assess not only higher brain functions but brainstem and spinal cord activity and spontaneous respiration as well. The accumulating scientific evidence indicates that patients who meet the Harvard criteria will not recover and on autopsy will be found to have brains which are irreversibly damaged.[131] These findings support the conclusion that the

---

[128] *See, e.g.,* MEDICAL PROGRESS, note 121 *supra,* at 69-74 (remarks of Drs. G.P.J. Alexandre, J. Hamburger, J.E. Murray, J.P. Revillard & G.E. Schreiner); *Updating the Definition of Death,* MED. WORLD NEWS, April 28, 1967, at 47; Beecher, *Ethical Problems Created by the Hopelessly Unconscious Patient,* 278 NEW ENG. J. MED. 1425 (1968). The University of Mississippi transplanters also reported that it was uncertainty about when a patient could safely be declared dead which led them to use a chimpanzee, rather than a human, as the source of the heart in their 1964 operation. Hardy, Chavez, Kurrus et al., *Heart Transplantation in Man,* 188 J.A.M.A. 1132 (1964).

[129] In addition to Beecher, the committee consisted of nine other physicians, a historian, a lawyer, and a theologian, all Harvard University faculty members.

[130] Ad Hoc Committee of the Harvard Medical School to Examine the Definition of Brain Death, *A Definition of Irreversible Coma,* 205 J.A.M.A. 337 (1968) [hereinafter cited as *Irreversible Coma*].

[131] In the largest single study of patients with flat E.E.G.'s of 24-hours' duration, which involved 2,639 comatose patients without anesthetic doses of c.n.s. depressants, not one recovered. Silverman, Masland, Saunders & Schwab, *Irreversible Coma Asso-*

criteria may be valid for determining that death has occurred. The Beecher Committee's views were well received in the medical community,[132] but some physicians have raised questions. David Rutstein of the Harvard Medical School, for example, expressed concern over "this major ethical change which has occurred right before our eyes . . . with little public discussion of its significance."[133]

Rutstein's concern, echoed by laymen,[134] has unfortunately not been met with the necessary response. This is not to say, however, that public bodies have not considered the issue. But their actions have apparently been motivated largely by requests from members of the medical profession, particularly transplanters, who fear that existing, judicially framed standards for determining death may expose them to civil or criminal liability.[135] To

---

ciated with Electrocerebral Silence, 20 NEUROLOGY 525 (1970). In an unreported study on 128 individuals who fulfilled the Harvard clinical criteria, postmortem examinations showed their brains to be destroyed. Unpublished results of E. Richardson, reported in Task Force on Death and Dying, Institute of Society, Ethics and the Life Sciences, *Refinements in Criteria for the Determination of Death: An appraisal*, 221 J.A.M.A. 48 (1972) [hereafter cited as *Refinements in Criteria*].

132 *See generally Refinements in Criteria*, note 131 *supra*. One member of the Beecher Committee recently observed that "[s]ince publication of the report, the clinical recommendations have been accepted and followed on a worldwide basis in a most gratifying fashion." Curran, *Legal and Medical Death: Kansas Takes the First Step*, 284 NEW ENG. J. MED. 260 (1971).

133 Rutstein, *The Ethical Design of Human Experiments*, 98 DAEDALUS 523, 526 (1969). *See also*, Rot & van Till, *Neocortical Death after Cardiac Arrest*, 2 LANCET 1099 (1971), wherein leaders of the Netherlands Red Cross Society's Organ Transplantation Committee argue that only "total absence of the brain's functional capacity" and not "irreversible coma" indicates that death has occurred and state the Dutch position that the Harvard criteria "are grounds for stopping treatment and letting the patient die," but not for declaring death. *Id.* at 1099-1100.

134 *See, e.g.*, Arnold, Zimmerman & Martin, *Public Attitudes and the Diagnosis of Death*, 206 J.A.M.A. 1949 (1968) [hereinafter cited as Arnold]; Biörck, *When is Death?* 1968 WIS. L. REV. 484, 490-91 [hereinafter cited as Biörck]; N.Y. Times, Sept. 9, 1968, at 23, col. 1 (quoting Drs. F.C. Spencer & J. Hardy); *The Heart: Miracle in Cape Town*, NEWSWEEK, Dec. 18, 1967, at 86-87. *Cf.* Corday, *Life-Death in Human Transplantation*, 55 A.B.A.J. 629, 632 (1969):

[C]ertain actions by transplant surgeons in establishing time of death on death certificates and hospital records have shaken public confidence. Coroners have denounced them in the press for signing a death certificate in one county when the beating heart was removed a day later in a far-off city. The public wonders what the "item" was that was transplanted across the state line and later registered as a person in the operating room record.

135 *See, e.g.*, Taylor, *A Statutory Definition of Death in Kansas*, 215 J.A.M.A. 296 (1971) [hereinafter cited as Taylor], in which the principal draftsman of the Kansas statute states that the law was believed necessary to protect transplant surgeons against the risk of "a criminal charge, for the existence of a resuscitated heart in another body should be excellent evidence that the donor was not dead [under the 'definition' of

eliminate that danger, the Kansas legislature in 1970 adopted a statute "defining death" in the alternate as occurring when "in the opinion of a physician, based on ordinary standards of medical practice, there is the absence of spontaneous respiratory and cardiac function and . . . attempts at resuscitation are considered hopeless" or "there is the absence of spontaneous brain function."[136] Statutes adhering closely to the Kansas model have been introduced in Florida, Illinois, and Wisconsin, and adopted in Maryland; differently worded statutes have been enacted in California and West Virginia.[137]

The routine manner in which these bills have been handled and the failure of the legislators to generate a general discussion of the issue among themselves are regrettable because the "defining" of death goes beyond physicians' sphere of competence. The belief that "defining death" is purely a medical matter has been frequently expressed, and not just by physicians.[138] Indeed, when a question concerning the moment at which a person died has arisen in litigation, common law courts have generally regarded this as "a question of fact" for determination at trial on the basis (partially but not exclusively) of expert medical testimony.[139] Yet the standards which are

---

death then existing in Kansas] until the operator excised the heart." *Cf.* Kapoor, *Death & Problems of Transplant,* 38 MANIT. B. NEWS 167, 177 (1971). The specter of civil liability was raised in *Tucker v. Lower,* a recent action brought by the brother of a heart donor against the transplantation team at the Medical College of Virginia; the case is discussed *infra* at pp. 213-15.

[136] Law of Mar. 17, 1970, KANSAS SESSIONS LAWS, ch. 378 (1970); *codified* at KAN. STAT. ANN. §77-202 (Supp. 1971).

[137] MARYLAND SESSIONS LAWS, ch. 693 (1972); Florida House Bill No. 551 (1972) —failed; Wisconsin Sen. Bill No. 550 (1971)—adjourned; Illinois House Bill No. 1586 (1971)—adjourned; CAL. SESSIONS LAWS, ch. 1524 (1974); W. Va. House Bill 1356 (March 14, 1975). *See also* note 161 *infra.*

[138] *See, e.g.,* Kennedy, *The Kansas Statute on Death: An Appraisal,* 285 NEW ENG. J. MED. 946, 947 (1971) [hereinafter cited as Kennedy]; Berman, *The Legal Problems of Organ Transplantation,* 13 VILL. L. REV. 751, 754 (1968); Sanders & Dukeminier, note 53 *supra,* at 409; NATIONAL CONFERENCE OF COMMISSIONERS ON UNIFORM STATE LAWS, HANDBOOK AND PROCEEDINGS OF THE ANNUAL CONFERENCE 192 (1968). *Cf.* Sadler, Sadler & Stason, *The Uniform Anatomical Gift Act: A Model for Reform,* 206 J.A.M.A. 2501 (1968). The *ad hoc* Harvard Committee, made up largely of physicians, came to the same conclusion. *See Irreversible Coma,* note 130 *supra,* at 339.

[139] *See* Thomas v. Anderson, 96 Cal. App. 2d 371, 215 P.2d 478 (1950). In that appeal, the court was called upon to decide whether the trial judge had erred in holding inapplicable to the case a provision of the California Probate Code based on the Uniform Simultaneous Death Act which provided for the equal distribution of the property of two joint tenants "where there is no sufficient evidence that they have died otherwise than simultaneously." The court cited Black's Law Dictionary (3d ed.) definition that "death is the cessation of life; the ceasing to exist; defined by physicians as a total stoppage of the circulation of the blood, and a cessation of the animal and

applied in arriving at a conclusion, although based on medical knowledge, are established by the courts "as a matter of law."[140]

Thus while it is true that the application of particular criteria or tests to determine the death of an individual may call for the expertise of a physician, there are other aspects of formulating a "definition" of death that are not particularly within medical competence. To be sure, in practice, so long as the standards being employed are stable and congruent with community opinion about the phenomenon of death, most people are content to leave them in medical hands.[141] But the underlying extramedical aspects of the "definition" become visible, as they have recently, when medicine departs

---

vital functions consequent thereon, such as respiration, pulsation, etc.," and went on to observe that "death occurs precisely when life ceases and does not occur until the heart stops beating and respiration ends. Death is not a continuing event and is an event that takes place at a precise time." *Id.* at 375, 215 P.2d at 482. It concluded that the "question of fact" as to which of the two deceased men died first had been correctly determined by the trial court in light of "sufficient evidence" given by non-medical witnesses concerning the appearance of the men on the evening in question.

[140] Smith v. Smith, 229 Ark. 579, 587, 317 S.W. 2d 275, 279 (1958). The Smiths, a childless couple who by will had each left his or her estate to the other, were involved in an automobile accident. Mr. Smith apparently died immediately, but when assistance arrived Mrs. Smith was unconscious, and she remained so in the hospital for seventeen days. Thereafter, Mr. Smith's administrator petitioned for the construction of the wills, alleging

That as a matter of modern medical science, your petitioner . . . will offer the Court competent proof that the Smiths lost their power to will at the same instant, and that their demise as earthly beings occurred at the same time in said automobile accident, neither of them ever regaining any consciousness whatsoever.

Id. at 582, 317 S.W.2d at 277. The Supreme Court of Arkansas upheld the trial court's dismissal of the petition as a matter of law on the ground that "it would be too much of a strain on credulity for us to believe any evidence offered to the effect that Mrs. Smith was dead, scientifically or otherwise, unless the conditions set out in the [Black's Law Dictionary (4th ed.)] definition existed." *Id.* at 586-87, 317 S.W.2d at 279. The court took "judicial notice that one breathing, though unconscious, is not dead," *id.* at 589, 317 S.W.2d at 281, and concluded that Mrs. Smith's death was therefore not simultaneous with her husband's.

Cf. In re Estate of Schmidt, 261 Cal. App. 2d 262, 67 Cal. Rptr. 847 (1968). *Schmidt,* like *Thomas* and *Smith,* involved an inheritorship issue under the Uniform Simultaneous Death Act. The appellate tribunal found that there was sufficient eye-witness testimony by laymen to support the trial court's conclusion that Mrs. Schmidt survived her husband by some minutes, and it found no fault in the use of the Black's Law Dictionary "definition of death" despite the argument that it "is an anachronism in view of the recent medical developments relating to heart transplants," since there was no evidence that the deceased were resuscitable. *Id.* at 273, 67 Cal. Rptr. at 854.

[141] *See* Arnold, note 134 *supra,* at 1950, in which the public's "nearly complete acceptance" of professional practice in this century until cardiac transplantation began is contrasted with the great concern manifested in the nineteenth century and earlier, largely because of fear of premature burial before embalming became routine.

(or appears to depart) from the common or traditional understanding of the concept of death. The formulation of a concept of death is neither simply a technical matter nor one susceptible of empirical verification. The idea of death is at least partly a philosophical question, related to such ideas as "organism," "human," and "living." Physicians *qua* physicians are not experts on these philosophical questions, nor are they experts on the question of which physiological functions decisively identify a "living, human organism." They, like other scientists, can suggest which "vital signs" have what significance for which human functions. They may, for example, show that a person in an irreversible coma exhibits "total unawareness to externally applied stimuli and inner need and complete unresponsiveness,"[142] and they may predict, when tests for this condition yield the same results over a 24-hour period, that there is only a very minute chance that the coma will ever be "reversed."[143] Yet the judgment that "total unawareness . . . and complete unresponsiveness" are the salient characteristics of death, or that a certain level of risk of error is acceptable, requires more than technical expertise and goes beyond medical authority.

There are a number of potential means for involving the public in this process of formulation and review, none of them perfect. The least ambitious or comprehensive is simply to encourage discussion of the issues by the lay press, among civic groups, and in the community at large. This public consideration might be directed or supported through the efforts of national organizations, such as the American Medical Association, the National Institutes of Health, or the National Academy of Sciences. The recently empanelled National Commission for the Protection of Human Subjects could also generate public discussion of the need and purposes of a "definition of death." Yet as important as it is to ventilate the issues in public meetings, studies and discussions alone may not be adequate to the task. They cannot by themselves dispel the ambiguities which will continue to leave decisionmakers and the public in doubt about the permissible and proper way to decide whether an artificially maintained, comatose "patient" is still alive.

A second alternative, reliance upon the judicial system, goes beyond the clarification of popular attitudes and could provide an authoritative opinion that might offer some guidance for decisionmakers. Reliance on judge-made law would, however, neither actively involve the public in the decision-making process nor lead to a prompt, clear, and general "definition" of death. The courts cannot speak in the abstract prospectively but must await litigation. This can also involve considerable delay and expense, which may

---

[142] *Irreversible Coma,* note 130 *supra,* at 337.
[143] *See* note 131 *supra.*

be detrimental for both the parties and society. The need to rely on the courts reflects an uncertainty in the law which is unfortunate in an area where private decisionmakers (namely physicians) have to make quick and irrevocable decisions. A doubtful legal standard means that the rights of many of the participants are endangered. In such circumstances, a person's choice of one course over another may depend more on his willingness to test his views in court than on the relative merits of the courses of action.[144]

A more fundamental difficulty with the judicial route is that courts operate within a limited compass (the facts and contentions of a particular case) and with limited expertise. They have neither the staff nor the authority to investigate or to conduct hearings in order to explore such issues as the public's opinion or the scientific merits of one "definition" rather than another. Consequently, a judge's decision may merely reflect the opinions expressed by the medical experts who appear before him. Indeed, those who believe that the "definition of death" should be left in the hands of physicians favor the judicial route over the legislative on the assumption that the courts will approve "the consensus view of the medical profession"[145] in the event of a lawsuit by a relative (or, perhaps, by a revived "corpse"). Thus, to leave the task of articulating a new set of standards to the courts is not completely satisfactory, if one believes that the formulation of such standards (as opposed to their application in particular cases) goes beyond the authority of the medical profession.

To be sure, uncertainties in the law are inevitable and are more readily tolerated if they do not involve matters of general applicability or of great moment. Yet the question of whether and when a person is dead is an issue that cannot escape the need for legal clarity. Therefore, it is not surprising that, although they would be pleased simply to have the courts endorse

----

144 For example, suppose that transplant surgeons were willing to employ a neurological definition of death, although most other physicians continued to use the "traditional" definition because of the unsettled nature of the law. If (*ex hypothesis*) the surgeons were less averse to the risks of testing their position in litigation, either because of their temperament, training, or desire for success, their "courage" could lead to patients being declared dead "prematurely" according to the traditional standard.

145 Kennedy, note 138 *supra*, at 947. Kennedy's reliance on a medical "consensus" has a number of weaknesses, which he acknowledges at least implicitly: (1) there may be "a wide range of opinions" held by doctors, so that "there need not necessarily be only one view" on a subject which would be supported by the medical community, in part because (2) the "usual ways" for these matters to be "discussed and debated" are not very clear or rigorous since (3) the "American medical profession is not all that well regulated" unlike its British counterpart and (4) is not organized to give "official approval" to a single position ŏr (5) to give force to its decision, meaning (6) that "the task will be assumed by some other body, most probably the legislature." *Id.*

their views, members of the medical profession are doubtful that the judicial mode of lawmaking offers them adequate protection.[146] There is currently no certainty that a doctor would not be liable, criminally or civilly, if he ceased treatment on a person found to be dead according to the Harvard Committee's criteria but not according to the "complete cessation of all vital functions" test presently employed by the courts. Although such "definitions" were adopted in cases involving inheritors' rights and survivorship[147] rather than a doctor's liability for exercising his judgment about when a person has died, physicians have with good reason felt that this provides them with slim grounds for confidence that the courts would not rely upon those cases as precedent.[148] On the contrary, there is every reason to expect that the courts would seek precedent in these circumstances. Adherence to past decisions is valued, because it increases the likelihood that an individual will be treated fairly and impartially; it also removes the need to relitigate every issue in every case. Most importantly, courts are not inclined to depart from existing rules because to do so may upset the societal assumption that one may take actions, and rely upon the actions of others, without fear that the ground rules will be changed retrospectively.[149]

The impact of precedent as well as other problems with relying on the judicial route to a new definition were made apparent in *Tucker v. Lower*,[150] the first case to present the question of the "definition of death" in the context of organ transplantation. Above all, this case demonstrates the uncertainty inherent in the process of litigation, which "was touch and go for the medical profession"[151] as well as for the defendants. *Tucker* involved a $100,000 damage action against Drs. David Hume and Richard Lower and other defendant doctors on the Medical College of Virginia

---

[146] *See, e.g.,* Taylor, note 135 *supra,* at 296; Arnold, note 134 *supra,* at 1954; Corday, *Definition of Death: A Double Standard,* HOSPITAL TRIBUNE, May 4, 1970, at 8; Halley & Harvey, *On an Interdisciplinary Solution to the Legal-Medical Definitional Dilemma in Death,* 2 INDIANA LEGAL F. 219, 227 (1969).

[147] *See* notes 139 & 140 *supra. Cf.* Gray v. Sawyer, 247 S.W. 2d 496 (Ky. 1952).

[148] *See* Taylor, note 135 *supra,* at 296. *Compare* Kennedy, note 138 *supra,* at 947.

[149] "[R]ules of law on which men rely in their business dealings should not be changed in the middle of the game. . . ." Woods v. Lancet, 303 N.Y. 349, 354 (1951). It must be admitted, however, that such principles usually find their most forceful articulation when the court is about to proceed on the counter-principle that when necessary the common law will change with the times to achieve justice. (In *Woods,* by way of illustration, the New York Court of Appeals overruled its prior decision in Drobner v. Peters, 232 N.Y. 220 [1921], in order to permit a child to sue for prenatal injuries.)

[150] Tucker v. Lower, No. 2831 (Richmond, Va., L. & Eq. Ct., May 23, 1972).

[151] 15 DRUG RES. REP., June 7, 1972, at 1.

transplant team, brought by William E. Tucker, whose brother Bruce's heart was removed on May 25, 1968, in the world's seventeenth human heart transplant. The plaintiff claimed that the heart was taken without approval of the next-of-kin and that the operation was begun before Bruce had died. On the latter point, William Tucker offered evidence that his brother was admitted to the hospital with severe head injuries sustained in a fall and that after a neurological operation he was placed on a respirator. At the time he was taken to the operating room to have his organs removed "he maintained vital signs of life, that is, . . . normal body temperature, normal pulse, normal blood pressure and normal rate of respiration."[152] Based on the neurologist's finding that Bruce Tucker was dead from a neurological standpoint, the respirator was turned off and he was pronounced dead. The defendants moved to strike the plaintiff's evidence and for summary judgment in their favor, but the trial judge denied the motions.

> The function of This Court is to determine the state of the law on this or any other subject according to legal precedent and principle. The courts which have had occasion to rule upon the nature of death and its timing have all decided that death occurs at a precise time, and that it is defined as the cessation of life; the ceasing to exist; a total stoppage of the circulation of the blood, and a cessation of the animal and vital functions consequent thereto such as respiration and pulsation. . . .
> This court adopts the legal concept of death and rejects the invitation offered by the defendants to employ a medical concept of neurological death in establishing a rule of law.

• • •

> If the jury concludes that the decedent's life was terminated at a time earlier than it would ordinarily have ended had all reasonable medical efforts been continued to prolong his life, then it will be allowed to assess damages not only for the pecuniary loss, if any, sustained by the statutory beneficiary, but also for the loss, if any, of the decedent's society as well as solatium to the beneficiary for his sorrow and mental anguish caused by the death.[153]

When the judge sent the case to the jurors, however, he permitted them to consider all possible causes of death (*i.e.,* injury to the brain as well as cessation of breathing or heartbeat), and a verdict was returned for the defendants. Unfortunately, the discrepancy between the judge's ruling and his subsequent instructions to the jury did little to resolve the legal uncertainty. The plaintiff has announced that he plans to appeal to the Supreme

---

[152] Tucker v. Lower, note 150 *supra* (denying defendants' motion for summary judgment).

[153] *Id.*

Court of Virginia,[154] and the creation of a clear and binding rule will depend on the action of the appellate tribunal.[155]

Some further clarification of the present legal definition of death may be forthcoming in California from the trials of two persons accused, respectively, of murder and vehicular homicide; in each case the defendant claims that he cannot be tried for killing his victim because the latter's heart was removed for transplantation at the Stanford Medical Center.[156] For the moment, however, these cases merely provide further indications of the harm to society in an ill-defined rule on such an important issue.

In declining the defendants' suggestion that he adopt a standard based on neurological signs, the judge in the *Tucker* case stated that application for "such a radical change" in the law should be made "not to the courts but to the legislature wherein the basic concepts of our society relating to the preservation and extension of life could be examined and, if necessary, reevaluated."[157] A statutory "definition" of death has notable advantages as an alternative to a judicial promulgation. Basically, the legislative process permits the public to play a more active role in decisionmaking and allows a wider range of information to enter into the framing of criteria for determining death. Moreover, by providing prospective guidance, statutory standards could dispel public and professional doubt and could provide needed reassurance for physicians and patients' families, thereby reducing both the fear and the likelihood of litigation for malpractice (or even for homicide).

The legislative alternative also has a number of drawbacks, however. Foremost among these is the danger that a statute "defining" death may be badly drafted. It may be either too general or too specific, or it may be so poorly worded that it will leave physicians or laymen unsure of its intent. There is also the danger that the statutory language might seem to preclude future refinements that increasing medical knowledge would introduce into the tests and procedures for determining death. The problem of bad draftsmanship is compounded by the fact that a statute once enacted may be difficult to revise or repeal, leaving the clarification of its intent and meaning to the slow and risky process of litigation.[158] An additional practical

---

[154] N.Y. Times, May 27, 1972, at 15, col. 5; *id.*, June 4, 1972, at 7, col. 1.

[155] As one medical journal, which favors legislative action by way of a "definition," accurately observed about the decision of the Richmond court: "It applies only to cases coming before that court and can be reversed on appeal or overridden by contrary decisions handed down in higher courts." 15 DRUG RES. REP., June 7 1972, at 1.

[156] *See* Capron, *To Decide What Dead Means*, N.Y. Times, Feb. 24, 1974, at 6, col. 4.

[157] Tucker v. Lower, note 150 *supra*.

[158] The general durability of statutes has the backhanded advantage, however, of emphasizing for the public as well as for legislators the importance of a thorough thrashing out of the issues in hearings and legislative debates.

problem is the possibility that the content of statutes enacted may reflect primarily the interests of powerful lobbying groups (*e.g.,* the state medical society or transplant surgeons), rather than carefully considered, independent public analysis and judgment.[159]

On the other hand, the legislative route may reduce the likelihood that conflicting "definitions" of death will be employed in different jurisdictions in this country. Theoretically, uniformity is also possible in judicial opinions, but it occurs infrequently. If the Uniform Anatomical Gift Act provides any precedent, there is every reason to believe that the Commissioners on the Uniform State Laws are well situated to provide leadership in achieving an intelligent response to changes in medical procedure.[160] In sum, then, if legislators approach the issues with a critical and inquiring attitude, a statutory "definition" of death may be the best way to resolve the conflicting needs for definiteness and flexibility, for public involvement and scientific accuracy.[161]

The need for a "redefinition" of death reflects not only the ever-increasing medical capabilities to maintain "life," but uncertainties in the medical profession about the use of these life-prolonging capabilities in many situa-

---

[159] Ian Kennedy has suggested the further danger that a statutory "definition" rather than protecting the public may leave it vulnerable to injury from physicians who "by liberal interpretation and clever argument" might take actions "just within the letter if not the spirit of the law." Kennedy, note 138 *supra,* at 947. Certainly, if doctors wish to be devious, they probably can be. Yet it is far from clear why they are likely to "think twice," as Kennedy asserts, about departing from a generalized "consensus view" of the medical profession (which may, or may not, eventually be adopted by the courts) if they would cavalierly violate a clear statute. Legislation will not remove the need for reasoned interpretation—first by physicians and perhaps then by judges—but it can restrict the compass in which they make their choices to one which has been found acceptable by the public.

[160] For a detailed discussion of the national acceptance of the Act, see Sadler, Sadler & Stason, *Transplantation and the Law: Progress Toward Uniformity,* 282 NEW ENG. J. MED. 717 (1970). See also Brickman, *Medico-Legal Problems with the Question of Death,* 5 CALIF. W.L. REV. 110, 122 (1968)—urging Commissioners to draft a uniform act on "the procedures for determining death."

[161] Further elaboration on this subject, and a proposed model statute to "define" death, are presented in Capron & Kass, *A Statutory Definition of the Standards for Determining Human Death: An Appraisal and a Proposal,* 121 U. PA. L. REV. 87 (1972), on which much of the foregoing discussion was based. In March 1975 West Virginia adopted the model statute proposed in that article; *see* note 137 *supra.* The House of Delegates of the American Bar Association (ABA) recently adopted a policy statement "defining" death, which was offered as a possible statute in light of the conflicting bills presently pending in fourteen states. The ABA "definition" is phrased solely in terms of an irreversible, total cessation of brain function. 43 U.S.L.W. 2362 (1975). The ABA proposal thus avoids the problems of the Kansas-Maryland approach pointed out in the article by Capron and Kass, and follows the alternative approach discussed there. 121 U. PA. L. REV. at 112-13.

tions. In the past, physicians were almost universally oriented "to the nearly absolute 'commandment' to combat . . . death,"[162] which was seen as a medical defeat. This gave physicians a great deal of assurance to their "saving" of life at almost any cost to the patient, to society, or to the pursuit of other values.

> This nearly absolute commitment to preserve life strongly insulated medical ethics from any ethical system or complex that did not place a commensurate emphasis upon the value of preserving life, and thereby firmly grounded the autonomy of medical ethics.[163]

With the emergence of what Parsons and his colleagues term "a relativized ethic"[164] among physicians, the old assurance about when to fight death has been eroded. Thus, physicians not only have to confront the choice on more personal grounds, but they possess less authority in asserting the primacy of their choices against those made by other groups in society.

D. CONCLUSION

Throughout this chapter we have emphasized two major issues: First, the importance of careful policy formulation in the catastrophic disease process and, second, the need for a variety of individuals and groups, with diverse values, to be involved in this process. We have also sought to illustrate the sorts of problems—for example, the delineation and funding of research and therapy, the selection of donors and recipients, and the definition of death—which require resolution. Moreover, we have tried to make specific suggestions which should be taken into account in the process of formulation and to show why these issues require thought and decision not only by members of the biomedical profession but by others as well.

We recognize that our discussion and recommendations have been premised not only on the value of involving the public in decisionmaking but also on the value of open, "visible" decisions. In the weighing of relative risks, the danger of arbitrariness in "low visibility" decisionmaking seems to us to exceed the demoralizing effects that may come from the public formulation of policy which leads to the selection of "one individual to live and thereby doom[s] others to death."[165] In the long run, the obscuring of the basis for decisions can only lead to fear and misunderstanding, as well as to abuse.

---

[162] Parsons, Fox & Lidz, *The "Gift of Life" and Its Reciprocation*, 39 Soc. Research 367, 395 (1972).

[163] *Id.*

[164] *Id.* at 402.

[165] Note, *Scarce Medical Resources*, 69 Colum. L. Rev. 620, 622 (1969).

CHAPTER NINE

The Administration of Major Medical Interventions

In the preceding chapter we did not attempt to discuss all the policies which require formulation. Instead we submitted some of the most important issues facing the catastrophic disease process—the definition of research and treatment, allocation of resources, selection of treatment recipients and of organ donors—to a more detailed analysis in order to demonstrate the importance of and need for careful and open formulation of the policies which are to guide medical decisionmaking. Recently NIH's Artificial Heart Assessment Panel came to similar conclusions with respect to the problems created by the impending development of a totally implantable artificial heart:

> Although the issues of human experimentation raised by the artificial heart are in no real sense unique, the prospect of clinical trials of the artificial heart does give rise to a unique occasion for reconsideration of the manner in which basic principles are formulated and implemented. If, as appears likely, the artificial heart system developed by the Federal Government with public funds is the system first available for human trials, a persuasive case can be made that the government has an obligation to ensure that this device is used in human experiments in an orderly and proper manner. If this obligation is recognized, it follows that the government has a responsibility (1) to pursue development of the device in a manner that strikes an appropriate balance between technical and medical objectives and broad societal consideration; (2) to ensure that clinical experiments will be properly conducted, with appropriate informed consent, in a manner that reconciles the objective

219

of therapeutic results with expeditious perfection of the device; and (3) to ensure that clinical experiments will be conducted in a manner that abuses neither patient-subjects nor the interests of society as a whole.

Accomplishment of these broad objectives involves the efforts and contributions of not only the scientific, engineering, and medical disciplines, but also of other disciplines reflecting the broad ethical and societal interests that are at stake. . . . The general policy of the National Heart and Lung Institute seems to be to use a number of small advisory bodies, each responsible for guidance on a fragment of the overall artificial heart program. Consideration of each set of issues seems, therefore, to be isolated from consideration of other issues. Because, as we approach the stage of human experimentation, these compartmentalized areas become increasingly interrelated, with a need for effective feedback and cross-fertilization, much could be gained by creation of a single new group, broadly constituted and representative of the full scope of technical, medical, and societal issues, to participate in the formulation of basic policies and principles, to monitor and evaluate further developments, and to recommend changes in the scope and direction of various efforts in the light of new data.[1]

In this and the next chapters the focus shifts to the administration and review stages of the catastrophic disease process. We believe that optimal functioning at the stages of administration and review will to a great extent be determined by the care which has been taken in formulating policies. Thus we have spent considerable time in delineating the latter and will now only present some of the major issues that require consideration, for the details will be shaped significantly by the way in which basic policies have been specified.

Once policies are better formulated, decisionmakers at the administration stage should be able to appreciate with greater certainty not only the limits within which they may operate but also the extent of their freedom to operate. A clearer articulation of policy and procedures should also help in identifying those policies which prove unworkable or overly burdensome (a task of the review process which is the topic of Chapter Ten) and are thus in need of reformulation. Although adherence to formulated policies will impose constraints on decisionmakers at the stage of administration, they should remain constantly alert to the danger of increasing inflexibility, always present in bureaucratic endeavors, and seek modification in existing practices whenever this pernicious problem comes to their attention.

The question of who should participate in the process of medical decisionmaking has generated much disagreement, often under the assump-

---

[1] ARTIFICIAL HEART ASSESSMENT PANEL, NATIONAL HEART AND LUNG INSTITUTE, U.S. DEP'T OF HEALTH, EDUCATION & WELFARE, THE TOTALLY IMPLANTABLE ARTIFICIAL HEART 181-183 (1973).

tion that what was being talked about was participation at the stage in the process that we call "administration." This debate has focused on the role of "insiders" and "outsiders" and has led to alternative recommendations. On the one hand, the traditional viewpoint of physicians and scientists that "insiders" ought to be permitted to make all the decisions was forcefully stated by Dr. Owen Wagensteen:

> I . . . worry over getting people into this field on the fringes, who do not really know much about the heart of the problem—the conscionable, dedicated, experienced people who are working day by day with the problem—these are the people who can speak knowledgeably and who can and must be trusted.
> . . . If you are thinking of theologians, lawyers, philosophers, and others to give some direction here for the ongoing research and for the development in this field, I cannot see how they could help. I would leave these decisions to the responsible people doing the work.[2]

On the other hand, dissatisfaction with existing "peer group review" mechanisms mandated by the Public Health Service, has led some commentators to urge broader representation of "outsiders." In his memorandum for our project, Bernard Barber wrote:

> [E]xternal control mechanisms are also necessary for a socially responsible profession because the consequences of its performances and power are too important to the outsiders for them to give up all control over their fate. We now paraphrase Clemenceau's old aphorism, "War is too important to be left to the generals," in many ways: Medicine is too important to be left to the scientists, and biomedical research is too important to be left to the biomedical researchers. . . .
> [R]eview procedures for the "experiment" phase should have much larger proportions of expert peers, of "insiders" to a profession, since that is the phase when the esoteric aspects of the research and treatment are most at issue. Even in this phase, however, . . . the use of outsiders has been *recommended* to scrutinize the research protocols for proper ethical conformity on the issues of informed voluntary consent and the risk-benefit ratio. . . .
> As research and treatment move along the spectrum from purely "experimental" toward the "allocative" phase, it seems to me that a greater admixture of "outsiders" is required to make ethical decisions. The esoteric problems become more standardized and there is less need for diverse "insiders" consideration. It is the "allocative" problems and their associated moral decisions that come more and more to the fore, so that the decisions are

---

[2] *Hearings on S.J. Res. 145 (National Commission on Health Science and Society) before the Subcomm. on Gov't Research of the Senate Comm. on Gov't Operations,* 90th Cong. 2d Sess., at 100 (1968) [hereinafter cited as *National Commission on Health Science and Society*].

more and more matters to be decided by representatives of society and government, who are more and more in control of the scarce resources which are in excess demand and have to be allocated according to some social and ethical criteria. Such "outsiders" are in a better position to make demands on the larger social and political process for enlarging the available resources. . . .[3]

In our view both positions have merit. We seek to promote increased representation by "outsiders" in the formulation of policy and yet to avoid interference by "outsiders" in the day-to-day activities which professionals are called upon to perform. Thus, our proposals do not leave the ordering of the entire catastrophic disease process solely to professional control, as advocated by some. In the light of the many decisions that have impact far beyond areas of professional expertise or concern, such a position seems untenable. This reality is appreciated by most of the severest critics of "outside" participation once they are pressed beyond their initial response.

In basic policy deliberations on how to guide the administration of both experimentation and therapy, persons from outside biomedicine have an important role to play in representing and championing those values which affect individual and societal rights and interests. Professionals have other goals to pursue and cannot be expected, even had their training and experience so prepared them, to encompass all these roles. Thus it is at the formulation stage that "outsiders" can make a most effective and much needed contribution. Once policies are set, the immediate participants, physician-investigators and patient-subjects, should be permitted to reach their own accommodations with as little interference as possible. Though additional controls will be necessary, it may be most effective for these to be administered by peers of the primary participants, since infringements of authority imposed by colleagues are generally better tolerated than those coming from outside.

A. ADMINISTRATION AT THE LOCAL LEVEL— THE INSTITUTIONAL ADVISORY COMMITTEE

In light of the division of authority we propose for the various decision-making stages, the purposes of any substantive and procedural controls at the stage of "administration" must be identified. We believe there are three purposes for giving "outsiders" authority at this stage in decisionmaking:

1. to *assist* physician-investigators and patient-subjects with the decisions they have to make;

---

[3] Barber, *The Structure, Functions and Efficacy of Peer Review Committees in the Experimental and Allocative Phases of Clinical Treatment*, at 15, 17-19 (1972) [Appendix D].

2. to *supervise* decisionmaking between physician-investigator and patient-subject; and

3. to *advocate* reformulation of policies whenever they become too burdensome and inflexible (a task which is also part of the first and third stages of the process).

Our analysis of the assignment of decisionmaking authority among the several participants is applicable alike to catastrophic disease treatment and to other areas of biomedical research and therapy. Although the previous chapter's discussion was of necessity confined to the formulation of policies about catastrophic diseases (since they are the specific topic of our report), many of the recommendations of this chapter are framed in more general terms since the same structure can be used for a variety of substantive problems. Indeed, the basic decisionmaking bodies in our scheme are the "Institutional Advisory Committees"[4] (IAC), which are intended to be capable of passing on projects outside the catastrophic disease area as well as within it.

The Department of Health, Education and Welfare's *Institutional Guide* suggests that the "appropriate institutional committee . . . may be an existing one such as a board of trustees, medical staff committee. . . ."[5] We disagree. The overall function of the Institutional Advisory Committee should be assigned to a new committee[6] and not to one which is already burdened with other distinct functions. To make the IAC part of another committee would simply pay insufficient respect to the many complex issues it will have to confront and resolve. Furthermore, the composition of existing committees may be inappropriate. Membership in the IAC should be drawn up with an eye to fulfilling the purposes of the committee. These

---

[4] A term frequently used at present is "Institutional Review Committee." We altered that for the following reasons: (a) the term "review" is slightly misleading, since the committees' primary function is to *preview* a course of action before it has taken place, rather than to review it and its consequences, as we use the term "review" in describing the third stage of the process; (b) although the committees usually have the official power to say "aye" or "nay" to a protocol, their overall function is to give advice to members at the institution on how such interventions ought to be handled; and (c) since we describe the role and membership of the IAC's in different terms than those usually associated with the Institutional Review Committees, a change of title helps to avoid confusion.

[5] U.S. DEP'T OF HEALTH, EDUCATION & WELFARE, INSTITUTIONAL GUIDE TO DHEW POLICY ON PROTECTION OF HUMAN SUBJECTS (1971) [hereinafter cited as INSTITUTIONAL GUIDE].

[6] Given the structure and functioning we envision for an IAC, we do not think that its duties should even be given (or assumed to be fulfilled) by existing "Peer Review" or "Clinical Investigations" committees. The establishment of an IAC suggests, however, that there would probably be no further need for a separate committee of the type now constituted under PHS or FDA regulations.

are most easily kept in mind by subdividing the IAC's specialized functions into three parts: a protocol approval group, a subject advisory group, and an appeals group.

1. Protocol Approval Groups

The heart of each Institutional Advisory Committee will be its Protocol Approval Group (PAG) which will be responsible for approving, disapproving, or offering suggestions for modification in protocols for experimental and therapeutic interventions which come within the policies on risk and consent formulated earlier in the process (as described in Chapter Eight). The PAG's task will be to apply the rules and policies already set down, but this should not be a matter of "clock work" or mere routine. Realistically, even if policy formulation proceeds with much more rigor, it is unlikely that it will result in directives that settle all issues faced by the PAG. This does not suggest, however, that Protocol Approval Groups set policies themselves, although they may be given some discretion in light of local institutional conditions and so permit experimentation with a variety of alternative policies that are still consistent with the general directives. This sort of flexibility is vital if the PAG's are to operate effectively and secure the services of thoughtful, devoted members. The danger posed by discretion and its potential for abuse (*i.e.*, that a local PAG will deviate substantially from the generally accepted norms) is reduced by the review provided first by its own Institutional Advisory Committee and then, through avenues described in the succeeding chapter, by national bodies.

a. Composition. Membership in the Protocol Approval Group should consist primarily of professionals with competence in biomedicine. This reflects the committee's function, which is to scrutinize protocols in light of the policy guidelines and directives, to evaluate whether the procedure should be undertaken, and to give advice to the physicians and scientists involved. In most instances these group members will be members of the institution's faculty and staff. However, when the presence of more than one institution in a locality permits it, having some people from one center serve on another's PAG would provide valuable cross-fertilization. Such an arrangement would also mean that some of the PAG members are "outsiders" in the sense of being free of the personal ties and biases of the institution's own employees, while maintaining the biomedical expertise that characterizes "insiders."

A basic question about the PAG's composition is whether it should also include "lawyers, clergymen, or laymen" to provide the group with the "competencies necessary to judge the acceptability of project or activity in terms of institutional regulations, relevant law, standards of professional practice, and community acceptance."[7] Such members, often suggested by commentators[8] and now required by the FDA, are clearly necessary to implement community values—but this should occur in the formulation stage rather than in administration. Consequently, it is our view that the PAG need include only enough "outsiders" to provide the requisite sensitivity and ability to understand the relevant policy formulations.[9] One area requiring particular care is that of the consent procedures; the PAG should include persons, be they laymen or professionals, with the competence and sensitivity to scrutinize consent forms and procedures in order to maximize the probability that patients and subjects will understand what is being asked of them. One novel source for such members could be from among convalescing patients or former patients whose term on the PAG should be for a limited period of time only, to preclude their becoming bureaucratized and to bring a fresh outlook to the group's proceedings. From the review of the PAG's decisions and from its interaction with the Subject Advisory Group, refinements in the guidelines for consent may be expected to emerge.

b. Structure. Depending on the size of the institution, the Protocol Approval Group may carry out all its functions as a whole or it may wish to form subgroups, although overall jurisdiction should probably remain with the entire group. An imaginative way of lightening the burden on group members and of spreading understanding of the group's activities throughout the institution is suggested by the practices of the Committee on Human Welfare and Experimentation at the University of California Medical Center in San Francisco:

> The Committee realized that the number of applications, the diversity of subject matter and the seriousness of the task would preclude meaningful review of consistent and high quality by a small fixed group. Therefore, the Committee established itself as parent group to three-man ad hoc review committees it appointed for each submitted protocol. Members of the parent

---

[7] Food and Drug Administration, *Institutional Committee Review of Clinical Investigations of New Drugs in Human Beings*, 36 FED. REG. 5037, 5038 (1971); *see* 21 C.F.R. §130.3 (1972).

[8] *See, e.g.,* Barber, *The Structure, Functions and Efficacy of Peer Review Committees in the Experimental and Allocative Phases of Clinical Treatment* (1972) [Appendix D].

[9] If legal advice is required, we believe it is preferable to seek it from the institution's regular counsel rather than from any lawyers who happen to be on the PAG, since they are there as members of the group and not in their distinct professional capacity as attorneys. On the other hand, it would seem legitimate to us for the function undertaken by lawyers or members of the institution's administration who serve on the PAG to be that of interpreters of regulatory language and as recorders of the "precedents" established by the group through its successive decisions.

committee could review some applications and take "administrative action," or they could serve on ad hoc committees. Members of the ad hoc groups were chosen by the Committee on Human Welfare and Experimentation from the faculty at large. Each member was chosen for his objectivity, morality, expertise in some area related to the research protocol, ability to communicate critical information to the investigator and lack of personal involvement in the research project.

• • •

The chairmen of ad hoc committees were asked to file a written report to the parent committee within 10 days of its assignment to the ad hoc committee. Disagreement by any member on any of the six points used for review was interpreted as a potential disapproval and required that the parent committee transmit recommendations for revision to the investigator. Re-examination of the revised protocol by the parent committee could then result in approval. If the ad hoc group disapproved unanimously of any of the six points, revision became mandatory, and the protocol could be accepted only with the unanimous approval of the ad hoc committee. In response to disapproval, an investigator could withdraw the request, alter the protocol to comply with recommendations or request another ad hoc committee that would review the protocol de novo. No more than two ad hoc committees could review an unaltered protocol.[10]

c. Functions. Once there has been better formulation of the substantive and procedural criteria for risktaking, risk-benefit equations, consent, selection of recipients and donors, and so forth, which are to guide the evaluation of research protocols, the burden of the evaluation process ought to be lessened. In the light of the expected greater specificity and clarity, which can also be communicated to individual physician-investigators, protocols should be easier to evaluate. Indeed, some groups might experiment with having physician-investigators "pre-screen" their own protocols. Those whose authors felt they raised no questions under the relevant guidelines could be passed upon more expeditiously; when a physician felt less sure, his protocol could be given a more thorough evaluation. It would, of course, be necessary to avoid "overconfidence" on the part of physicians, and the least question raised about an "easy" protocol should lead to its getting a complete evaluation. If such doubts prove to be well founded, the physician who submitted the protocol should be briefed on his apparent misunderstanding of the relevant guidelines and his future submissions should be given more careful scrutiny.

---

[10] Melmon, Grossman & Morris, *Emerging Assets and Liabilities of a Committee on Human Welfare and Experimentation,* 282 NEW ENG. J. MED. 427, 428 (1970) [hereinafter cited as Melmon].

In order to determine whether a proposed intervention satisfied relevant risk-benefits standards,[11] it will be necessary for the PAG to determine the adequacy of the research design and the contributions which the intervention is likely to make to scientific knowledge. The greatest controversies between physician-investigators and the Protocol Approval Groups will probably arise on these two points. Although interrelated, they are distinct issues and should be evaluated separately. Any questions about either should be carefully set forth in writing by the PAG so that the physician-investigator can study them and make appropriate modifications in design or forward them with his rebuttal to an appeal board for further consideration. The appeal board will, of course, also have to rule on any controversy about scientific merits, and we shall have more to say about this later.

A further function of the PAG's, and of their parent IAC's generally, is to inform all personnel at their institutions at appropriate intervals, and at a minimum once at the beginning of each academic year, about the duties and obligations imposed on them whenever they engage in investigative endeavors. They should also be acquainted with the procedures and composition of the IAC and its subgroups. Current practice at many institutions is limited to merely informing the staff by letter about the obligation to submit protocols for review or to describing briefly this requirement in the hospital's procedural handbook. This is not sufficient, in our opinion. A general meeting, or even better small workshops, should be convened from time to time at which members of the PAG not only explain in detail its requirements but also acquaint physician-investigators more fully with the underlying reasons for the procedures it has established. This educational function has been neglected and its absence has contributed to the alienation between physician-investigators and the existing institutional review committee. Face-to-face discussions, focused around presentations of the problems encountered by the Protocol Approval Groups when evaluating protocols, could clear up many misconceptions or at least convey an appreciation of the duties they have to perform. Such interchanges could also give valuable feedback to the members of PAG's about the difficulties faced by physician-investigators and lead in turn to modifications in administrative practices. Moreover, these educational gatherings may stimulate some of the participants to explore the complex problems posed by investigative

---

[11] The most recent promulgations by HEW, in the section on risks and benefits, require that the committee "carefully weigh the known or foreseeable risks to be encountered by subjects, the probable benefits that may accrue to them and the probable benefits to humanity that may result from the subject's participation in the project or activity." INSTITUTIONAL GUIDE, note 5 *supra*, at 6. While we hope, and expect, that the guidelines formulated as suggested in Chapter Eight will add greater specificity to this preachment, the difficulty mentioned in the text will remain.

medicine, and valuable scholarly contributions may result from such pursuits.

A final function of each PAG is to assure itself that the interventions being carried out are consistent with the protocols it has approved. The basically collegial nature of the PAG should place it in a good position to counsel and admonish physician-investigators who wittingly or unwittingly disregard proper procedures. In addition, the Protocol Approval Group should ask physician-investigators to notify it immediately about significant modifications in research protocols as well as about complications which had not been expected at the initiation of the investigation. Such information will permit the PAG to reconsider its prior approval if necessary and provide valuable feedback about weaknesses in the evaluation process. Upon completion of each project, the group should also require a summary from the physician-investigators setting forth, *inter alia,* significant discrepancies between the initial protocol and subsequent experiences.

Present guidelines view the monitoring of ongoing projects as "an essential part of the review process [including] systematic review of projects at fixed intervals or at intervals set by the committee commensurate with the project's risk. . . ."[12] We do not believe that monitoring needs to be carried out at all times for all projects at all institutions. Instead, it appears to us that spot checks of selected interventions (randomly chosen) to determine compliance with their protocols and absence of unforeseen risks would be as effective and much more conserving of the scarce time of PAG members. Should these spot checks reveal widespread deviations from the group's expectations, better education of physician-investigators about their responsibilities, more careful evaluation of protocols and of their sponsors' capabilities and past performance, and routine monitoring of all projects (at least for a while) would be indicated.

Experience with existing institutional review committees has shown that a few investigators do not submit protocols for prior approval.[13] If adequate procedures have been formulated to permit expedited or summary approval of a protocol in an emergency (properly defined), there should be no reason for physician-investigators to proceed without approval. Should such a situation come to the attention of a PAG, whether informally or through its spot-check activities, it must deal with two questions, separate albeit related. First, it must review the project and decide whether it would have been approved if properly submitted; if the protocol would not have been approved, the PAG must determine whether the project should be halted or if it can be made acceptable through modification. Second, the

---

12 INSTITUTIONAL GUIDE, note 5 *supra,* at 8.
13 *See, e.g.,* Melmon, note 10 *supra,* at 430.

PAG should consider the physician's explanation for his failure to follow proper procedures. Having provided him with a hearing, it may then wish to refer his case to the review body for the imposition of previously promulgated sanctions, such as censure or denial of research privileges. The general topic of sanctions, and particularly the role which professional journals can play, is discussed in the following chapter.

2. Subject Advisory Groups

Procedures should also be created for the establishment of Subject Advisory Groups (SAG) to aid patient-subjects in decisionmaking. The composition of these groups should be a mixed one and include both professionals and laymen. Their availability for consultation ought to be made known to patient-subjects whenever they are invited to participate in biomedical interventions within the purview of the Institutional Advisory Committee and should be clearly repeated on the consent form. The SAG should also communicate to the PAG recurrent problems it encounters in the administration of consent procedures; as necessary, these observations should also be considered by the organization charged with reviewing the process and reformulating policies.

We do not lightly suggest the creation of another subgroup within the Institutional Advisory Committee, since we have no desire to overburden the process with excessive bureaucracy.[14] Yet the experience to date with

---

[14] Recently HEW has proposed the creation of special "Protection Committees" for research with children and prisoners. The functions of these committees are much more extensive than those proposed by us; they overlap and duplicate responsibilities assigned by HEW to other committees charged with protecting the subjects of research. For example with respect to research on prisoners, the proposed regulations state:

... The primary function of the Protection Committee is to provide supplementary judgment by overseeing the selection of subjects who may be included in a research project to assure that their consent is as voluntary as possible under the conditions of confinement.

Consent is a continuing process. To assure the voluntariness of consent, subjects must be able to withdraw from the research project without prejudice. Each Protection Committee shall establish such a withdrawal mechanism.

The duties of the Protection Committee, therefore, shall include:

1. Reviewing the information given the potential subjects, with special attention to: adverse effects, the importance of reporting all deviations from normal function, the continuing option of withdrawing from participation at any time, and the identification of a member of the committee who will be available, at reasonable intervals upon request, for consultation regarding the research project. All of this information shall appear on the consent form, a copy of which will be given to each participant. ...

2. Overseeing the process of selection of subjects who may be included in the re-

consent procedures indicates that present means do not provide patient-subjects with adequate protection. A sociologist recently studied the inter-actions between physician-investigators and their patient-subjects at a university hospital; his interviews with patient-subjects revealed among other things that

> 20 subjects (of 51) were not aware that they were experimental subjects until their participation in the study was well under way. Most of these subjects learned of the existence of the study during the interviews done for my research. [M]any more subjects . . . while aware of the research had significant gaps in their understanding of the project and consented on a more or less uninformed basis. These included women who had no knowledge of whether there were alternatives to participation, women who did not know that two drugs were involved, women who did not know of the double-blind nature of the study (it was not part of the research design to withhold this information) and women who were not aware of the fetal monitoring procedures and extra blood samples required by the research.[15]

Clearly, the major need is for more complete and comprehensible information to be communicated to patients. With better education and more dedication, physician-investigators may handle this task adequately. One way of encouraging them to do so would be to have them audio or video taperecord their information-giving and consent-receiving sessions with patient-subjects. This could provide an extremely useful supplement to their written records, for use by the PAG in its spot checks and by reviewing bodies considering the results, particularly if allegations of uninformed consent were raised.

Yet even when physician-investigators have mended their ways and auditing procedures are in effect, we believe there is a role for a group not directly involved with an intervention to be available to patient-subjects. Creating an opportunity for someone in addition to physician-investigators to talk with patient-subjects does not suggest a lack of trust in the investi-

---

search, to the extent stipulated in the recommendation of the Organizational Review Committee. . . .

3. Visiting the institution on a regular basis to invite questions, to monitor the progress of the research, and to assess the continued willingness of subject participation. . . .

4. Maintaining records of its activities including contacts initiated by subjects in the project between regular site visits. These records shall be made available to the agency upon request. . . .

38 FED. REG. 31744 (November 16, 1973).

[15] Gray, *Some Vagaries of Consent* in J. KATZ WITH THE ASSISTANCE OF A. CAPRON AND E. GLASS, EXPERIMENTATION WITH HUMAN BEINGS 660 (1970) [hereinafter cited as KATZ].

gators' integrity; rather, it recognizes the reality that investigators cannot help but plead, however unconsciously, their interests in the research and therefore will find it difficult to safeguard fully the interests of their subjects. Subjects may wish to turn to a disinterested party for additional advice or help to sort out their feelings about participating in the proposed project.

To a certain extent some medical personnel already fill this role, albeit by default. We believe there is need for a more organized system, so that some people regard it as their assignment to counsel patient-subjects in this regard and answer their questions, rather than it being an extraneous duty which they may perform if they are so inclined. Formalizing the arrangement somewhat may also invest the members of the SAG with more stature in the eyes of patient-subjects. One mechanism along these lines has been established by the Massachusetts General Hospital in Boston:

> A safeguard is to be found in the practice of having at least two professionally qualified persons involved in experimental situations: First, there is the physician or other person concerned with the care of the subject; his primary interest is the subject's welfare. It is of utmost importance in experimental situations involving children or incompetent individuals that this person serve as the subject's advocate. Second, there is the investigator whose interest is the sound conduct of the investigation. Perhaps too often a single individual attempts to encompass both roles.[16]

Although we agree with the intention expressed here—protecting patient-subjects—we are doubtful that this procedure will be sufficient to make patient-subjects into informed decisionmakers. We wonder whether the treating physician can advise his patient about becoming a research subject or whether with children or incompetent individuals he can "serve as the subjects' advocate." Although the treating physician's personal knowledge and understanding of his patients may give him insight into the best ways to communicate with them, the mutual ties between physician and patients may make both the informing and consenting aspects of "informed consent" more difficult; thus, it would be better if a less involved physician or a lay person were available for that purpose. Moreover, once the project has been initiated it would be advisable to give total responsibility for the care of patient-subjects to the physician-investigator, for if this role is split the danger is great that neglect will occur, because each one may expect the other to take charge. Instead, the representative of the SAG (physician or lay person depending on the type of biomedical procedure) can explain to the patient, or to the parents or guardians of an incompetent, what the procedure is all about, answer all questions, and make sure that the patient

[16] MASSACHUSETTS GENERAL HOSPITAL, HUMAN STUDIES: GUIDING PRINCIPLES AND PROCEDURES 13 (1970) [hereinafter cited as MASS. GENERAL GUIDELINES].

or guardian is aware of the consequences of participation. Thus, the role of SAG members is to inform but not to make judgments for patient-subjects. In their advisory, one-to-one capacity, they should never allow themselves to be placed in the position of answering the ultimate question, "Should I participate?"

A much more ticklish problem is raised when the SAG is called upon to decide whether a patient-subject's consent should be honored. Dr. Carl Fellner has observed, for example, that at present, the decision whether or not to permit kidney transplantation from a living donor rests with the physician's evaluation of the donor's voluntariness and freedom from undue pressure.[17] While we do not believe that physician-investigators should have the authority to pass on consent in this way, we also doubt that in most cases this role should be shifted to the SAG. Occasionally, however, questions will be raised about consent which cannot be overcome by a SAG's merely counseling the patient-subject further and providing him with more information about the proposed intervention.[18] It may become necessary for the SAG to suggest the need for policy formulations in this area which would specify the grounds (short of a judicial finding of incompetence) for holding a potential subject's consent inoperative. The principles of self-determination and autonomy would weigh heavily against any interference with a patient-subject's consent. The subject would in such circumstances at least have the right to appeal this determination as discussed in the next section.

Not all patient-subjects may wish to seek out representatives of the Subject Advisory Group, for some may be satisfied with the information obtained from physician-investigators. But patient-subjects should be well apprised of the availability of these representatives prior to their participation in projects which have to be submitted to the PAG because of the risk involved or because of the problems anticipated with obtaining valid consent. Patient-subjects may also wish to avail themselves of the SAG's services when they begin to wonder whether continuation of the intervention is worth the pain and suffering they have to endure. At such time, the Subject Advisory Group assumes the important function of administering the procedures formulated for the cessation of experimental treatments. With

---

[17] *See* Fellner, *The Genetically Unrelated Living Kidney Donor: Unemployed and Unwanted* (consultant's memorandum) (1972) [Appendix E].

[18] Such occasions should arise less frequently than at present because under our proposals SAG's will be better guided by policies formulated at the national level. For example, during the trial in the Detroit Psychosurgery Case questions were raised about the adequacy of the existing subject protection committee. To a large extent the inadequate protection provided by the members of this committee to John Doe rested on their lack of clarity over the policies which ought to guide their deliberations.

terminal patients, such interruption may permit death to occur more quickly, so the SAG must be sensitive to the distinction between terminating an intervention and active euthanasia, not yet sanctioned by society.[19] In making this distinction, reference may be made to the patient's right to have refused the intervention in the first place. In these circumstances, the Subject Advisory Group has a duty to ascertain that the patient-subject appreciates as fully as he can the implications of his decisions to terminate and that his relatives are also provided with necessary information and counseling. If the SAG determines that the patient-subject should not or cannot terminate the intervention, he and his relatives should be advised of their right to appeal to the appeal board or if necessary to the courts.

3. Appeals Groups

This brings us to the third specialized subdivision of the Institutional Advisory Committee, namely its appellate arm. The Appeals Group would be charged with resolving disagreements between physician-investigators and patient-subjects and the PAG and SAG; it could also hear an appeal brought by the chief of the relevant hospital service.[20] We do not believe there is need for an elaborate set of rules to govern Appeal Groups' proceedings. Simply stated, an Appeals Group would decide whether the relevant advisory group had made accurate factual determinations and applied the correct policy formulations; this would be determined by examining the advisory group's reasons for its determination in light of whatever points and countervailing evidence the objecting party wanted to introduce.

Appeals could be decided by panels of five, constituting the Appeals Group or drawn from its membership if the Appeals Group is larger. Membership in each panel should be chosen to bring expertise relevant to the issues raised by the objecting party. For example, appeals involving the

---

[19] For an introduction to the literature on these issues, *see* KATZ, note 15 *supra*, at pp. 702-718, 1072-1082.

[20] *Cf.* MASS. GENERAL GUIDELINES, note 16 *supra*, at 13:

It is the responsibility of the Chief of Service to decide whether to accept the advice of the Committee on Research or to refer the matter to the General Director and the Trustees for a definitive decision. The Trustees may seek the advice of its Advisory Committee on Research and the Individual in the unlikely event of disagreement among those concerned.

As indicated in the text, we think that the right to appeal should be held by others besides the Chief of Service. Moreover, we doubt that a hospital board of trustees is the most appropriate appellate body, since its longstanding and complex institutional involvements and interactions may not permit its members either to be impartial or to give the appearance of fairness so essential to the functioning of an appeal board.

adequacy of research design would be heard by professionals including well recognized research scientists. Members for such panels should probably not be connected with the particular institution in order to assure impartiality and objectivity. These qualities are more difficult to achieve if the appeals board is composed of members chosen from the same institutions as the physician-investigator because of the real or felt impact of intimate friendships and rivalries on decisionmaking. An appeal questioning the risks to which patient-subjects will be exposed or possibly detrimental consequences for society ought to be heard by a panel which includes laymen who are sensitive to the relevant aspects of the policy guidelines. Further appeals may also be taken to a national panel, as described hereafter.[21]

4. Overview—The Functions of the Institutional Advisory Committee

Most of our comments have been directed to the roles which will be played by the three working arms of the Institutional Advisory Committee, so we perceive a need to pause here to give a fuller view of our conception of the IAC itself. Its primary function is to serve as the umbrella body for all matters dealing with biomedical innovation at its institution. On its shoulders falls the general responsibility of educating and sensitizing the institution's staff and of making sure that policy formulations and revisions are communicated to the staff and particularly to the members of the groups that will be applying them.

The process of communication should not be only one way, however. The IAC also has the responsibility of assuring that adequate information is available to the reviewing bodies and, in particular, that the "larger issues" raised by the biomedical enterprise are addressed publicly. The history of hemodialysis has placed in stark relief the moral and professional problems created by the insufficiency of resources to provide adequate treatment to sufferers from certain chronic renal diseases. These problems are not limited to hemodialysis but affect other medical conditions as well; in addition, they are more serious in some localities than in others. Physician-investigators should not be shouldered with the responsibility of carrying these burdens in silence or of waging individual campaigns to remedy these situations. They should instead be able to apprise the local Institutional Advisory Committee of these problems. The members of the IAC's will gradually accumulate a great deal of experience about the administration of these problems. Moreover, the IAC's will be able to bring those issues which require not only more prolonged exploration but also the advice of "outsiders" to the attention of the national policy formulation board. It is our impression that in the past physicians concerned with these issues

---

[21] *See* pp. 337-338 *infra.*

had no one to turn to, especially at the local level, and often gave up in frustration to the detriment of the profession, patients, and society.

B. ADMINISTRATION AT THE NATIONAL LEVEL

The scheme which we have suggested relies primarily on policy formulation and review by broadly based groups at the national level and policy administration at the local level largely by biomedical professionals. There are also administrative matters which arise at the national level, however, and we turn briefly now to a consideration of some of these.

1. Selection of Treatment Recipients

In discussing the formulation of policy on recipient selection, we emphasized the need to make established treatments available on an equitable basis rather than depending on a physician's capacity to exert influence on behalf of his patient with a local hospital or the like. While limitations on resources may lead to local variations in the availability of treatment—and *should* lead to variations in the case of treatments which are still experimental—such fortuitous factors as location and initial treating facility ought not affect whether a patient gets needed care. Thus, each patient has the right to be included in a national program, such as the one outlined in Chapter Eight which relies on a combination of medical screening and random selection mechanism to select treatment recipients. Administratively, this system would require procedures for the direct, confidential registration of eligible patients. The system could operate directly between the individual's physician and the national registry, since there would be no role for a local selecting body. It ought also to be confidential, since it would involve an extension of the physician-patient relationship. Special legislation and regulation would be needed to protect the confidentiality of the data submitted. Making sure that physicians are only submitting qualified patients would be the responsibility of those operating the national registry, through special examining physicians who conducted spot checks on applicants or through intake officials at the centers where treatment (*e.g.*, hemodialysis) is actually administered.

A national system for the allocation of donor organs would also be advisable. Such systems have been established for cadaver organs in Western Europe and around Paul Terasaki's computerized tissue-typing facility at UCLA. As histocompatibility becomes better understood—and provided that it is not rendered unnecessary by completely safe and effective immunosuppressives—the need for better administrative mechanisms becomes more acute.

Present organ-sharing arrangements are informal and nonbinding. "Once the kidneys are obtained, how they are distributed is currently a matter mostly of who salvaged the kidneys."[22] Although it is true under the Uniform Anatomical Gift Act that physicians act as "recipients" of cadaver organs, it is clear that the intent of the Act was that they were only trustees and that they need be given no personal control over who receives the organs. Therefore, there should be no legal impediments to moving beyond the present informal systems, such as that operated out of UCLA. More than 500 organs have already been shared among more than 90 transplant centers through the UCLA tissue-matching and recipient registry, but the nonmandatory nature of the system creates problems of its own. Less than the best matches occur for two reasons. First, participating transplant centers typically share only one kidney from the cadaver and keep the other for one of "their own" patients. Second, a center which has shared a kidney gets a "credit" which places it in a preferential position for receiving future kidneys from other centers.

The emphasis on the "ownership" of the donated kidney thus biases the choice of the recipients according to the center at which they are awaiting treatment rather than solely according to the medical probabilities (*e.g.,* closeness of tissue type, surgical success record of physician performing the operation, etc.). As techniques of organ preservation and tissue matching are perfected, there is no excuse for a continuation of a system which relies on arbitrary, nonmedical factors in the assignment of scarce resources such as cadaver organs.[23] If a transplant center wishes to participate in a national organ-sharing arrangement, in order to increase the range of tissue types it can offer to patients, it should be obliged to share all the cadaver organs which become available to it. We are not persuaded of the danger that physicians' motivation to seek cadaver organs will be destroyed if the organs are going to be shared with the best-matched patients at other hospitals. The greater supply of, and better chances with, such organs will provide sufficient motivation for physicians, who—like potential donors and their families—will be made more aware of organ donation as a con-

---

[22] Terasaki, *Organ Transplantation* (consultant's memorandum), at 3 (1972) [Appendix K]. The informal system of organ sharing has nevertheless been remarkably successful, although a much greater degree of organization and cooperation would be needed to produce an adequate supply of cadaver kidneys. By 1972 nearly half of all cadaver kidneys transplanted were obtained from other hospitals (600 shared within the same city and 455 shared between cities). A wide, national pool of donors and recipients is particularly necessary to avoid mismatches caused by lymphocytotoxins. *See* Opelz & Terasaki, *National Utilization of Cadaver Kidneys for Transplantation,* 228 J.A.M.A. 1260 (1974).

[23] *See* Terasaki, Wilkinson & McClelland, *National Transplant Communications Network,* 218 J.A.M.A. 1674-78 (1971).

tribution to an important national need with the potential of saving many lives.

2. Research v. Therapy

An example of a national administrative decision of a very different type would be the need to decide when an intervention designated as "research," in the sense discussed in Chapter Eight, has become "therapeutic." Although basic policies on this and similar matters will have been established previously at the formulation stage, these policies are not self-executing. Thus, national bodies must keep abreast of the progress of catastrophic disease research and treatment in order to determine, *inter alia,* when a procedure which had been available only on a limited "research" basis should be more widely offered or whether a procedure which had called for review by the local Institutional Advisory Committees should be regarded as no longer needing protocol approval.

3. Appeals

Another important function for the national body will be the resolution of appeals from local Institutional Advisory Committee decisions. Present HEW guidelines make no provision for appeals, and committees can deprive physician-investigators of federal support (and, in effect, funding from other sources as well) without recourse. Bernard Barber and his colleagues have suggested that this may not only hinder the acquisition of knowledge but also undermine the legitimacy of the entire decisionmaking process.[24] In most instances it is expected that the physician-investigator (or, where appropriate, the patient-subject or his representative) will be satisfied with the local decision, will accept the necessary modifications, or will not desire to expose to further and wider scrutiny a protocol repeatedly found ethically or scientifically deficient. But where there is desire for an appeal, that avenue should be open. The appellant should be allowed to file papers

---

[24] We have heard researchers object to peer review as they know or understand it because they believe that research proposals having real potential for medical scientific advances, or even "pioneering breakthroughs," frequently either are not or will not be approved by those who sit on institutional review committees. The reasons for these rejections they are especially concerned about do not involve the ethical defectiveness of the proposals. Rather they include local institutional politics and conflicts as well as resistance to innovations just because they depart from accustomed ways of scientific thinking and proceeding.

B. BARBER, J. LALLY, J. MAKARUSHKA & D. SULLIVAN, RESEARCH ON HUMAN SUBJECTS 156 (1973) (footnote omitted). *See also* TUSKEGEE SYPHILIS STUDY AD HOC ADVISORY PANEL, U.S. DEP'T OF HEALTH, EDUCATION & WELFARE, FINAL REPORT 44 (1973).

specifying the grounds for his objection and supporting his position. The local committee may be satisfied that the minutes of its Protocol Approval Group and Appeals Group adequately dispose of the appellant's contention or they too may file a specific reply. Where necessary, the national body may choose to have an oral presentation of evidence and arguments, but it is likely that a decision will usually be rendered on the written submissions. On the basis of handling appeals, the national body may apprise its members who are in charge of the "review" process that certain policies are in need of reformulation because they are causing repeated misunderstanding at the local level.

CHAPTER TEN

Review of Decisions and Consequences

In addition to an appellate procedure for disputes or disagreements over the conduct of individual research projects, as described in the foregoing chapter, adequate functioning of the catastrophic disease decisionmaking process also requires the creation of procedures for evaluating the decisions which have been reached and their consequences. The mechanisms of appeal and reconsideration discussed previously were concerned with the resolution of issues which arise at what we term the stage of "administration" in decisionmaking—that is, they involve the application of formulated policies to specific medical interventions. Means for after-the-fact review are also needed if the wisdom and efficacy of existing policies is not to go unquestioned. Moreover, a policy or practice which has not been the subject of criticism or disagreement among the participants may nevertheless be in need of alteration. All outcomes—and not just those which are noticeably "harmful"—should be reviewed to keep policy formulations flexible and up-to-date.

In this chapter we examine the third stage in the catastrophic disease process which seeks to provide an opportunity for evaluating the consequences of the decisions made at the two prior stages. The mechanisms of review fall into two groups: those which look toward policy reformulation through a broad input of data on a nonadversary basis, and those which in addition to providing data for the reformulation process are primarily concerned with the adjudication of individual cases and the compensation of injured parties. Both types of review mechanism are designed to control

239

the catastrophic disease process in the sense not only of limiting but also of modulating, improving, and facilitating it. But they differ in their primary purposes and therefore in the qualifications and authority of the persons selected to conduct the review process.

The first mechanism attempts solely to facilitate an examination of the outcome of decisionmaking so that policies in need of reformulation can be reexamined and administrative procedures in need of improvement can be revised. It seeks to accomplish these goals through a broad input of information and value judgments from a great many segments of the profession and society and thus both "insiders" and "outsiders" should participate in this process. To be effective, it requires that any impediments to a free examination of practices be removed or at least minimized, recognizing that this will not be totally effective since real and imaginative fears of the results of scrutiny will lead to some witting and unwitting withholding of data. It also requires that procedures be developed so that what is learned from the data collected will be utilized and not dissipated. The creation of committees and procedures for these purposes has been a long neglected aspect of medical decisionmaking.

The second mechanism similarly seeks to obtain data for purposes of evaluation but does so through the process of adjudicating claims brought by the participants in the process against one another. Since such adjudication can lead to the imposition of sanctions, the tendency to withhold data will be considerable. Moreover, in any controversy data may be unconsciously withheld or distorted in order to champion one's cause, and these considerations impose limits on the usefulness for review of data thus obtained. Yet the catastrophic disease review process must offer some devices for imposing sanctions, and much can still be learned from the information obtained during adjudication. Needless to say, before sanctions can even be considered, it must be clear to the participants what kind of acts could lead to their imposition, both for reasons of fairness and because unanticipated sanctions would do nothing to enforce or support the policies and procedures which are intended to be promoted.

A. REVIEW THROUGH THE EXAMINATION OF DATA

It seems advisable that the group charged with formulating policy should play the major role in the nonadjudicatory review of decisions and their consequences. Since the entire catastrophic disease process can only benefit from intermittent reformulation of policies, it is this group that can best utilize this data. We have already suggested that the members of the policy-making group also must formulate policies with respect to review and the input of information about what has actually transpired so as to permit them constantly to improve on their promulgations.[1] Finally, the policy-making group should have no sanctioning authority, although it will be the body to formulate policies with respect to the enforcement of its promulgations and the imposition of sanctions.[2] In certain circumstances it may pass information on to the appropriate sanctioning body when it deems this necessary. Such a step could, we realize, interfere with its primary functions of data gathering and policy reformulation, but we believe it is necessary for the group to have this power in certain extreme situations. Without such authority, intolerable conflicts of conscience may develop among the group members. Over time, as the reviewing arm of the policymaking group gathers experience, the need for it to intervene in the sanctioning proce-

---

[1] Title II, Part B, of the National Research Act of 1974 provides for the creation of a National Advisory Council for the Protection of Subjects of Biomedical and Behavioral Research after July 1, 1976, to administer and review the policies formulated by the present National Advisory Commission. Among its responsibilities, the Council shall

(B) review policies, regulations, and other requirements of the Secretary governing such research to determine the extent to which such policies, regulations, and requirements require and are effective in requiring observance in such research of the basic ethical principles which should underlie the conduct of such research and, to the extent such policies, regulations, or requirements do not require or are not effective in requiring observance of such principles, make recommendations to the Secretary respecting appropriate revision of such policies, regulations, or requirements; and

(C) review periodically changes in the scope, purpose, and types of bio-medical and behavioral research being conducted and the impact such changes have on the policies, regulations, and other requirements of the Secretary for the protection of human subjects of such research.

Pub. L. No. 93-348, §211 (July 12, 1974) (amending §217 of the Public Health Service Act).

[2] The Tuskegee Syphilis Study *Ad Hoc* Advisory Panel observed that the HEW guidelines on enforcement "are written in permissive and general language." TUSKE-GEE SYPHILIS STUDY AD HOC ADVISORY PANEL, U.S. DEP'T OF HEALTH, EDUCATION & WELFARE, FINAL REPORT 36 (1973). After quoting 1-40-50 (E) on sanctions in the HEW Grants Administration Manual Chapter 1-40 (1971), the Panel concluded:

These enforcement guidelines delegate sole responsibility for the detection of failures to comply to the Division of Research Grants. But staff members of the DRG are probably the last persons to hear of any infractions once they have occurred, and then only when, as in the Tuskegee Study, they are of major proportions. Indeed, no procedures have been established to require institutional review committees to report to HEW any evidence on noncompliance. Moreover, HEW has made no efforts to define categories of noncompliance which should lead to the imposition of sanctions which should be imposed in particular cases. Finally, institutional review committees and HEW are not authorized to take disciplinary action, except for the Secretary's prerogative to terminate grants or make the investigator or his institution ineligible to receive future funds.

dures will decrease markedly, because it will be able to propose corrective measures based on what it has learned about the reasons for improper practices not having been picked up earlier, before they were uncovered by the policymaking body.

In addition to the "review" role played by the general formulating group, a number of other groups can make a contribution to the data gathering and evaluating process. These will include biomedical journals, the popular press, the professions, legislatures, and administrative bodies.

1. Editors of Biomedical Journals

In Chapter Seven we discussed the debate about the function of biomedical journals in the catastrophic disease decisionmaking process.[3] We believe that the major function of these journals begins at the review stage and that this function should be devoid of any sanctioning authority. Some commentators have suggested that journals should refuse to publish "unethical" papers otherwise of scientific merit, but this would diminish the opportunity to appraise research practices. Indeed, the editors of journals should encourage such appraisals by requiring authors in the section on methods to give a detailed account about the way subjects were selected, the precautions they took, the procedures which were followed for the evaluation of protocols, and the like. It should no longer suffice merely to state that "informed consent was obtained" or that "the Helsinki Declaration was followed." Rather, the article should detail, among other things, what problems were encountered, how many subjects refused to consent or interrupted participation and their reasons, the steps taken to remedy these difficulties, and so forth. Much can be learned from such data. For example, the assertion that there were no problems when others would expect some to occur under the stated circumstances would lead readers, including those officially involved in the review process, to wonder why none were encountered; one British researcher told us that whenever none of the prospective subjects refuses to participate in one of his research projects, he begins to wonder about the way he has gone about obtaining consent, since he believes that some refusals are inevitable. In addition to requiring all articles to be of appropriate scientific merit and to contain a statement on procedures as outlined, the editors should discuss on the editorial page whatever "ethical problems" are raised by a particular project and in certain situations specifically invite others, from both inside and outside the profession, to comment on controversial practices. Moreover, whether a manuscript is accepted for publication or not, whenever the editors find themselves with serious doubts about the propriety of a particular study, and the behavior

---

[3] *See* pp. 122-24 *supra.*

of the physician-investigators raises the question of imposition of sanctions, it becomes the duty of the editors to bring this to the attention of the relevant sanctioning body.[4]

2. Journalists

The important role which the news media can play in educating the public about research practices and in exposing abuses has already been noted.[5] Unfortunately, after a few days of making headlines many biomedical events pass into obscurity, pushed aside by accounts of other pressing issues and events. It should be the function of the reviewing arm of the policymaking group to make inquiries into such reports. Of course, this does not suggest that every "sensational" newspaper story has to be followed up and that discretion cannot be employed in sorting out which revelations need be pursued and which can be dropped. The increasing trend toward responsible science reporting by qualified science workers should make this task easier.

3. Legislators

Legislatures, particularly Congress, have from time to time taken an active interest in reviewing the consequences of medical interventions.[6] Generally, this has occurred in moments of crisis when a particularly unfortunate event, such as the elixir-sulfanilamide tragedy of 1938, the thalidomide incident of 1962, or the revelations in 1972 of the cancer radiation studies and Tuskegee syphilis experiments, led to congressional hearings. Even though these hearings were conceived in and held during periods of crisis, much thoughtful testimony was forthcoming concerning the strengths and weaknesses of medical research practices. These legislative hearings usually lead to modifications in biomedical practices, either at the initiative of the professions as a result of the legislative scrutiny or directly through legislative action. This mechanism of review consequently gives elected representatives of the public a powerful influence on medical decisionmaking. More recently these efforts have been joined by public interest groups, such as "Nader's Raiders" and the Health Law Project, who through their investigations and recommendations have sought to influence legislators to enact new legislation to control medical practices.

Perhaps the reviewers, in these instances members of Congress, should not have immediately passed legislation—becoming thereby simultaneously formulators of policy—but should instead have asked others to make

---

[4] *See* Katz, *Editorial Rewritten*, 22 CLIN. RES. 10-11 (1974).

[5] *See* pp. 144-48 *supra.*

[6] *See* pp. 129-30 *supra.*

recommendations to them first with respect to policies that would improve medical decisionmaking. This would, however, have required a mechanism for convening a group charged with the responsibility of formulating policy; beyond the National Academy of Sciences or the National Research Council such an expert, interdisciplinary public policy group did not and does not yet exist. If such a group is ever constituted, it will include as part of its task formulating proposals for new federal legislation to be submitted to Congress for action. Such procedures may facilitate more desired participation of all interest groups in legislative decisionmaking rather than the prevalent indirect influence exerted through testimony at hearings.

4. Professions

Careful study of congressional hearings, investigative studies published in journals, and the deliberations of institutional advisory groups are other potentially powerful review mechanisms which have not been sufficiently utilized by the professions themselves. The study of such documents could be of great educational value as well in preparing medical and other students for the professional tasks that lie ahead of them.[7] The intensive studies of these by students and teachers alike could also lead to the publication of scholarly papers which point to existing problems in the formulation and administration of the catastrophic disease process and propose new ways of resolving these complex issues. In his pioneering article, *Ethics and Clinical Research*,[8] Dr. Henry K. Beecher made use of this device by carefully examining 100 consecutive research studies published in an "excellent journal" during one year and then basing his conclusions about ethical and unethical research practices on these findings. Studies and recommendations initiated and promulgated by the profession could create a better climate for a larger measure of control being exercised by the professions themselves rather than being entirely imposed on them from the outside.

---

[7] In 1973, Senator Jacob Javits introduced a bill (S.974) in the Senate which sought to provide funds for such an educational effort. The bill

would authorize special project grants for medical schools to develop and operate programs which provide increased emphasis on the ethical, social, moral, and legal implications of advances in biomedical research and technology. . . .

The bill . . . provides the opportunity for our Nation's medical schools to develop the appropriate program curriculums regarding ethical, moral, and social issues to meet the need—the protection of human subjects at risk in medical research and improved understanding of the consequences and implications for the individual and society of the advances in biomedical science—and through their own initiative and leadership construct an appropriate continuing professional institutional activity to safeguard human subjects in research.

118 *Congressional Record* S3114 (February 22, 1973).

[8] Beecher, *Ethics and Clinical Research*, 274 NEW ENG. J. MED. 1354 (1966).

5. Medical Common Law

The review process would be further enhanced if, beyond the study of existing materials, the deliberations of the committees charged with administration, including appeals, were eventually published. Guido Calabresi has outlined the implications of such a proposal:

The best way of testing lay reaction to particular experiments—indeed, the best way of broadening the inputs to the committees—lies in another device: publication of the cases decided by the committees. Such cases could well be anonymous (at least at first). They could be collected and published in much the same way that decisions of the courts are collected. The reports on any case could include, first, a factual part describing, among other things, the experience of the experimenter, the antecedent tests in non-human subjects, the major risks perceived, the scientific gains perceived possible, the availability of subsequent controls to limit the risks, the origin and life expectancy of the subjects, and the nature of the consent and the manner in which it was obtained; and, second, a jurisprudential section containing the decision of the committee (whether favorable or unfavorable), together with the principal arguments for and against the decision reached.

Such published cases would soon become the subject of intense study both inside and outside the medical profession. Analyses in learned journals by lawyers, doctors, and historians of science would inevitably follow. These would undoubtedly re-argue the more important or pathbreaking cases. If law cases are any guide, the analyses would sometimes conclude that the cases were wrongly decided, but frequently that they were rightly decided but for the wrong reasons. To the extent that Law Reviews consider themselves courts of last appeal beyond the highest courts in the land, so would the learned journals in which this *giurisprudenza* would be dissected. From all this, a sense of what society at large deems proper in medical experiments might well arise. This sense would, in turn, guide the committee and make their decisions more sophisticated. The result would not only be better thought-out decisions, but also a more complex system of controls, which, in effect, took into account much broader sources of information as to societal values. . . .[9]

These opinions should not only be published but also preserved and consulted so that they can become precedents for future opinions and lay the basis for newly articulated counterprecedents as the need arises. This eventually will give us something like a medical common law, analogous to what has worked so well for the legal profession. A medical common law rooted in precedent yet flexible and responsive to the needs of changed

---

[9] Calabresi, *Reflections on Medical Experimentation in Humans*, 98 DAEDALUS 387, 400-01 (1969).

situations and new problems would be a valuable component of any mechanism of review.[10]

B. REVIEW INVOLVING ADJUDICATION AND SANCTIONS

There is much value in a review process which is prospective and focuses on a reformulation of policies and procedures in light of experience. But the catastrophic disease process needs more than data collection, for there will be instances in which the violation of existing rules and standards will require the imposition of sanctions or the compensation of injured persons. Such functions can be fulfilled by groups drawn largely from the ranks of the professions or by the courts.

1. Review by Administrative and Professional Bodies

In the preceding chapter we suggested that each Protocol Approval Group should monitor the operation of catastrophic disease projects at its institution by having physician-investigators notify it of complications and by spot checking projects randomly to determine whether there are deviations from compliance.[11] Any substantial violations should be reported to the national bodies charged with review, either on a government-wide basis or separately within each grant-making agency. Depending on the severity of the transgression and the intentionality with which the physician-investigator acted, we believe the promulgated sanctions should include censure,, fines, and suspension of the right to receive government funds for research. Needless to say, special statutory authorization would be necessary for the national body to have such powers. The legislation would also have to spell out the procedural rights enjoyed by the physician and extent of judicial review available to the parties; it is our belief that judicial scrutiny can be limited to an appellate court determination that the review body has not abused its discretion.

Besides these national review mechanisms there is also a place for local and state professional organizations to scrutinize decisions and their consequences. The medical standards in a particular area, embodied in codes, guidelines or even in statutes,[12] may provide grounds for action by local professional authorities before the national review body would find sanc-

---

[10] *See generally* Jaffe, *Law as a System of Control*, 98 DAEDALUS 406 (1969).

[11] *See* p. 228 *supra.*

[12] *See, e.g.,* such proposed statutes as New York Assembly Bill 1837, *A Bill to Amend the Education Law, in Relation to Scientific Research on Human Subjects, to Provide for the Advancement of Such Research through the Protection of its Subjects, and to Establish a State Board on Human Research* (introduced Jan. 13, 1971).

tions to be justified under its own standards. Censure, revocation or suspension of license, or imposition of a monetary penalty are examples of the sanction which might be employed in such a situation.

2. Review by Courts

In this book, we have analyzed a series of problems which arise from research on and treatment of catastrophic diseases, and we have attempted to suggest some solutions for these problems. We recognize that all our recommendations taken together amount only to a "model of successive approximations,"[13] by which the extent of harm can be limited but never entirely eliminated. Thus, in some instances participants in the process—most especially patient-subjects and their relatives—are still going to suffer injuries.

The need for a case-by-case determination of liability for injuries would be eliminated if a system of compensation without fault were instituted as has been suggested by a number of commentators.[14] If such a compensation scheme were coupled with sanctions meted out under a system such as the ones described in the preceding subsection, both aims now sought by tort law—deterrence of harmful conduct and recovery by the persons injured—would be accomplished. Until a system of full compensation is developed,[15] the courts will continue to bear the primary burden of adjudicating claims arising from the catastrophic disease process. The difficulties with a judicial resolution of the issues raised is suggested by *Karp v. Cooley*,[16] the action brought against Dr. Denton Cooley and his colleagues by the widow of the first (and thus far only) recipient of an artificial heart. The case, which was decided in the physicians' favor, reflects the narrow way in which questions of liability arising from innovative medical treatment are dealt with by judges confined by traditional legal doctrines and reluctant to question the competence or judgment of eminent research physicians.[17] This is not to suggest that the judiciary should have no role in reviewing the catastrophic disease process. But it can be of greatest service once legal rules become more responsive to the realities of the physician-patient relationship and

---

[13] *See* Capron, *Legal Considerations Affecting Clinical Pharmacological Studies in Children,* 21 CLIN. RES. 141, 144-49 (1973).

[14] *See, e.g.,* Ladimer, *Protection and Compensation for Injury in Human Studies,* in EXPERIMENTATION WITH HUMAN SUBJECTS 247 (P. Freund ed. 1970); Calabresi, note 9 *supra,* at 395-400; Havighurst, *Compensating Persons Injured in Human Experimentation,* 169 SCIENCE 153 (1970).

[15] The development of a compensation scheme is a duty of the National Commission for the Protection of Human Subjects of Biomedical and Behavioral Research.

[16] 349 F.Supp. 827 (S.D. Tex. 1972); *aff'd,* 493 F. 2d 408 (5th Cir. 1974).

[17] *See* R. C. FOX & J. SWAZEY, THE COURAGE TO FAIL 149-211 (1974).

courts coordinate their own findings and review mechanisms with those of other participants in the process.

C. CONCLUSION

We regard conscientious efforts by all the participants at the review stage as crucial to the proper functioning of the entire process. Review might be less important if it were possible to design a system for developing new treatments for catastrophic diseases, selecting patient-subjects, and so forth, which operated with mathematical precision, causing no unexpected results, and closely serving the value preferences which guided the initial design of the system. But even in such a system it would be necessary to monitor the results to assure compliance with expectations. Moreover, we do not believe that such an "ideal" but impersonal system is possible. Rather, the catastrophic disease process we have described is populated with real people, who act on the basis of values, training, and goals of their own and of the groups to which they belong. In attempting to combat catastrophic disease they display great ingenuity, perseverance, and even courage, but also self-interest and thoughtlessness. Since we believe that the "who" of the system is so important and that the policies and procedures formulated will at best be approximations of what is most desirable, we cannot emphasize too strongly the need for diligence and creativity in reviewing the results of today in order to formulate better policies for tomorrow.

Table of Sources

(Page references in this volume are indicated by boldface numbers.)

Abel, J.J., L.G. Rowntree & B.B. Turner, On the Removal of Diffusible Substances from the Circulating Blood of Living Animals by Dialysis, 5 J. Pharmacol. Exp. Ther. 275 (1914), **35.**

ACS–NIH Organ Transplant Registry, Human Heart Transplantation (Dec. 3, 1967–June 4, 1974) (1974), **50, 52, 66.**

ACS–NIH Organ Transplant Registry, Third Scientific Report, 226 J.A.M.A. 1211 (1973), **10.**

ACS–NIH Organ Transplant Registry Newsletter (Spring 1972), **43.**

ACS–NIH Organ Transplant Registry Newsletter (Spring 1974), **13, 14, 44, 66.**

Ad Hoc Committee of the Harvard Medical School to Examine the Definition of Brain Death, A Definition of Irreversible Coma, 205 J.A.M.A. 337 (1968), **120, 207, 209, 211.**

Ad Hoc Task Force on Cardiac Replacement, National Heart Institute, U.S. Dept. of Health, Education & Welfare, Cardiac Replacement: Medical, Ethical, Psychological and Economic Implications (1969), **9, 10, 14, 134.**

Advisory Committee to the Renal Transplant Registry, The Ninth Report of the Human Renal Transplant Registry, 220 J.A.M.A. 253 (1972), **200-201, 203.**

Advisory Committee to the Renal Transplant Registry, The Tenth Report of the Human Renal Transplant Registry, 221 J.A.M.A. 1495 (1972), **44, 49.**

Advisory Committee to the Renal Transplant Registry, The Eleventh Report of the Human Renal Transplant Registry, 226 J.A.M.A. 1197 (1973), **47.**

Alexander, S., Who Decides Who Lives, Who Dies, Life, Nov. 9, 1962, **160, 168, 191, 192.**

Altman, L.K., Artificial Kidney Use Poses Awesome Questions, N.Y. Times, Oct. 24, 1971, at 1, col. 6, **144.**

————. Cost of Kidney Therapy: Two Fundamental Questions Raised, N.Y. Times, Jan. 23, 1973, at 21, col. 1, **31.**

American Medical Association, Opinions and Reports of the Judicial Council
    (1969), **121, 163, 164.**
Arnold, J.D., I.F. Zimmerman & D.C. Martin, Public Attitudes and the Diagno-
    sis of Death, 206 J.A.M.A. 1949 (1968), **208, 210, 213.**

Bailey, G.L., C.L. Hampers, J.P. Merrill & P.A. Paine, The Artificial Kidney
    at Home: A Look Five Years Later, 212 J.A.M.A. 1850 (1970), **39.**
Bar Council Report on Organ Transplant, 3 Brit. Med. J. 716 (1971), **201.**
Barber, B., The Structure, Functions and Efficacy of Peer Review Committees
    in the Experimental and Allocative Phases of Clinical Treatment (1972),
    222, 225.
Barber, B., J. Lally, J. Makarushka & D. Sullivan, Experimenting with Humans:
    Problems and Processes of Social Control in the Bio-Medical Research
    Community (unpublished manuscript, 1971), **127.**
————. Research on Human Subjects: Problems of Social Control in Medical
    Experimentation (1973), **55, 62, 70, 73, 118, 124, 125, 126, 128, 165, 237.**
Beecher, H.K., Ethical Problems Created by the Hopelessly Unconscious
    Patient, 278 New Eng. J. Med. 1425 (1968), **207.**
————. Ethics and Clinical Research, 274 New Eng. J. Med. 1354 (1966), **59,
    244.**
Berlin, I., Two Concepts of Liberty (1958), **81.**
Bessman, S.P., The Legal Problems of Organ Transplantation, 13 Vill. L. Rev.
    751 (1968), **209.**
Bessman, S.P. & J.P. Swazey, Phenylketonuria: A Study of Biomedical Legisla-
    tion, in Human Aspects of Biomedical Innovations 49 (E. Mendelsohn, J.
    Swazey & I. Travis eds. 1971), **150.**
Bilinsky, R.T., A. Morris & H.R. Klein, Satellite Dialysis: An Economic Ap-
    proach to the Delivery of Hemodialysis Care, 218 J.A.M.A. 1809 (1971),
    39.
Billingham, R.E., L. Brent & P.B. Medawar, Actively Acquired Tolerance of
    Foreign Cells, 172 Nature 603 (1953), **42.**
Billingham, R.E. & W. Silvers, The Immunobiology of Transplantation (1971),
    45-46, 48.
Biörck, G., When is Death? 1968 Wis. L. Rev. 484, **208.**
Blachly, P.H., Can Organ Transplantation Provide an Altruistic-Expiatory Al-
    ternative to Suicide? 1 Life-Threatening Behavior 6 (1971), **205.**
Blagg, C.R., R.D. Hickman, et al., Home Hemodialysis: Six Years Experience,
    283 New Eng. J. Med. 1126 (1970), **95.**
Blaiberg, P., Looking at My Heart (1968), **97.**
Blum, W. & H. Kalvern, Public Law Perspectives on a Private Law Problem
    (1965), **143.**
Braybrooke, D. & C. Lindblom, A Strategy of Decision (1963), **159.**
Brewer, L.A., Cardiac Transplantation: An Appraisal, 205 J.A.M.A. 691 (1968),
    174.
Brickman, M.J., Medico-Legal Problems with the Question of Death, 5 Calif.
    W. L. Rev. 110 (1968), **216.**

British National Health Service, Advice on the Question of Amending the Human Tissue Act 1961 (Cmnd. 4106, 1969), **198-199.**

Burnett, F.M., The Clonal Selection Theory of Acquired Immunity (1959), **42.**

Cahn, E., Drug Experiments and the Public Conscience, in Drugs in Our Society 255 (P. Talalay ed. 1964), **104.**

Calabresi, G., Reflections on Medical Experimentation in Humans, 98 Daedalus 387 (1969), **136, 245, 247.**

————. The Costs of Accidents (1970), **89, 143.**

————. Memorandum (1970), **179, 180, 183, 185, 186, 188, 191-193.**

Calland, C., Iatrogenic Problems in End-Stage Renal Failure, 287 N. Eng J. Med. 334 (1972), **12.**

Calne, R.Y., The Rejection of Renal Homograft: Inhibition in Dogs by 6-mercaptopurine, 1 Lancet 417 (1960), **46.**

Calne, R.Y. & J. Murray, Inhibition of the Rejection of Renal Homografts in Dogs by BW 57-322, 12 Surg. Forum 118 (1961), **46.**

Cannon, J.A. & W.P. Longmire, Studies of Successful Skin Homografts in the Chicken, 135 Annals Surg. 60 (1952), **42.**

Cantor, N.L., A Patient's Decision to Decline Life-Saving Medical Treatment, 26 Rutgers L. Rev. 228 (1973), **105, 108.**

Capron, A.M., Informed Consent in Catastrophic Research and Treatment, 123 U. Pa. L. Rev. 340 (1974), **149.**

————. The Law of Genetic Therapy, in The New Genetics and the Future of Man 133 (M. Hamilton ed. 1972), **59.**

————. Legal Considerations Affecting Clinical Pharmacological Studies in Children, 21 Clinical Research 141 (1973), **109, 112, 247.**

————. Legal Rights and Moral Rights, in Ethical Issues in Human Genetics 221 (Hilton, et al. eds. 1973), **103.**

————. To Decide What Dead Means, N.Y. Times, Feb. 24, 1974, at 6, col. 4, **215.**

Capron, A.M. & L.R. Kass, A Statutory Definition of the Standards for Determining Human Death: An Appraisal and a Proposal, 121 U. of Pa. L. Rev. 87 (1972), **25, 31, 216.**

Castelnuovo-Tedesco, P., Cardiac Surgeons Look at Transplantation—Interviews with Drs. Cleveland, Cooley, DeBakey, Hallman and Rochelle, 3 Seminars in Psychiatry 5 (1971), **69.**

Committee on Chronic Kidney Disease, U.S. Bureau of the Budget, Report (1967), **16.**

Compulsory Removal of Cadaver Organs, 69 Colum. L. Rev. 693 (1969), **197, 199.**

Corday, E. Definition of Death: A Double Standard, Hospital Tribune, May 4, 1970, **213.**

————. Life-Death in Human Transplantation, 55 A.B.A.J. 629 (1969), **208.**

Crafton, J., Doc: Ethics Made Me Save Heart Man, Daily News (N.Y.), Jan. 29, 1972, at 5, col. 1, **107.**

Crammond, W.A., Renal Homotransplantation: Some Observations on Recipients and Donors, 113 Brit. J. Psych. 1223 (1967), **203.**

Crane, D., Social Aspects of the Prolongation of Life (1969), **25.**

Crane, D. & D. Matthews, Heart Transplantation Operation: Diffusion of a Medical Innovation (1970), **52.**

Curran, W.J., A Problem of Consent: Kidney Transplantation in Minors, 34 N.Y.U.L. Rev. 891 (1959), **94, 204.**

————. Governmental Regulation of the Use of Human Subjects in Medical Research, 98 Daedalus 542 (1969), **72, 73, 126, 136.**

————. Legal and Medical Death: Kansas Takes the First Step, 284 N. Eng. J. Med. 260 (1971), **208.**

Curran, W.J. & H.K. Beecher, Experimentation in Children, 210 J.A.M.A. 77 (1969), **111.**

Curtis, F.K., J.J. Cole, B.J. Fellows, et al., Hemodialysis in the Home, 11 Trans. Am. Soc. Artif. Intern. Organs 7 (1965), **39.**

Daube, D., Transplantation: Acceptability of Procedures and the Required Legal Sanctions, in Ethics in Medical Progress: With Special Reference to Transplantation 198 (G.E.W. Wolstenholme & E.M. O'Connor eds. 1966), **110, 204, 207.**

Davis, K., Discretionary Justice: A Preliminary Inquiry (1969), **165.**

Dormont, M.J., Les Problèmes Moraux de la Transplantation d'Organs, 154 Bull. Acad. Nat. Med. (Paris) 623 (1970), **201.**

Duff, R. & A. Hollingshead, Sickness and Society (1968), **28, 98.**

Dukeminier, J., Jr., Supplying Organs for Transplantation, 68 Mich. L. Rev. 811 (1970), **196, 197, 198, 199.**

Dukeminier, J. & D. Sanders, Organ Transplantation: A Proposal for the Routine Salvaging of Cadaver Organs, 379 N. Eng. J. Med. 413 (1968), **198.**

Dunsford, I., et al., A Human Blood-Group Chimera, 2 Brit. Med. J. 81 (1953), **42.**

Eisindrath, R.M., R.D. Guttman & J.E. Murray, Psychological Considerations in the Selection of Kidney Transplant Donors, 129 Surg. Gynec. & Obstet. 243 (1969), **203.**

Experience with Human Heart Transplantation: Proceedings of the Cape Town Symposium, 13-16 July 1968 (H.A. Shapiro ed. 1969), **51, 52.**

Federal Panel Urges Reform to Diminish Malpractice Suits, N.Y. Times, Apr. 18, 1972 at 20, col. 4, **149.**

Feifel, The Function of Attitudes toward Death, in Death and Dying: Attitudes of Patient and Doctor (G.A.P. Symposium #11) 632 (1965), **101.**

Fellner, C.H., Altruism Revisited: The Genetically Unrelated Living Kidney Donor (consultant's memorandum) (1972), **201-203.**

————. The Genetically Unrelated Living Kidney Donor: Unemployed and Unwanted (1972), **63, 98, 232.**

Fellner, C.H. & J.R. Marshall, Kidney Donors: The Myth of Informed Consent, 126 Am. J. of Psychiatry 1245 (1970), **55, 91, 98, 202.**

———. Twelve Kidney Donors, 206 J.A.M.A. 2703 (1968), **202.**

Fellner, C.H. & S.H. Schwartz, Altruism in Disrepute, 284 N. Eng. J. Med. 282 (1971), **63, 98.**

First Ann. John F. Kennedy Symposium on Recent Significant Developments in Medicine and Surgery (1968), **69.**

Folkman, A., Transplacental Carcinogenesis by Stilbestrol, 285 New Eng. J. Med. 404 (1971), **170.**

Fox, A.S., Heart Transplants: Treatment or Experiment? 159 Science 374 (1968), **146, 171.**

Fox, R.C., Experiment Perilous (1959), **56, 60-61.**

———. A Sociological Perspective on Organ Transplantation and Hemodialysis, 169 Ann. N.Y. Acad. Sci. 406 (1970), **64, 65, 69, 70, 71, 72.**

———. Some Social and Cultural Factors in American Society Conducive to Medical Research on Human Subjects, 1 Clin. Pharm. & Therap. 423 (1960), **90.**

Fox, R.C. & J.P. Swazey, The Courage to Fail (1974), **29, 55, 64-66, 68, 149, 247.**

Fox, T.S., The Ethics of Clinical Trials, 28 Medico-Legal J. 132 (1960), **122, 123.**

Franklin, B.A., Chairmen of Two Senate Committees Urge a Federal Inquiry into Fatal Coal Mine Explosion in Kentucky, N.Y. Times, Jan. 3, 1971 at 34, col. 1, **24.**

———. U.S. Lags in Effort to Implement Mine Safety Law, N.Y. Times, March 23, 1970 at 15, col. 1, **24.**

Freud, A., The Doctor-Patient Relationship, in Katz, with the assistance of A. Capron & E. Glass, Experimentation with Human Beings 642 (1972), **67.**

Freund, P.A., Legal Framework for Human Experimentation, 98 Daedalus 315 (1969), **88.**

Friedman, E.A., & S.L. Kountz, Impact of H.R.-1 on the Therapy of End Stage Uremia, 288 New Eng. J. Med. 1286 (1973), **16, 95.**

From a Correspondent, 1 The Lancet 1394 (1961), **70.**

Gail, M.H., Does Cardiac Transplantation Prolong Life: A Reassessment, 76 Ann. Intern. Med. 815 (1972), **51.**

Glass, E.S., Restructuring Informed Consent: Legal Therapy for the Doctor-Patient Relationship, 79 Yale L. J. 1533 (1970), **81, 86.**

Glasser, B. & A. Strauss, Awareness of Dying (1965), **93.**

Gray, B., Some Vagaries of Consent, in Katz with the assistance of A. Capron & E. Glass, Experimentation with Human Beings (1972), **230.**

Griffiths, J. & R.E. Ayres, A Postscript to the Miranda Project: Interrogation of Draft Protestors, 77 Yale L. J. 300 (1967), **98.**

Halberstam, I., The Doctor's New Dilemma: "Will I Be Sued?," N.Y. Times, Feb. 14, 1971, § 6 (Magazine) at 8, **149.**

Halley & J.D. Harvey, On an Interdisciplinary Solution to the Legal-Medical Definitional Dilemma in Death, 2 Indiana Legal F. 219 (1969), **213.**

Hamburger, J., Protection of Donor Rights in Renal Transplantation, in Biomedical Science and the Dilemma of Human Experimentation 44 (V. Fattorusso ed. 1967), **63.**

Hamburger, J., et al., A Declaration of the International Society of Transplantation, 12 Transplant. 77 (1971), **201.**

Hamburger, J., J. Vaysse, J., Crosnier, et al. Renal Homotransplantation in Man after Radiation of the Recipient: Experience with Six Patients since 1959, 32 Am. J. Med. 854 (1962), **45.**

————. Transplantation d'un rein entre jumeaux non monozygotes après irradiations du receveur: Bon functionnement au quatrième mois, 67 Presse Med. 1771 (1959), **45.**

Hamilton, M. ed., The New Genetics and the Future of Man (1972), **59, 161.**

Handler, P. ed., Biology and the Future of Man (1970), **167, 168.**

Hardy, J.D. & C.M. Chavez, The First Heart Transplant in Man: Historical Reexamination of the 1964 Case in the Light of Current Clinical Experience, 1 Transplant Proc. 717 (1969), **109.**

Hardy, J.D., C.M. Chavez, F.D. Kurrus, et al., Heart Transplantation on Man, 188 J.A.M.A. 1132 (1964), **50, 207.**

Havighurst, C.C., Compensating Persons Injured in Human Experimentation, 169 Science 153 (1970), **247.**

Hearings on Competitive Problems in the Drug Industry before the Subcommittee on Monopoly of the Senate Committee on Small Business, 91st Cong., 1st Sess. (1969), **148.**

Hearings on Death with Dignity, An Inquiry into Related Public Issues, Before Senate Special Committee on Aging, 92d Cong., 2d Sess. (1972), **25.**

Hearings on H.R. 8395 before the Subcommittee on the Handicapped of the Senate Committee on Labor and Public Welfare, 92d Cong. 2d. Sess., pt. 1 at 310-50 (1972), **151.**

Hearings on S.J. Res. 145 (National Commission on Health Science and Society) before the Subcommittee on Government Research of the Senate Committee on Government Operations, 90th Cong., 2d Sess. (1968), **132, 133, 152, 154, 182, 206, 221.**

The Heart: Miracle in Cape Town, Newsweek, Dec. 18, 1967 at 86, **208.**

Henderson, L.J. Physician and Patient as a Social System, 212 New Eng. J. Med. 819 (1935), **99.**

Hendin, D., Death as a Fact of Life (1973), **107.**

Hessel, S.J., Heart·Transplants and Public Information, 278 New Eng. J. Med. 797 (1968), **146.**

Hilton, B. et al., eds., Ethical Issues in Human Genetics (1973), **103, 161.**

Hinton, J.M., The Physical and Mental Distress of the Dying, 32 Q. J. Med. 1 (1963), **102.**

Holden, C., Ethics: Biomedical Advances Confront Public, Politicians as well as Professionals with New Issues, 175 Science 40 (1972), **161, 162.**

Hollingshead, A.B. & F. Redlich, Social Class and Mental Illness (1958), **98.**

Holman, E., Protein Sensitization in Isoskingrafting, 38 Surg., Gynec. & Obstet. 100 (1924), **41.**

Hoover, R. & J.F. Fraumeni, Risk of Cancer in Renal Transplant Recipients, 2 Lancet 55 (1973), **49.**

Jaffe, L.L., Law as a System of Control, 98 Daedalus 406 (1969), **142, 246.**

Janis, I.L., Psychological Stress: Psychoanalytic and Behavioral Studies of Surgical Patients (1958), **100.**

Jonas, H., Philosophical Reflections on Experimenting with Human Subjects, 98 Daedalus 219 (1969), **75, 168.**

Kapoor, Death and Problems of Transplant, 38 Manit. B. News 167 (1971), **209.**

Kass, L., A Caveat on Transplants, Washington Post, Jan. 14, 1968, at B-1, col. 1, **147, 183.**

Katz, A., Process Design for Selection of Hemodialysis and Organ Transplant Recipients (1972), **194.**

Katz, J., Editorial Rewritten, 22 Clin. Res. 10 (1974), **123, 243.**

————. The Education of the Physician-Investigator, 98 Daedalus 480 (1969), **61.**

————. Human Experimentation, 275 New Eng. J. Med. 790 (1966), **122.**

————. The Regulation of Human Research—Reflections and Proposals, 21 Clin. Res. 787 (1973), **88.**

Katz, J., with the assistance of A. Capron & E. Glass, Experimentation with Human Beings (1972), **23, 59, 60, 67, 74, 77, 147, 163, 230, 233.**

Kelman, H.C., The Rights of the Subject in Social Research: An Analysis in Terms of Relative Power and Legitimacy, 27 Am. Psych. 989 (1972), **28.**

Kennedy, I.M., The Kansas Statute on Death: An Appraisal, 285 New Eng. J. Med. 946 (1971), **209, 212, 213, 216.**

Kessler, F., Contracts of Adhesion: Some Thoughts about Freedom of Contract, 43 Colum. L. Rev. 629 (1943), **85.**

Kidd, A.M., Limits of the Right of a Person to Consent to Experimentation on Himself, 117 Science 211 (1953), **90.**

Kübler-Ross, E., On Death and Dying (1969), **93, 101, 114.**

Küss, R., M. Legrain, G. Mathe, et al., Etude de quatre cas d'irradiation totale par le cobalt radioactif (A des doses respectives de 250, 400 et 600 rads.), 7 Rev. Franc. Etudes Clin. Biol. 1028 (1962), **45.**

Ladimer, I., Protection and Compensation for Injury in Human Studies in Experimentation with Human Subjects 247 (P. Freund ed. 1970), **247.**

Langmuir, A.D., New Environmental Factor in Congenital Disease, 284 New Eng. J. Med. 912 (1971), **170.**

Lasswell, H.D., The Decision Procéss (1956), **92.**

————. The Political Science of Science, 50 Am. Pol. Sci. Rev. 961 (1956), **160.**

Lasswell, H.D. & M. McDougal, Law, Science and Policy: The Jurisprudence of a Free Society, in Katz with the assistance of A. Capron & E. Glass, Experimentation with Human Beings (1972), **32.**

Law of March 17, 1970, Kansas Sessions Laws, ch. 378 (1970); codified in Kan. Stat. Ann. § 77-202 (Supp. 1971), **209.**

Lazarus, J.M. & C.L. Hampers, Renal Transplantation—1972, 76 Ann. Intern. Med. 504 (1972), **47.**

Lecatsas, G., Papopavirus in Urine after Renal Transplantation, 241 Nature 343 (1973), **49.**

Levine, R., Ethical Consideration in the Publication of the Results of Research Involving Human Subjects, 21 Clin. Res. 763 (1973), **122.**

Lindblom, C.E., New Decision-Making Procedures Governing Research on and Treatment of Catastrophic Diseases (1970), **159, 182.**

————. The Science of "Muddling Through," 29 Pub. Admin. Rev. 79 (1959), **32.**

Lindner, A., B. Charra, D.J. Sherrard & B.H. Scribner, Accelerated Atherosclerosis in Prolonged Maintenance Hemodialysis and Cardiovascular Disorders, 290 New Eng. J. Med. 697 (1974), **12.**

Lower, R.R., R.C. Stofer, E.J. Hurley, E. Dong, R.B. Cohn & N.E. Shumway, Successful Homotransplantation of the Canine Heart after Anoxic Preservation for Seven Hours, 104 Am. J. Surg. 302 (1962), **51.**

Massachusetts General Hospital, Human Studies: Guiding Principles and Procedures (1970), **122, 126, 231, 233.**

Matte, P.J., Law, Morals and Medicine: A Method of Approach to Current Problems, 13 J. For. Sci. 318 (1968), **159.**

Mead, M., Research with Human Beings: A Model Derived from Anthropological Field Practice, 98 Daedalus 361 (1969), **83.**

Medical Report: Malpractice Crisis, 38 Ins. Counsel J. 521 (1971), **149.**

Melmon, K.L., M. Grossman & R.C. Morris, Emerging Assets and Liabilities of a Committee on Human Welfare and Experimentation, 282 New Eng. J. Med. 427 (1970). **165, 226, 228.**

Merrill, J.P., J.E. Murray, J.H. Harrison, E.A. Friedman, J.B. Dealy & G. J. Damin, Successful Homotransplantation of the Kidney between Non-Identical Twins, 262 New Eng. J. Med. 1251 (1960), **45.**

Merrill, J.P., J.E. Murray, J.H. Harrison & W.E. Guild, Successful Homotransplantation of the Human Kidney between Identical Twins, 160 J.A.M.A. 277 (1956), **43.**

Merrill, J.P., E. Schupak, E. Cameron, et al., Hemodialysis in the Home, 190 J.A.M.A. 468 (1964), **39.**

Merton, R.K., Some Preliminaries to a Sociology of Medical Education, in The Student Physician 7 (R. Merton, G. Reader, & P. Kendall eds. 1957), **118.**

Michaelson, M.G., Book Review of Cooley: The Career of a Great Heart Surgeon, N.Y. Times, Apr. 7, 1973, Sec. 7 (Book Review), at 23, **2.**

Minetree, H., Cooley: The Career of a Great Heart Surgeon (1973), **135.**

Mintz, M., Are Birth Control Pills Safe? Some Doctors Doubt that the Drug Has Been Tested Well Enough for Possible Side Effects, Washington Post, Dec. 19, 1965 at E-1, col. 1, **147**.

————. The Therapeutic Nightmare (1965), **148**.

Minutes of the Cape Town Meeting, Medical World News, Aug. 9, 1963, **171**.

Moore, F.D., Scientists and Surgeons, 176 Science 1100 (1972), **170**.

————. Transplant: The Give and Take of Tissue Transplantation (1972), **13, 36, 37, 40, 41, 45, 110**.

Murray, J.E., R.E. Wilson, N.L. Tilney, et al., Five Years Experience in Renal Transplantation with Immunosuppressive Drugs: Survival, Functioning, Complications, and the Role of Lymphocyte Depletion by Thoracic Duct Fistula, 168 Annals Surg. 416 (1968), **48**.

NAS Board on Medicine, Statement on Cardiac Transplantation, 18 News Report of the National Academy of Sciences (March 1968), **165, 173**.

National Conference of Commissioners on Uniform State Laws, Handbook and Proceedings of the Annual Conference (1968), **209**.

National Research Act, Pub. Law No. 93-348 (1974), **75, 161-162, 241**.

New York Assembly Bill 1837, A Bill to Amend the Education Law, in Relation to Scientific Research on Human Subjects, to Provide for the Advancement of Such Research through the Protection of Its Subjects, and to Establish a State Board on Human Research (introduced Jan. 13, 1971), **246**.

Nomos VII – Rational Decision (C. Friedrich ed. 1964), **92**.

Nora, J.J., D.A. Cooley, et al., Rejection of the Transplanted Human Heart: Indexes of Recognition and Problems of Prevention, 280 New Eng. J. Med. 1079 (1969), **172**.

Nuremberg Code, 2 Trials of War Criminals before the Nuremberg Military Tribunals 181 (1948), **14**.

Oken, D., What to Tell Cancer Patients: A Study of Medical Attitudes, 175 J.A.M.A. 1120 (1961), **100, 101**.

Opelz, G. & P.I. Terasaki, National Utilization of Cadaver Kidneys for Transplantation, 228 J.A.M.A. 1260 (1974), **236**.

Organ Transplantation, 223 J.A.M.A. 320 (1973) [editorial], **47**.

Owen, R.D., Immunogenetic Consequences of Vascular Anastomoses between Bovine Twins, 102 Science 400 (1945), **42**.

Page, I., The Ethics of Heart Transplantation: A Personal View, 207 J.A.M.A. 109 (1969), **145, 146**.

Pappworth, M., Human Guinea Pigs (1967), **59**.

Parsons, T., Research with Human Subjects and the "Professional Complex," 98 Daedalus 325 (1969), **84**.

————. The Social System (1951), **71**.

Parsons, T., R.C. Fox & V.M. Lidz, The "Gift of Life" and its Reciprocation, 39 Social Research 367 (1972), **94, 217**.

Physician's Duty to Warn, 75 Harv. L. Rev. 1445 (1962), **99.**

Plant, M., An Analysis of "Informed Consent," 36 Fordham L. Rev. 639 (1968), **81.**

President's Commission on Heart Disease, Cancer and Stroke, A National Program to Conquer Heart Disease, Cancer and Stroke (1964), **133, 176.**

Principles of Medical Ethics, in American Medical Association, Opinions and Reports of the Judicial Council vii (1969), **119, 121.**

Proceedings of the Conference on the Ethical Aspects of Experimentation on Human Subjects (Daedalus–National Institutes of Health, 1967), **99.**

Prosser, W., Handbook of the Law of Torts (1971), **125.**

Protection of Human Subjects Act (H.R. 7724), 118 Cong. Rec. S16335 (Sept. 11, 1973), **75.**

Ramsey, P., The Patient as Person (1970), **83, 172.**

Rapaport, F.T. & J. Dausset, Ranks of Donor-Recipient Histocompatibility for Human Transplantation, 167 Science 1260 (1970), **48.**

Remington, C., An Experimental Study of Man's Genetic Relationship to Great Apes, By Means of Interspecific Hybridization, in Katz with the assistance of A. Capron & E. Glass, Experimentation with Human Beings 461 (1972), **74.**

Renal Failure: The Agony and the Ecstacy, 222 J.A.M.A. 829 (1972) [editorial], **12.**

Report of the Committee on Chronic Kidney Disease [the Gottschalk committee] (1967), **134, 151.**

Richardson, E., Refinements in Criteria for the Determination of Death: An Appraisal, 221 J.A.M.A. 48 (1972) [unpublished results, reported in Task Force on Death and Dying, Institute of Society, Ethics and Life Sciences], **208.**

Rosenbaum, M.E., The Effect of Stimulus and Background Factors on the Volunteering Response, 53 J. Abnormal and Soc. Psych. 118 (1956), **94.**

Rosenfeld, A., The Second Genesis (1969), **161.**

Rot, A. & H.A.H. Van Till, Neocortical Death after Cardiac Arrest, 2 Lancet 1099 (1971), **208.**

Rugaber, W., F.D.A. Will Require Drug Test Review, N.Y. Times, Aug. 13, 1969, at 1, **147.**

_____. Prison Drug and Plasma Projects Leave Fatal Trail, N.Y. Times, July 29, 1969 at 1, **147.**

Rutstein, D.D., The Ethical Design of Human Experiments, 98 Daedalus 523 (1969), **208.**

Sadler, A.M., B.L. Sadler & E.B. Stason, Transplantation and the Law: Progress toward Uniformity, 282 New Eng. J. Med. 717 (1970), **216.**

_____. The Uniform Anatomical Gift Act: A Model for Reform, 206 J.A.M.A. 2501 (1968), **209.**

Sadler, A.M., B.L. Sadler, E.B. Stason & D.L. Stickel, Transplantation: A Case for Consent, 280 New Eng. J. Med. 862 (1969), **198.**

Sadler, H.H., Summary Notes on a Clinical Decision-Making Model (1972), **93, 94, 115, 201.**

Sadler, H.H., L. Davison, C. Carroll & S.L. Kountz, The Living, Genetically Unrelated Kidney Donor, 3 Sem. Psych. 86 (1971), **55, 93, 146, 201.**

Salpukas, Caution Is Urged in Psychosurgery, N.Y. Times, Apr. 6, 1973, at 24, col. 4, **161.**

Sanders, D. & J. Dukeminier, Medical Advance and Legal Lag: Hemodialysis and Kidney Transplantation, 15 U.C.L.A. L. Rev. 357 (1968), **181, 197, 198, 209.**

Sarton, G., A History of Science (1952), **67.**

Scarce Medical Resources, 69 Colum. L. Rev. 620 (1969), **217.**

Schonberg, Informed Consent, 230 J.A.M.A. 38 (1974), **92.**

Schwartz R. & W. Dameshek, Drug Induced Immunological Tolerance, 183 Nature 1682 (1959), **46.**

Schwartz, R., W. Dameshek & J. Donovan, The Effects of 6-mercaptopurine on Homograft Reactions, 39 J. Clin. Invest. 952 (1960), **46.**

Schwartz, R., J. Stack & W. Dameshek, Effect of 6-mercaptopurine on Antibody Production, 99 Proc. Soc. Exp. Biol. Med. 164 (1958), **46.**

Scribner, B.H., Ethical Problems of Using Artificial Organs to Sustain Human Life, 10 Trans. Am. Soc. Art. Organs 209 (1964), **205.**

—————. The Problem of Patient Selection for Treatment with an Artificial Kidney (1972), **37.**

Senate Joint Resolution 75, 92d Cong., 1st Sess., 117 Cong. Rec. 3710 (Mar. 24, 1971), **130-132.**

Shaldon, S., Experience to Date with Home Hemodialysis, Proceedings of Working Conference on Chronic Hemodialysis (1966), **39.**

Shapiro, D.L., The Choice of Rulemaking or Adjudication in the Development of Administrative Policy, 78 Harv. L. Rev. 921 (1965), **165.**

Silverman, D., R.L. Masland, M.G. Saunders & R.S. Schwab, Irreversible Coma Associated with Electrocerebral Silence, 20 Neurology 525 (1970), **207-208.**

Simmons, R.B., K. Hickey, C.M. Kjellstrand & R.L. Simmons, Family Tension in the Search for a Kidney Donor, 215 J.A.M.A. 909 (1971), **203.**

Smith, H.W., Therapeutic Privilege to Withhold Specific Diagnosis from Patient Sick with Serious or Fatal Illness, 19 Tenn. L. Rev. 349 (1946), **99.**

Social Security Act Amendments of 1972, Pub. L. No. 92–603, 86 Stat. 1329 (1972), **15, 183.**

Stewart, W.H. (Surgeon General), Memorandum to Heads of Institutions Conducting Research with Public Health Grants (Feb. 8, 1966), **125, 164.**

Swazey, J.P. & R.C. Fox, The Clinical Moratorium: A Case Study of Mitral Valve Surgery, in Experimentation with Human Subjects 315 (P. Freund ed. 1969), **55, 56, 75-76.**

Taylor, L.F., A Statutory Definition of Death in Kansas, 215 J.A.M.A. 296 (1971), **208, 213.**

Terasaki, P.I. Organ Transplantation (1972), **236.**

Terasaki, P.I., M.R. Mickey, D.P. Singal, K.K. Mittal & R.P. Patel, Stereotyping
   for Homotransplantation: XX, Selection of Recipients for Cadaver Donor
   Transplants, 279 New Eng. J. Med. 1101 (1963), **48.**
Terasaki, P.I., G. Wilkinson & J. McClelland, National Transplant Communica-
   tions Network, 218 J.A.M.A. 1674 (1971), **49, 196-197, 236.**
Thomas, N., One Victim's Kidneys Aid Pair: Transplants Performed Here,
   Boston, N.H. Register, Feb. 13, 1971, at 1, col. 3, **145.**
Thompson, T., Hearts: Of Surgeons and Transplants, Miracles and Disasters
   along the Cardiac Frontier (1971), **145.**
Thornsby, E., Human Major Histocompatibility System, 18 Transplant Rev. 51
   (1974), **48.**
Titmuss, R.M., The Gift Relationship: From Human Blood to Social Policy
   (1971), **197.**

Ullmann, E., Experimentelle Nierentransplantation, 15 Wiener Klinische Wo-
   chenschrift 1 (Mar. 13, 1902), **39.**
U.S. Dep't of Health, Education, and Welfare, Artificial Heart Assessment
   Panel, National Heart and Lung Institute, The Totally Implantable Arti-
   ficial Heart: Economic, Ethical, Legal, Medical, Psychiatric and Social
   Implications (1973), **9, 220.**
U.S. Dep't of Health, Education, and Welfare, Food and Drug Administration,
   Institutional Committee Review of Clinical Investigation of New Drugs
   in Human Beings, 36 Fed. Reg. 5037 (1971), **150, 164, 225.**
————. Notice of Proposed Rulemaking, 34 Fed. Reg. 13552 (1969), **147.**
U.S. Dep't of Health, Education, and Welfare, Public Health Service, The Insti-
   tutional Guide to DHEW Policy on Protection of Human Subjects (1971),
   as amended, 39 Fed. Reg. 18914 (1974), **59, 86, 112, 128, 155, 223, 227,
   228.**
U.S. Dep't of Health, Education, and Welfare, Tuskegee Syphilis Study Ad Hoc
   Advisory Panel, Final Report (1973), **237, 241.**
————. Protection of the Individual as a Research Subject (1969), **125, 128,
   164.**
Updating the Definition of Death, Med. World News, Apr. 28, 1967, **207.**
Uphoff, D.E., Alteration of Homograft Reaction by A-methopterin in Lethally
   Irradiated Mice Treated with Homologous Marrow, 99 Proc. Soc. Exp.
   Biol. Med. 651 (1958), **46.**

Veatch, R.M., The Medical Model: Its Nature and Problems, 1 Hastings Center
   Studies 59 (No. 3, 1973), **113.**

Waltz, J.R. & T.W. Scheunemann, Informed Consent to Therapy, 64 N.W.U.
   L. Rev. 628 (1969), **87.**
Weisman, A.D., The Patient with a Fatal Illness: To Tell or Not to Tell? 201
   J.A.M.A. 153 (1967), **102.**
Welt, L., Reflections on the Problems of Human Experimentation, 25 Conn.
   Med. 75 (1961), **126.**

What Price Transplanted Organs?, Med. World News, (June 28, 1968), **134, 135, 183.**

Woodford, F.P., Ethical Experimentation and the Editor, 286 New Eng. J. Med. 892 (1972), **123.**

Woodruff, M.F.A., Can Tolerance in Homologous Skin Be Induced in the Human Infant at Birth? 4 Transplant. Bull. 26 (1957), **42.**

Woodruff, M.F.A. & B. Lennox, Reciprocal Skin Grafts in a Pair of Twins Showing Blood Chimerism, 2 Lancet 476 (1959), **42.**

Woodruff, M.F.A. & L.O. Simpson, Induction of Tolerance to Skin Homografts in Rats by Injection of Cells from the Prospective Donor Soon after Birth, 36 Brit. J. Ex. Path. 494 (1955), **42.**

World Medical Association, Declaration of Helsinki, 271 New Eng. J. Med. 473 (1964), **14, 119, 163, 164.**

Zarday, Z., F.J. Veith, M.L. Gliedman & R. Soberman, Irreversible Liver Damage after Azathioprine, 222 J.A.M.A. 690 (1972), **46.**

Zeckhauser, R., Some Thoughts on the Allocation of Resources in Biomedical Research [Occasional Paper No. 4, Office of Assistant Secretary for Planning and Evaluation, DHEW] (1967), **176.**

————. Catastrophic Illness (1972), **180, 183, 186.**

Index

263

Printed in the United States
by Baker & Taylor Publisher Services

Printed in the United States
by Baker & Taylor Publisher Services